THE REAL
PALEO DIET
COOKBOOK

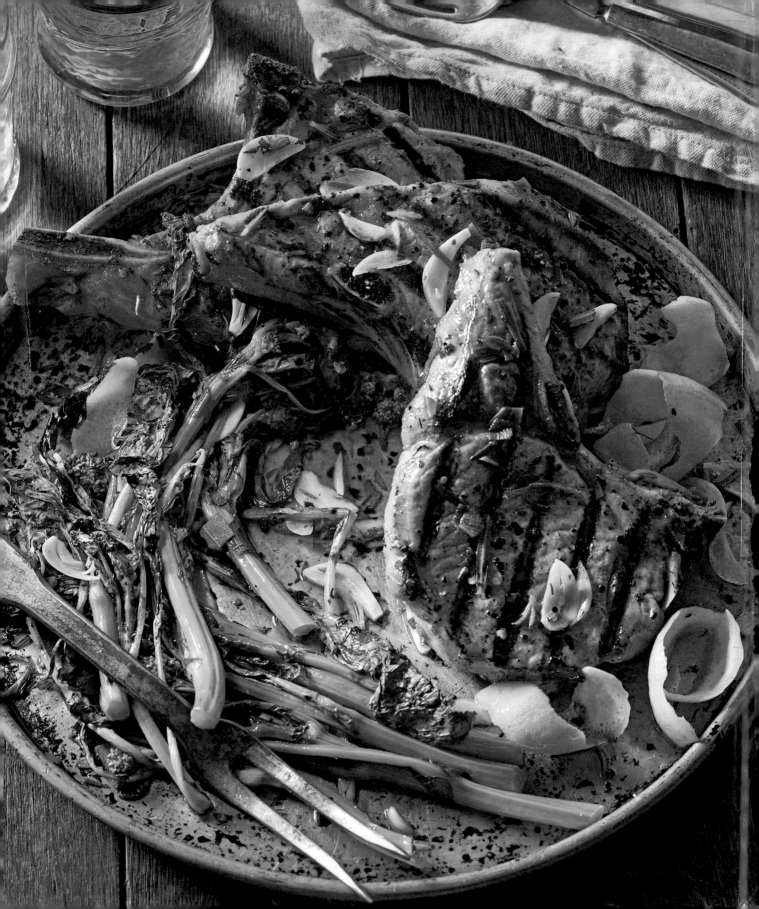

LOREN CORDAIN, PH.D.

THE REAL
PALEO DIET
COOKBOOK

HOUGHTON MIFFLIN HARCOURT
BOSTON · NEW YORK · 2015

FOR INFORMATION ABOUT PERMISSION TO REPRODUCE SELECTIONS
FROM THIS BOOK, WRITE TO PERMISSIONS, HOUGHTON MIFFLIN
HARCOURT PUBLISHING COMPANY, 215 PARK AVENUE SOUTH,
NEW YORK, NEW YORK 10003

WWW.HMHCO.COM

LIBRARY OF CONGRESS CATALOGING-IN-PUBLICATION DATA IS
AVAILABLE UPON REQUEST.

ISBN 978-0-544-30326-3 (HBK); 978-0-544-30327-0 (EBK)

BOOK DESIGN BY WATERBURY PUBLICATIONS, INC., DES MOINES, IOWA.

COVER PHOTOGRAPH: WATERBURY PUBLICATIONS, INC., PETER KRUMHARDT

C&C 10 9 8 7 6 5 4 3 2 1

PRINTED IN CHINA

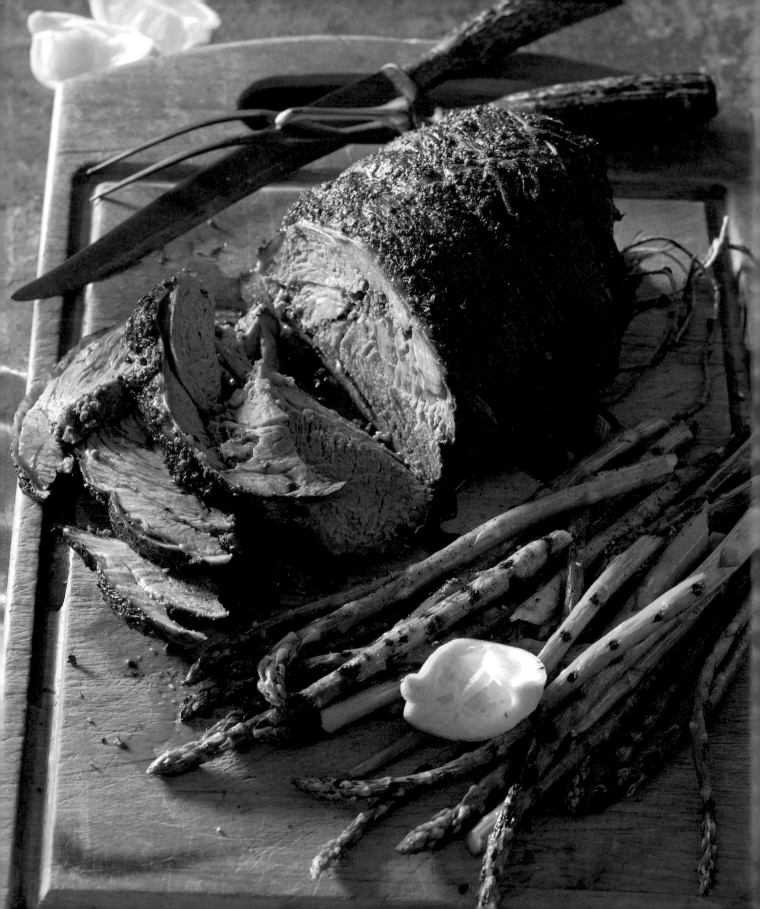

CONTENTS

ACKNOWLEDGMENTS

More than a decade has passed since the publication of my first book, *The Paleo Diet®*, in 2002. In the ensuing years "Paleo" has become a dietary concept known to the world. It is especially gratifying to have been involved early on in a nutritional idea that has positively changed people's lives throughout the world.

A talented and expert team has worked closely with me to create *The Real Paleo Diet® Cookbook*. Many thanks to my editor, Anne Ficklen, without whose insight and dedication to "Paleo," this book would not have materialized. Ken Carlson and Lisa Kingsley have been instrumental in coordinating the efforts of many talented people to produce the delicious recipes and colorful photos throughout this cookbook. Over the years, my wife, Lorrie, and my boys (now men) have supported me unconditionally as I wrote about The Paleo Diet®. I also am indebted to my literary agents, Channa Taub and Carol Mann, for their enthusiastic support and encouragement over the years. Most of all I want to acknowledge you, my dedicated Paleo audience, who "get it".

Thank you,
Loren Cordain, Ph.D.

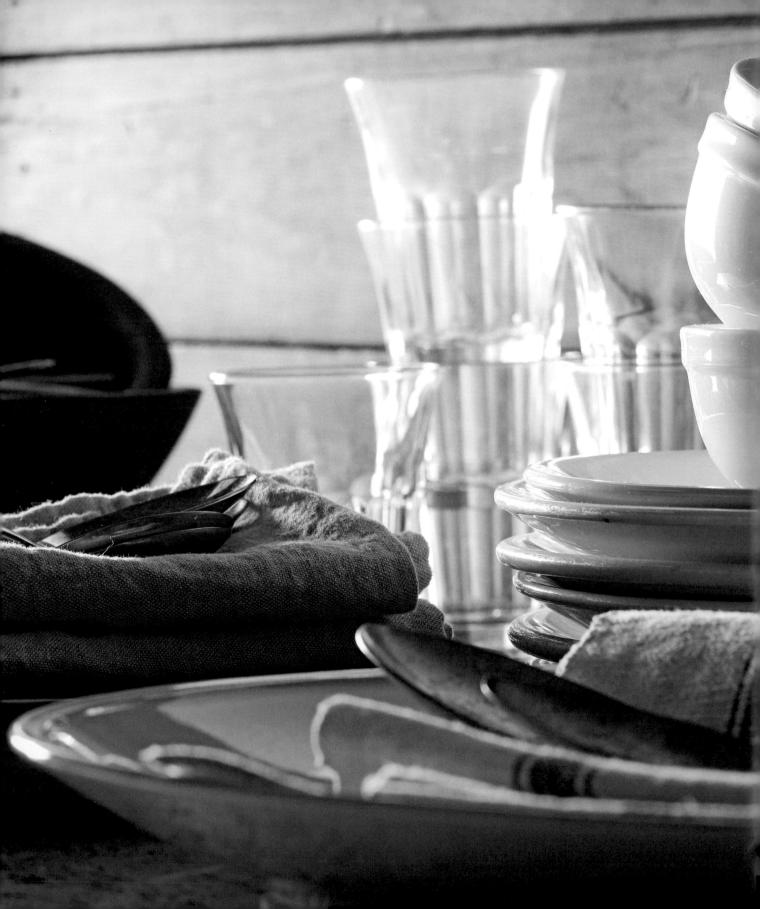

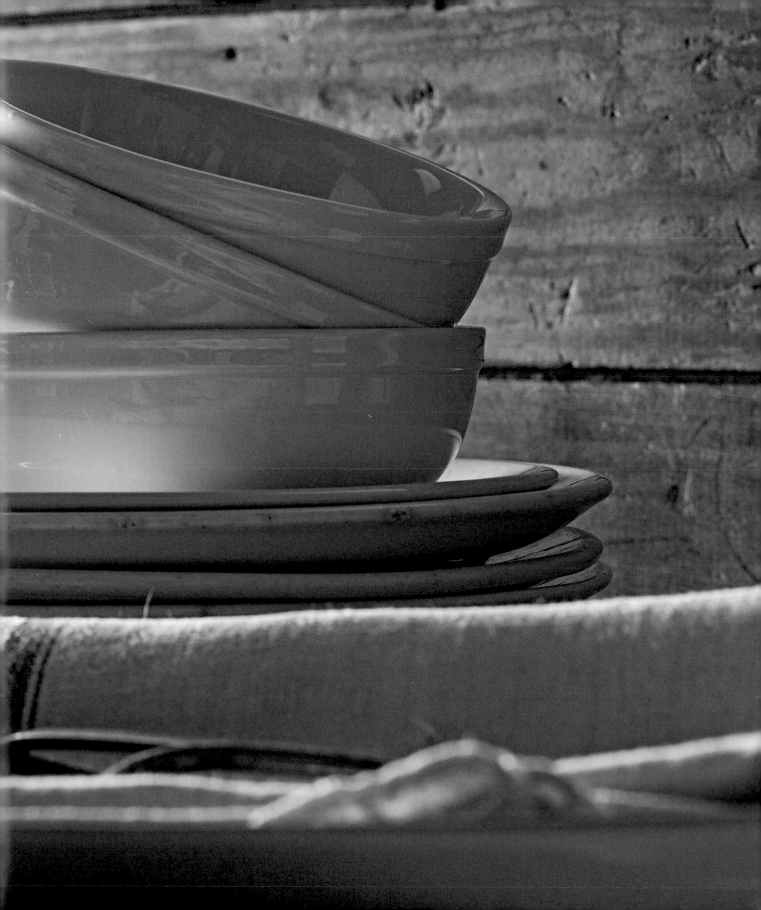

INTRODUCTION

When your interest is initially piqued by a new diet or cookbook, it is only natural to want to discover a bit more about the history of the topic—where it came from, why it currently exists, and where it may be going. Sometimes we can get up to speed more rapidly on a topic by starting in the present and going backward in time or, sometimes, vice versa. When it comes to The Paleo Diet® concept, I not only have the luxury of being able to personally travel backward in time to its very beginnings, but I am able to move forward in time to appreciate its current worldwide impact.

For me, The Paleo Diet® concept began on a crisp Colorado fall day in 1987 when I read a scientific paper by Dr. S. Boyd Eaton called "Paleolithic nutrition: a consideration of its nature and current implications," published two years earlier in the prestigious *New England Journal of Medicine*. This scientific article represented nothing less than the defining moment in my career, which set me off on a 30-year quest into what would become my life's work. My ensuing scientific and popular writings over the intervening years (www.thepaleodiet.com) have helped to define a worldwide concept now known as "The Paleo Diet®," a term I coined with my first book in 2002 and that was later revised in 2010.

So for those of you who are just starting to wrap your heads around The Paleo Diet®, let's fast forward to 2013–2014 and take a look at just how well-known "Paleo" has become to the general public. On a recent *Dr. Oz* show devoted entirely to diets, the good doctor introduced the broadcast by saying that "the number-one Google search of all diets in 2013 was for The Paleo Diet®." This show came only a few months after a previous broadcast in which Dr. Oz featured me and my first book, *The Paleo Diet®*, which had become a *New York Times* best seller and had been translated into more than 20 languages worldwide.

As you may expect, the global Paleo Diet movement has spawned an explosion of copycat books over the past several years. Look no further than amazon.com to literally see the hundreds of diets and cookbooks that manage to shoehorn the word "Paleo" into their titles.

In a way, all of these books are a good thing because they tend to get more and more people involved in a lifetime way of eating that may improve health and well-being while reducing the risk for chronic diseases. The downside of this situation is that many authors are poorly informed and frequently provide misleading information about food, recipes, and meals that are not "Paleo" by any stretch of the imagination. Accordingly, one of my primary goals in writing *The Real Paleo Diet® Cookbook* is to correct this glut of misinformation and give you the best and most scientifically accurate facts about which foods, ingredients, and recipes should be included in your Paleo Diet. But even more important, with *The Real Paleo Diet® Cookbook*, you will become privy to an incredible cornucopia of enticing and delectable foods and recipes designed and fully tested by a top-notch group of chefs and cooks.

PALEO PRINCIPLES

THE PALEO DIET® COMES FROM THE WORD "PALEOLITHIC," WHICH MEANS "THE OLD STONE AGE"—A PERIOD LASTING FROM THE APPEARANCE OF STONE TOOLS ABOUT 3 MILLION YEARS AGO TO THE BEGINNINGS OF AGRICULTURE AND ANIMAL HUSBANDRY 10,000 YEARS AGO. DURING THIS ERA, ALL OF OUR ANCESTORS LIVED AS HUNTER-GATHERERS AND OBTAINED EVERYTHING THEY ATE FROM WILD PLANT AND ANIMAL FOODS THAT COULD BE HUNTED, FISHED, OR FORAGED.

THE PALEO DIET® IN A NUTSHELL

Obviously, we can no longer live as hunter-gatherers, and few, if any of us, could ever eat wild plants and animals exclusively. When I first wrote *The Paleo Diet®* in 2002, it was never my intention for us to literally consume the foods hunter-gatherers ate, but rather for us to do our "foraging" in supermarkets and grocery stores and in our gardens. The primary goal of contemporary "Paleo Diets" is to mimic the food groups our ancestors ate by consuming commonly available foods found in grocery stores and supermarkets, while avoiding modern foods that hunter-gatherers rarely or never ate. This simple template I originally envisioned years ago eventually morphed into the worldwide phenomenon now known as The Paleo Diet®. By following this fundamental concept with only a few exceptions, you will join millions of people around the globe who now enjoy the health benefits of this lifetime nutritional plan, to say nothing of the delicious, living, "real" foods that will become part of this way of eating.

The Real Paleo Diet® Cookbook will become your guidepost to correct and scientifically accurate Paleo dieting as you and your family adopt the world's healthiest way of eating. The diet really is not a diet at all, but rather a lifetime program of eating that will maximize your health and well-being and help you to take weight off and keep it off. The Paleo Diet® is simplicity itself. Once you get a feel for it with the scrumptious recipes in *The Real Paleo Diet® Cookbook*, your choice of healthful "real" foods will become second nature. The recipes in *The Real Paleo Diet® Cookbook* show you how to make fantastically delicious meals without using refined sugars, refined grains, whole grains, trans fats, dairy food, and salt. You will learn how to avoid processed foods as you focus your grocery shopping in the outside aisles of the supermarket and avoid the center aisles, where most of the packaged, processed foods reside. Better yet, discover your local farmers' markets and learn where and when you can purchase grass-produced meats, poultry, and eggs. If you happen to have the time, space, and inclination, start your own garden. By following the recipes and cooking guidelines contained in *The Real Paleo Diet® Cookbook*, you will soon be preparing savory and delicious meals to be shared with family and friends.

BASIC FOODS AND FOODS TO AVOID

The diet Mother Nature intended for us is simple and uncomplicated. You don't have to count calories, measure portions, or worry about how much or how little to eat. The fundamental guidelines of The Paleo Diet® are amazingly easy to follow: fresh meats, poultry; fish, seafood, eggs, vegetables, fruits, and nuts. Let your appetite be your guide and eat until you are full at each and every meal. Protein is far and away the most satiating of all three macronutrients (fat, carbohydrate, and protein). When you adopt The Paleo Diet® your appetite will naturally self-regulate, and you will not have a desire to overeat because high-quality animal protein (meat, fish, seafood, and eggs) is consumed at nearly every meal. Protein-rich animal foods, along with low-glycemic index fresh fruits and vegetables, encourage the normalization of your blood sugar and insulin levels, which further helps to normalize your appetite. The health benefits of The Paleo Diet® are not to be overshadowed by the world-class flavors and textures of Mother Nature's "real" foods. As you first thumb through the gorgeous photographs in *The Real Paleo Diet® Cookbook*, stop and take time to randomly read any recipe that may catch your eye. Notice that these appealing meals are easily prepared from a wide range of foods and spices that barely differ from some of your favorite dishes—except that they are much healthier for you because they are devoid of added sugars, salt, bad fats, and refined grains.

In the next few pages, I will fully summarize the delicious, healthful foods that are front and center on The Paleo Diet® menu and those that should be avoided. The basic list of foods to eliminate or stay away from includes refined sugars, refined cereal grains, most refined vegetable oils, salt, whole grains, dairy foods, legumes, and most processed foods.

When you adhere to the straightforward dietary guidelines outlined in this section and later fully laid out in the delicious, trouble-free recipes in *The Real Paleo Diet® Cookbook,* you will lose weight, reduce your risk for the metabolic syndrome (high blood pressure, type 2 diabetes, and heart disease), autoimmune diseases, cancers, and nearly every other chronic illness that troubles the western world. Your sleep will improve, you will have even more energy throughout the day, and many people report a more positive mental outlook. More important, you won't feel hungry all day, because high-protein foods satiate the brain's appetite center. In *The Real Paleo Diet® Cookbook* you will discover an amazing wealth of stunning, truly delicious foods and recipes that will improve your vitality and put the odds on your side for leading a long, healthy life.

THE PALEO DIET® AND THE 85:15 RULE

Incorporated into The Paleo Diet® from the very get-go when I wrote the first edition of the book in 2002 was the 85:15 Rule. Most people eat about 20 meals per week, plus snacks. Accordingly, three non-Paleo meals per week represents 15 percent of your weekly meal total. Most people experience noticeable, positive health benefits at this level of compliance. Two non-Paleo meals per week would correspond to a 90:10 percent compliance, and a single non-Paleo meal per week would be a 95:5 percent compliance. The attractiveness of this approach is that you aren't required to abstain from your favorite foods entirely and forever. I advise Paleo Diet novices to begin at 85:15 for a few weeks and then steadily move toward 95:5 as you become accustomed to the diet. The flexibility of this strategy is that it permits a little cheating, without losing the diet's general health effectiveness. Many Paleo dieters report that once they ditch a favorite food, its reintroduction causes such ill effects that they simply lose their cravings for former junk food preferences.

THE PALEO DIET®: SPECIFIC DOS AND DON'TS

Fresh foods are best. When you decide to adopt The Paleo Diet®, one of the key ideas to keep in mind for all foods is freshness and quality. Always strive to eat your fruits, vegetables, meat, eggs, poultry, fish, and seafood as fresh as possible. The order of preference is almost always

1. fresh, 2. frozen, 3. dried, and 4. canned, bottled, or tinned. The fresher the food, the greater its nutritional value and vitamin and mineral content—to say nothing of how much better it tastes! This is a lesson that the world's great chefs and restaurants understand well. It is axiomatic in the best international cuisines that freshness, food quality, and good taste go hand in hand. Keep this lesson firmly in mind as you trade in your former jaded palate, accustomed to years of salted, sugary, processed foods, for the subtle and exquisite flavors of "real," living foods perfectly prepared. You can start with the delicious recipes in *The Real Paleo Diet® Cookbook.*

VEGETABLES

The guidelines for vegetables are simple—basically eat as much of these as you like—either fresh, lightly steamed, or prepared in the innovative recipes described in Chapter 7 (Salads, Slaws & Vegetable Sides). There are only a few vegetables that should be avoided on contemporary Paleo Diets. Potatoes are banned because they maintain a high glycemic index similar to refined grains that unfavorably influences your blood sugar and insulin concentrations. Corn is actually not a vegetable per se, but rather is a grain most frequently consumed as high glycemic load foods such as tortillas, tortilla chips, cornstarch, grits, hominy, and other processed items. All grains, whether whole or refined, are not on The Paleo Diet® menu. Although we frequently think of sweet peas, green beans, snap beans, and even alfalfa and bean sprouts as vegetables, they are actually legumes, which contain a variety of compounds called anti-nutrients that may have multiple adverse health effects, fully explained in my book *The Paleo Answer*. Similarly, all other legumes (kidney beans, lentils, lima beans, soybeans, pinto beans, navy beans, garbanzo beans, fava beans, black-eyed peas, etc.) should not be regularly consumed by Paleo dieters—particularly autoimmune disease patients—because of their high anti-nutrient load. So what is left? You name it—just about any other fresh vegetable you can find in the grocery store, ethnic market, farmer's market, or your backyard garden. Here is a partial alphabetic list of some Paleo-friendly veggies (some are technically fruits and some may be considered fresh herbs):

Arame	Avocado
Artichoke	Bamboo shoots
Arugula	Beet greens
Asparagus (green, purple, white)	Beets
	Bok choy

Broccoli
Brussels sprouts
Burdock root
Cabbage (green, red, savoy)
Capers
Carrots
Cauliflower
Celeriac (celery root)
Celery
Chayote
Chickweed
Chicory
Chives
Collard greens
Cucumber
Cucumber (English)
Daikon radish
Dandelion greens
Dill
Dulse
Eggplant
Endive
Fennel root
Fiddlehead
Garlic
Ginger
Green onions
Hearts of palm
Horseradish
Jerusalem artichoke
Jicama
Kale
Kohlrabi
Lamb's quarters
Leeks

Lemongrass
Lettuce (all varieties)
Lotus root
Mushrooms (all edible
  varieties)
Mustard greens
Nori
Onions
Parsley
Parsnip
Peppers (all varieties)
Pumpkin
Purslane
Radicchio
Radish
Rutabaga (Swedes)
Seaweed
Shallots
Spinach
Spinach (New Zealand)
Squash (all varieties)
Sweet potatoes
Swiss chard
Taro root
Tomatillos
Tomato
Turnip greens
Turnips
Wakame
Wasabi root
Water chestnut
Watercress
Water spinach
Yams
Yarrow

FRUITS

The ground rules for fresh fruits are pretty straightforward. If you are not overweight or obese and are healthy, eat as much of these wholesome foods as you please. Avoid canned fruits as they are typically packed in heavy syrups and have lost considerable nutrients during the canning process. One exception here is the tomato, which really is a fruit and not a vegetable. Canned tomatoes, tomato paste, and tomato sauce are permitted, but only if you can find brands that don't contain added salt. Dried fruits should be eaten with discretion as they can contain as much concentrated sugar as candy. If you are overweight or maintain a disease of insulin resistance (high cholesterol, high blood pressure, type 2 diabetes, or heart disease), you should completely avoid dried fruit and only consume "very high-" and "high"-sugar fruits in moderation as listed below.

DRIED FRUITS (*total sugars per 100 grams*)

EXTREMELY HIGH IN TOTAL SUGARS

Dried mango	73.0	Dried papaya	53.5
Raisins, golden	70.6	Dried pears	49.0
Zante currants	70.6	Dried peaches	44.6
Raisins	65.0	Dried prunes	44.0
Dates	64.2	Dried apricots	38.9
Dried figs	62.3		

FRESH FRUITS (*total sugars per 100 grams*)

VERY HIGH IN TOTAL SUGARS

Grapes	18.1	Mango	14.8
Banana	15.6	Cherries, sweet	14.6

HIGH IN TOTAL SUGARS

Apples	13.3	Purple passion fruit	11.2
Pineapple	11.9		

MODERATE IN TOTAL SUGARS

Kiwifruit	10.5	Cantaloupe	8.7
Pear	10.5	Peach	8.7
Pear, Bosc	10.5	Nectarine	8.5
Pear, D'Anjou	10.5	Jackfruit	8.4
Pomegranate	10.1	Honeydew melon	8.2
Raspberries	9.5	Blackberries	8.1
Apricots	9.3	Cherries, sour	8.1
Orange	9.2	Tangerine	7.7
Watermelon	9.0	Plum	7.5

LOW IN TOTAL SUGARS

Blueberries	7.3	Grapefruit, white	6.2
Starfruit	7.1	Guava	6.0
Elderberries	7.0	Guava, strawberry	6.0
Figs	6.9	Papaya	5.9
Mamey apple	6.5	Strawberries	5.8
Grapefruit, pink	6.2	Casaba melon	4.7

VERY LOW IN TOTAL SUGARS

Tomato	2.8	Avocado, Florida	0.9
Lemon	2.5	Lime	0.4
Avocado, California	0.9		

NUTS AND SEEDS

When people first try The Paleo Diet®, they frequently jump on the "nuts and seeds" bandwagon with great fervor, thinking that these foods are "natural," nutritious, and completely healthy. In part, they are correct, as most fresh nuts are excellent sources of monounsaturated fats, which may help to reduce blood cholesterol.

The downside to almost all nuts and seeds is that they are concentrated sources of omega 6-fatty acids (specifically linoleic acid) and contain little or no omega 3-fatty acids. Excessive dietary omega 6-fatty acids when omega 3-fatty acid intake is low tends to promote inflammatory conditions such as heart disease, cancer, and autoimmune diseases. There is no doubt that our hunter-gatherer ancestors would have relished nuts and seeds, but these foods were not consumed year-round to the exclusion of rich dietary sources of omega-3 fatty acids found in fish and animal foods. So the take-home message for contemporary Paleo dieters is this: Enjoy nuts and seeds but do not overdo them—and regularly include omega 3-fatty acids in your diet from such rich sources as salmon, mackerel, herring, sardines, and other fatty fish.

One final point: Peanuts are not nuts, but are actually legumes, and definitely should not be part of contemporary Paleo diets. Peanuts contain a number anti-nutrients that quickly enter our bloodstream and may cause allergies and autoimmune and heart diseases. Peanut allergy is one of the most common food allergies, as are other nut allergies. So be cautious with these foods and carefully listen to your body. Paleo-approved nuts and seeds include:

Almonds	Macadamia nuts
Betel nuts	Pecans
Brazil nuts	Pine nuts
Cashews	Pistachios (unsalted)
Chestnuts	Pumpkin seeds
Coconuts	Sesame seeds
Flaxseeds	Sunflower seeds
Hazelnuts (filberts)	Walnuts
Kola nuts	

SALAD AND COOKING OILS

For Paleo recipes, salad and cooking oils are to food ingredients a bit like mortar is to bricks—in both cases, neither works well alone but together they work magic. Salad and cooking oils are indispensable ingredients in Paleo recipes because they bring together flavors, aromas, consistencies, and textures in a cohesive, delectable manner greater than the sum of the individual food ingredients.

Unfortunately, vegetable oils were clearly not a component of Stone Age diets, simply because our hunter-gatherer ancestors did not have the technology to produce them. Nevertheless, a number of contemporary salad and cooking oils maintain nutritional qualities that are consistent with the fat profiles found in the wild plant and animal foods our Stone Age ancestors would have eaten. Below is a list of the six salad and cooking oils that I endorse for contemporary Paleo diets.

Before you start using these oils, it is absolutely essential to know that flaxseed and walnut oils should never be used for cooking. They contain high concentrations of polyunsaturated fats (PUFA), which make them quite fragile and therefore susceptible to oxidation and degradation that occurs to their structures when heated. Accordingly, only use flax and walnut oils in recipes and foods that are served cold or at room temperature. Coconut oil is the most stable oil when heated because of its high concentrations of saturated fats (SAT) and is a good choice for all-around cooking as well as baked items. Olive, macadamia nut, and avocado oils can be used both as cooking and salad oils because of their high amounts of monounsaturated fats (MUFA), which make them relatively stable at moderate cooking temperatures but also liquid at room temperatures. Note that except for olive oil, all other oils are a bit pricey. In the recipes calling for olive oil in *The Real Paleo Diet® Cookbook*, I recommend that you use extra virgin olive oil because it tastes better and has greater amounts of health-promoting phytochemicals than regular olive oil or virgin olive oil.

	ω6/ω3	% PUFA	% MUFA	% SAT
Flaxseed Oil	0.24	66.0	20.2	9.4
Walnut Oil	5.1	63.3	22.8	9.1
Macadamia Nut Oil	6.3	1.9	81.6	16.5
Avocado Oil	13.0	13.5	67.9	11.6
Olive Oil	13.1	8.4	72.5	13.5
Coconut Oil	no ω3	4.4	1.3	94.3

Abbreviations: ω 6/ω 3 (omega-6/omega-3 fats); PUFA (polyunsaturated fats); MUFA (monounsaturated fats); SAT (saturated fats)

Before we leave the topic of salad and cooking oils, you may be wondering about other common oils, including the following:

Canola	Sesame
Corn	Soybean
Cottonseed	Sunflower seed
Peanut	Wheat germ
Safflower	

None of these oils should be used in contemporary Paleo Diet recipes because of excessive concentrations of omega 6-fats (linoleic acid), anti-nutrients, and other unfavorable residual compounds. Furthermore they simply do not taste as good as the six Paleo-approved oils.

FRESH MEATS AND POULTRY

One of the more important factors of The Paleo Diet® is to consume fresh animal foods at almost every meal. If you have the choice, free-ranging, grass-fed, or pasture-produced beef, bison, pork, lamb, and poultry are best. Clearly these meats are more expensive than their feedlot and grain-produced counterparts, so check out your neighborhood farmer's market to connect directly with a rancher or farmer who has grass-fed meats, poultry, or eggs for sale. By not going through a middleman, you can save yourself considerable money—and if you have a freezer, buying meat in bulk by the quarter or half side can also save you cash. Jo Robinson's website (www.eatwild.com) is one of the best on the Web to help you find a farmer or rancher selling grass-produced animal products in your area.

Freezing does not significantly change the nutritional qualities of fresh meat and is a great strategy to buy meats in bulk at a reduced cost while simultaneously allowing you to maintain adequate supplies of meat on hand. The nutritional characteristics of feedlot-produced meats are generally inferior when contrasted to meat from grass-fed

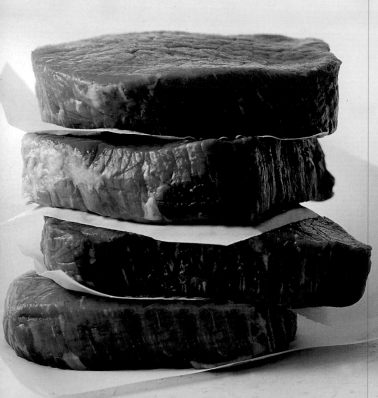

or free-ranging animals. This doesn't mean that you should completely avoid feedlot-produced meat and poultry. These meats are less expensive and can be a nourishing part of The Paleo Diet®, particularly if you purchase leaner cuts and also consume fatty fish like salmon, mackerel, herring, and others a few times a week. This dietary strategy will provide you with good sources of protein, iron, zinc, and B vitamins, while giving you sufficient long-chain omega-3 fats.

With The Paleo Diet®, you should try to consume about 55 % to 65 % of your daily calories from animal foods (beef, lamb, pork, poultry, fish, shellfish, organ meats, game meats, and eggs). Plant foods should comprise the balance. A general rule is to put a fist-size portion of meat or fish on your plate and then fill the rest with fruits and veggies. But as I mentioned earlier, you really shouldn't focus on how much you eat, but rather focus upon eating living, "real" foods and eat until you are full at each meal.

The only meats you should avoid are processed, salted, and canned meats, which are typically laced with additives and preservatives. Most of us know these meats quite well, but here is a partial list, just in case:

Bacon	Pork rinds
Bologna	Processed meats
Deli meats	Prosciutto
Frankfurters	Salami
Hams	Sausages
Hot dogs	Smoked, salted meats of
Link pork sausage	any kind
Lunch meats	Summer sausage

FRESH FISH, SEAFOOD, AND SHELLFISH

Fish, seafood, and shellfish maintain nutritional characteristics that in many ways are similar to the wild game meats and organs that were staples in our ancestors' Stone Age diets. Fish and seafood are rich sources of the beneficial omega-3 fatty acids known as EPA and DHA and are high in protein and B vitamins. You should try to include fatty fish (salmon, mackerel, herring, and sardines) about two to three times per week in your diet to obtain sufficient quantities of EPA and DHA. Avoid farm-raised fish—particularly tilapia. If possible and affordable, choose wild fish and seafood, and as with all other Paleo ingredients, the fresher, the better.

NON-PALEO INGREDIENTS

The popularity of The Paleo Diet® has spread to become a worldwide phenomenon, and as such it has been embraced by millions of people. Unfortunately, the correct dietary message has become diluted as hundreds of copycat books and thousands of websites and blogs deliver their individual messages, which frequently aren't always true to the best science about contemporary Paleo diets. So briefly, let me correct some of these mistakes. The Paleo Diet® generally should not include the following ingredients for staples and everyday food, though nut flours can be used in some recipes:

All cereal grains (*wheat, rye, barley, oats, rice, corn, millet, and sorghum*) *and cereal-like grains including amaranth, quinoa, chia seeds, and buckwheat* (*see my book* The Paleo Answer, *Chapter 6, as to why these items are excluded*)

Amalgamations of any or all of these ingredients, which can be employed, cooked, or combined in recipes by clever and innovative cooks to create a panoply of foods (*cookies, cakes, doughnuts, pastries, athletic bars, pancakes, "breads," wraps, etc.*) that have little to do with our ancestral diet. Think about fresh fruits, vegetables, meats, and fish—and you get the point!

Coconut sugars

Combinations of dried fruits, nuts, vegetable oils, sea salt, and honey—frequently called trail mix, gorp, or snack bars

Date sugars

Honey

Maple sugars

Molasses

Most refined vegetable oils (*except the list of 6 approved*)

Nut flours (particularly almond flour)

Raisin sugars

Sea salt

NON-PALEO FOODS TO CONSUME IN MODERATION

Because we clearly live in the 21st century and not in the Stone Age, it is impractical or impossible to consume only the Stone Age foods our ancestors ate. Nevertheless, a number of contemporary foods that you may enjoy will have little or no detrimental effect upon your health, particularly if they are consumed in moderation. Frequently, people are amazed to discover alcohol in this group.

No data suggests that Stone Age hunter-gatherers ever drank alcohol of any type. There is no doubt that alcohol abuse can impair our health, damage the liver, and increase our risk of developing many cancers. If you presently drink in moderation or take pleasure in an occasional glass of wine or beer, there's no requirement to give up this pleasure with The Paleo Diet®. In fact, moderate alcohol consumption may

significantly lower the risk of heart disease. When consumed in moderation, wine has been shown to have numerous positive health effects. A glass of wine before or during dinner may improve your insulin metabolism and increase satiety. Wine is also an appetizing ingredient that adds flavor to many Paleo Diet dishes, including meat, fish, poultry, and vegetable dishes. Feel free to cook with wine and spirits. The following items are non-Paleo. Enjoy them in moderation, but don't overdo:

Beer (*one 12-ounce serving*). Note: Try to purchase gluten-free beers.

Coffee

Nuts mixed with dried fruit (*no more than 4 ounces of nuts and 2 ounces of dried fruit a day, particularly if you are trying to lose weight*)

Spirits (*4 ounces*). Note: Stick to spirits distilled from non-gluten-containing grains (potato vodka, rum, 100% agave tequila, and brandy).

Tea

Wine (*two 4-ounce glasses*). Note: Cooking wines frequently contain salt.

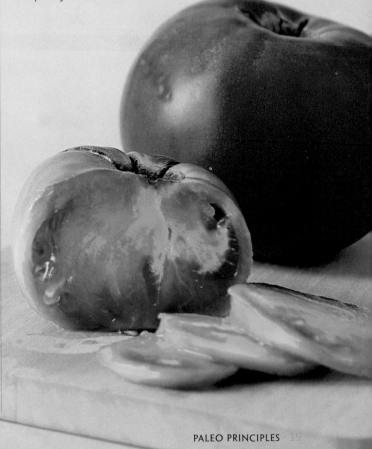

FLAVOR

AS YOU KNOW BY NOW, THE PALEO DIET® IS A SALT-FREE DIET. SALT IS NOT REQUIRED TO MAKE FOODS TASTE "GOOD." IN FACT, THE OPPOSITE IS TRUE—SALT DROWNS OUT THE FLAVOR OF FRESH FOOD. IF THE SUGGESTION THAT YOU COULD TRULY ENJOY A SALT-FREE DIET GIVES YOU PAUSE, BE ASSURED THAT THERE ARE MANY WAYS TO BUILD FANTASTIC FLAVOR IN FOODS WITHOUT SALT. ONE OF THE INCREDIBLE BENEFITS OF GETTING SALT OUT OF YOUR DIET WILL BE THE RESURGENCE OF YOUR TASTE BUDS AND NEW ENJOYMENT OF THE SUBTLE FLAVORS OF "REAL," LIVING FOODS.

SALT-FREE FOODS

On The Paleo Diet®, the only salt you will be getting is from naturally occurring salt found in meat, fish, seafood, eggs, vegetables, and nuts. This is all the salt you will ever need—just as Mother Nature intended. By complying with this dietary strategy, you will reduce your risk for high blood pressure, stroke, osteoporosis, heart disease, and many cancers. If you have been eating the standard American diet for your entire life, then you have been on a high-salt diet, perhaps without even knowing it.

Over time, you will not even miss it. Lightly steamed veggies, for instance, maintain delicate flavors and aromas that you may have never appreciated until your taste buds are freed from the yoke of this omnipresent and overpowering ingredient found in almost all contemporary foods and recipes. Enjoy the recipes in *The Real Paleo Diet® Cookbook* and you will be astonished that "real," living foods can be prepared in an exquisitely delicious manner that's completely free of salt.

Cooking with The Paleo Diet® doesn't mean that you need to eat bland, tasteless foods—far from it. On these pages we cover ingredients and techniques that build incredible flavor in foods without a single grain of salt. An added note: I don't recommend using any of the "lite salts" or potassium chloride salts because chloride, like sodium, has deleterious health effects.

HERBS

Walk through an herb garden and rub the leaves between your fingers and you will understand from the incredible aromas that arise how herbs add so much flavor to food. Their naturally occurring oils infuse foods with their essence. There are too many herbs to list here, but a few favorites include sweet Italian basil, oregano, thyme, rosemary, sage, parsley, cilantro, tarragon, Thai basil, and sage. Most can be used in both fresh and dried forms. In general, fresh herbs are added at the end of cooking and dried herbs are added at the beginning. In most recipes, you can substitute one for the other. A general rule is 1 teaspoon of dried herb for every 1 tablespoon of fresh. A scattering of fresh snipped herbs over the top of a dish right before serving adds both visual appeal and taste.

SPICES

The term "spice" refers to the seed, fruit, flower, root, or bark of a plant or tree. Cinnamon is made from the ground bark of the cassia tree. Ginger is a dried and ground root. Cumin, mustard, and fennel are all seeds that can be used whole or ground. Paprika is made from dried peppers (a fruit) and black pepper is a dried berry. Saffron—the most expensive spice in the world—is the dried, hand-picked stamen of a crocus. For convenience, commercially prepared ground spices are just fine, but if you have time and inclination, there is no substitute for the intense flavor and aroma of freshly ground spices—all you need is a mortar and pestle or an electric spice grinder. Check out our custom salt-free spice blends on page 324.

ALLIUM

While you might not recognize this term, you have no doubt used members of this plant family nearly every day in your cooking. Onions, garlic, shallots, leeks, chives, and scallions are all members of this botanical group and—to varying degrees, depending on their strength—contribute pleasantly pungent flavor and aroma to savory dishes of every stripe.

CITRUS

Citrus fruits such as lemon, lime, orange, and grapefruit are high in acid. Acid, in proper balance with fats and natural sugars, brightens the flavor in foods. Both the peels and juice can be used. A squeeze of fresh lemon right before serving is sometimes all a dish needs to take it from good to great.

CHILES

A compound called capsaicin is responsible for the heat encountered when your tongue comes in contact with a chile—or even the fraction of a chile. The more capsaicin a chile contains, the hotter it is. Although capsaicin is considered an irritant to mammals (which includes us humans) because it creates a burning in tissues, some of us can't seem to get enough of it. In just the right amounts, it simply creates a pleasantly warm sensation. People with autoimmune disease should proceed cautiously with chiles—particularly the hotter varieties that contain more capsaicin, which promotes a "leaky gut." In my book *The Paleo Answer,* I fully explain how a leaky gut may represent an important factor in promoting autoimmune diseases.

SPICY ROOTS

Ginger, horseradish, wasabi, and daikon are all roots that have head-clearing properties. They are frequently used freshly grated in marinades, stir-fries, and sauces.

VINEGAR

Like citrus, vinegar is an acid, which heightens flavor. In the past, I have suggested that vinegar should not be part of contemporary Paleo diets because it is a mixture (generally 5% acetic acid and water) of a compound that was not a regular component of ancestral Paleo diets. However, like the six vegetable oils I have recommended in this cookbook, the most recent research indicates that vinegar has few adverse health effects (and actually may improve blood sugar and insulin metabolism). Good vinegars include white vinegar, cider vinegar, white wine vinegar, red wine vinegar, balsamic vinegar, and rice vinegar. Because vinegar can substantially add to the flavor of contemporary Paleo recipes, I now fully endorse it—just make sure you purchase vinegars that are free from salt, sugar, and additives.

SEAWEED

Dried seaweeds such as arame, dulse, nori, and wakame all taste of the sea—briny and with a touch of minerals. Read the package for rehydration instructions, if that applies.

CARAMELIZATION

When naturally occurring sugars in fresh vegetables and fruits are heated to 300°F or higher, they turn brown and concentrate, which intensifies flavor without the addition of processed sugar. This process is related to the Maillard reaction, in which proteins in meat brown when exposed to high, dry heat. The thick, dark-brown crust created on the meat enhances appearance and flavor.

EQUIPMENT

I AM NOT A WORLD-CLASS CHEF, BUT I LOVE TO COOK AND FIDDLE AROUND IN OUR KITCHEN. I HAVE BEEN PREPARING MEALS FOR LORRIE AND MY THREE SONS FOR MORE THAN 20 YEARS. I KNOW WHAT IT TAKES TO COOK CONTEMPORARY, TASTY MEALS IN A FASHION THAT MIMICS THE FOOD GROUPS OUR STONE AGE ANCESTORS WOULD HAVE CONSUMED. I ONLY HAVE A FEW ABSOLUTES WHEN IT COMES TO COOKING UTENSILS—ONE IS GOOD KNIVES. YOU DON'T HAVE TO GO OUT AND BUY EVERYTHING ON THIS LIST, BUT A FEW KEY PIECES WILL MAKE COOKING FASTER AND MORE EFFICIENT.

ELIMINATE ALUMINUM

First, throw out all pots, pans, vessels, and baking sheets that have an aluminum surface. When we heat foods in aluminum pots or pans, tiny amounts of aluminum escape into our foods and ultimately find their way into our bodies. Although we don't totally understand how aluminum unfavorably affects human health, a number of scientific studies imply that it may damage the intestinal barrier, thereby promoting chronic low-level inflammation. Aluminum also seems to preferentially attach itself to brain and nervous tissue. It is still unclear if aluminum damages mental or nervous tissue function. I recommend that you get rid of all of your aluminum pots, pans, and cooking vessels and replace them with either Pyrex, ceramic, pottery, or stainless-steel.

Also, you should replace your plastic containers, storage jugs, and water bottles with glass, ceramic, pottery, or stainless-steel counterparts. Again, don't use aluminum. Plastic containers universally contain phthalates, BPA (bisphenol A), dioxins, and other compounds that leech into the foods and liquids stored in our plastic containers. These compounds may have adverse health effects.

BEYOND THE BASICS

These recommendations assume you have a basic set of saucepans, skillets, or sauté pans, spoons, spatulas, scrapers, and the like. Not every tool or appliance on this list is absolutely necessary—and some of them overlap—but most of them may prove very useful as you adopt The Paleo Diet®:

BAKING SHEETS: A couple large rimmed baking sheets— either 10×15 or 11×17—are indispensable for toasting nuts, roasting vegetables, and baking thin pieces of fish.

BLENDER: While most kitchens are equipped with a blender, a high-performance blender is a real boon for the Paleo cook. The best-known brands are Vitamix and Blendtec. Their specially designed blades and high-powered motors make silky-smooth soups, sauces, nut butters, and condiments and are especially helpful for making Dijon-Style Mustard (page 322) and Cashew Cream (page 327).

BOX GRATER: This four-sided grater has different surfaces on each side for coarse or fine grating, as well as slicing.

CUTTING BOARDS: Wood cutting boards won't dull your knives and are safe to use as long as you scrub them with hot soapy water and rinse and dry well. You might want to invest in two cutting boards so that one can be dedicated to raw meat and the other to fruits and vegetables.

DEHYDRATOR: To ensure that your dried fruits don't contain any sugar or sulfur dioxide, dry your own. A dehydrator can also be used to make veggie chips and homemade jerky.

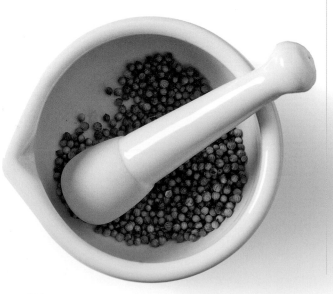

DUTCH OVEN: The rounded shape of this covered pot is ideal for long-simmering, moist-heat cooking, such as braising large roasts and meaty ribs—as well as for making soups and stews. The most useful Dutch ovens are between 5 and 8 quarts and are made of heavy, heat-conducting material, such as enameled cast iron.

EXTRA-LARGE SKILLET: For family-scaled one-dish meals that contain meat and vegetables—or simply for cooking several chops or steaks at once—this oversize pan is a must. Look for a 14-inch skillet (curved sides) or 6-quart sauté pan (straight sides).

FOOD PROCESSOR: This machine makes quick work of chopping large amounts of vegetables and is essential for making a variety of flavorful pestos (page 320).

GARLIC PRESS: Place a peeled garlic clove in the perforated cup of this tool and with squeeze of the handle, it's minced.

JUICER: Citrus juices are used in profusion in Paleo recipes, as both flavoring agents and in sauces, beverages, and marinades. Look for a generously sized citrus juicer that has a sharp point and a strainer for seeds and pulp.

JULIENNE PEELER: Run this peeler down root vegetables and summer or winter squash and in a flash get delicate vegetable strands for "noodles," slaws, or stir-fries.

KNIFE SHARPENER: Once you have high-quality knives, you want to keep them in good working order. A few swipes in an electric knife sharpener keeps your knives sharp and safe.

KNIVES: A vital component of all Paleo kitchens is high-quality cutlery. First-class stainless-steel knives are absolutely essential for cutting, chopping, and preparing the foods you and your family will eat when you adopt The Paleo Diet®. If you don't currently own first-rate cutlery, regard it as a lifetime investment for the health and well-being of you and your family. Look for high-quality stainless-steel knife sets that allow you the freedom to cut, chop, slice, and core all foods that are vital to this lifelong way of eating.

MANDOLINE SLICER: While there are very expensive ($250-plus) French-made versions of this tool, you can get a decent one for about $40. For quickly making uniform, paper-thin slices of root vegetables, zucchini "noodles," and matchstick or julienne-cut carrots, it's priceless.

MEAT GRINDER: The freshest ground meat and poultry is the stuff you grind yourself. You can also be sure it's made from the exactly the cuts you choose.

MEAT MALLET: Although the studded side of this tool isn't as necessary as it used to be for tenderizing tough cuts of meat, the smooth side is used to pound cuts of meat or poultry thinner for quick cooking or for stuffing and rollling.

MEAT THERMOMETER: Look for a digital instant-read thermometer. It looks like a large needle with a temperature gauge at one end. You simply poke it into the meat to get the internal temperature in seconds.

MICROPLANE ZESTER/GRATER: This narrow rasp grater makes quick work of zesting citrus and grating fresh nutmeg.

MORTAR AND PESTLE: Though this might be the closest to a Stone Age tool on this list, it is still relevant to the modern kitchen for crushing seeds and grinding spices. If you prefer, use an electric spice grinder.

NUT GRINDER: In both hand-cranked and electric versions, this tool allows you to effortlessly grind or chop nuts.

OVENPROOF SKILLET: Many dishes involving large chops or roasts quickly sear on the stovetop to create a nice exterior crust, then finish cooking in the oven to retain their juiciness. Cast-iron is an ideal material for this.

PARCHMENT PAPER: Line pans with this heat-tolerant paper to keep food from sticking. It's also essential for cooking "en papillote," or "in paper"—a moist-heat cooking technique that steams food in packets to retain nutrients and enhance flavor. (See page 247 for an example.)

ROASTING PAN: Look for a heavy pan that can accommodate large birds and roasts.

SALAD SPINNER: Quickly wash and spin-dry salad greens, herbs, and cooking greens (mustard, collards, and kale).

SLOW COOKER: If you plan on making slow-cooker versions of homemade broth or for fix-and-forget stews, brisket dishes, and roasts, this is essential to the busy Paleo cook.

STEAMER INSERT: A pop-up steamer insert fits into most large saucepans and can be used for steaming vegetables, fish, and poultry.

STOCKPOT: A large (8- to 10-quart) stockpot is essential for making your own stocks and broths, such as Beef Bone Broth (page 131) or Chicken Bone Broth (page 235).

WOK: This deep, bowl-shape pan is helpful if you are fond of stir-fries.

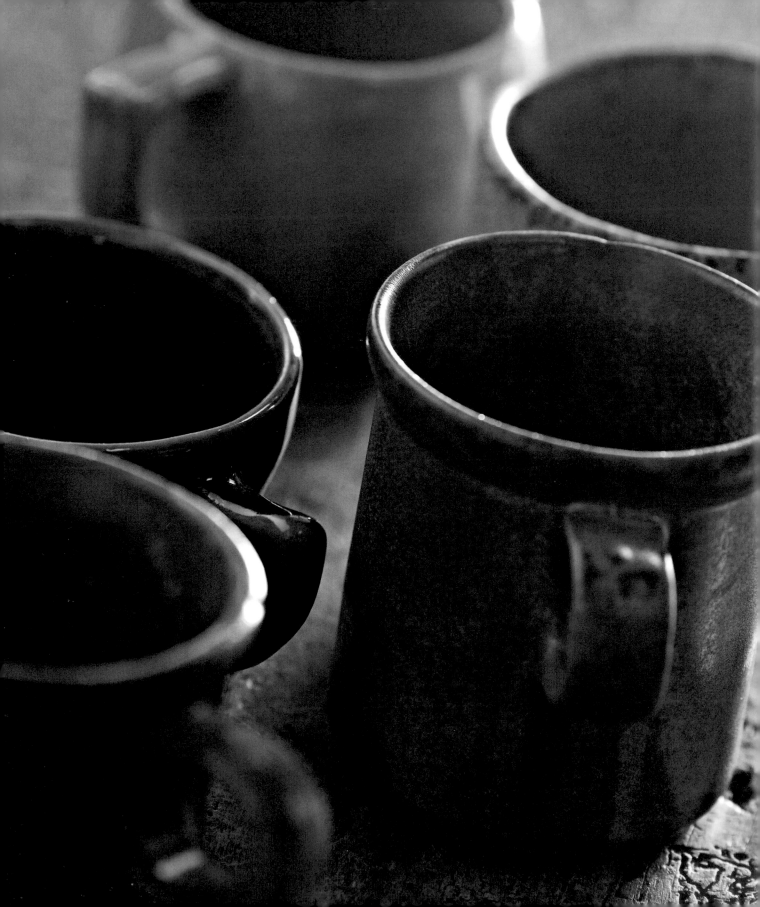

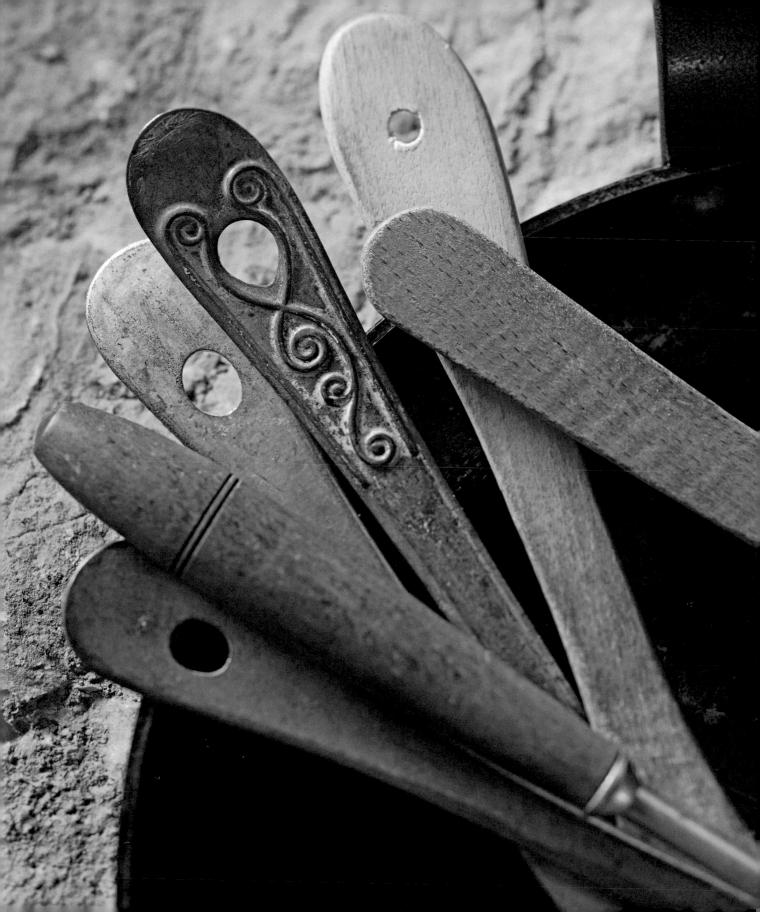

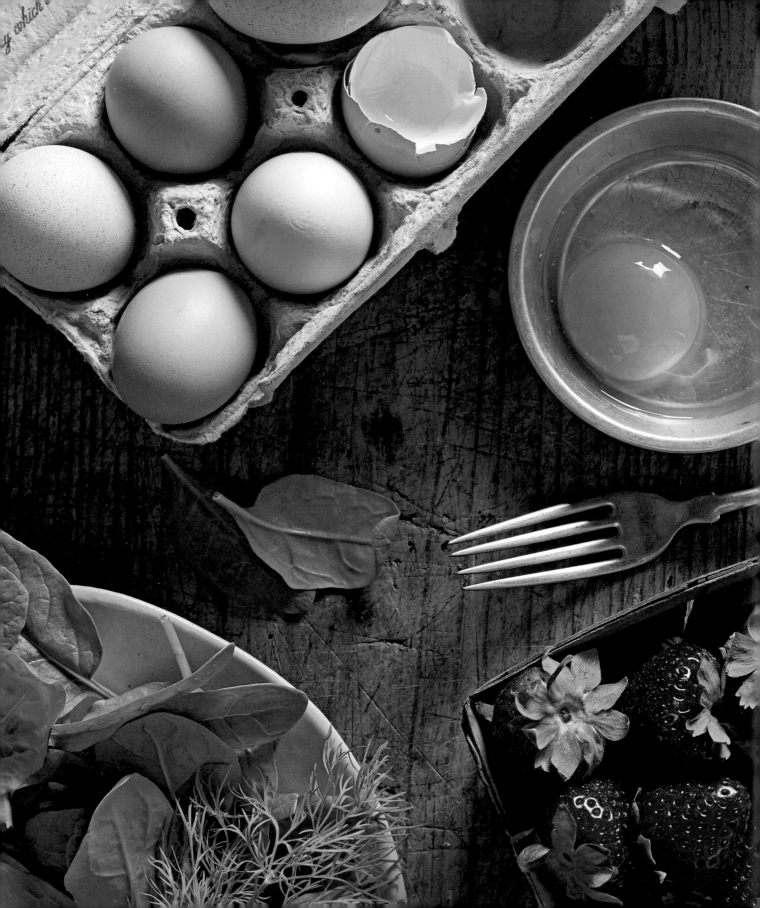

BREAKFAST & BRUNCH

My favorite time of the day is the early morning, particularly in the spring and summer. The air is so fresh and clear in Colorado that it just feels good to be alive. I normally like to start my days with exercise in one form or another. I have been a lifelong runner and swimmer, so these are my preferred choices for a workout first thing in the morning, but I also enjoy mountain biking. One of the best aspects of early-morning exercise is that it invigorates you for the rest of the morning—but it also gives you a great appetite for breakfast.

When I was a child growing up in Southern California in the 1950s and '60s, my mom would give me a couple choices for breakfast, which were then (and are now) pretty much the norm in America. Scrambled eggs; bacon or sausage; white bread toast with butter, jelly, or jam; and a glass of orange juice were frequently on the menu. On weekends she would make pancakes or waffles smothered in maple syrup and butter along with a glass of O.J. or milk. Back in those days, the junk food industry hadn't really geared up to the extent that it has today, so there weren't as many sugary breakfast cereals as there are now. Every few days Mom served us cold cereal along with white bread toast and O.J. Such were the halcyon, untroubled days of my youth. Little did I know that my breakfasts were generally high glycemic-index meals, loaded with refined cereal grains, sugar, and salt. These kinds of foods—pancakes, waffles, syrup, jam, jelly, white bread, processed breakfast cereals, and milk—represent the types of non-Paleo foods that have contributed to making Americans some of the fattest, unhealthiest people on the planet.

Mom actually did serve us at least one healthy breakfast food— eggs—that should be on your morning menu whenever you like. Eggs from free-ranging chickens would have been better still, but in those days, these items were rarely or never found in the supermarkets. Better than orange juice would have been fresh oranges. Better than bacon, sausage, or processed meats would have been pork chops or other fresh meats. But that was the 1950s and 1960s, and The Paleo Diet® movement was still 30 to 45 years in the future. We now have the knowledge to prepare and eat fantastically delicious breakfast foods which are, by the way, quite healthy. Check out any one of the following breakfasts designed and tested by our team of innovative chefs and cooks. I know you will enjoy them!

DRIED CHERRY-SAGE SCOTCH EGGS

PREP: 20 minutes   BAKE: 35 minutes   MAKES: 4 servings

THIS CLASSIC BRITISH PUB SNACK TRANSLATES INTO A PERFECT PALEO BREAKFAST. IF YOU MAKE THE HARD-COOKED EGGS AHEAD, THIS RECIPE GOES TOGETHER VERY QUICKLY—AND THEY PEEL MORE EASILY AS WELL. KEEPING A BOWL OF HARD-COOKED EGGS IN THE REFRIGERATOR IS A GREAT IDEA FOR QUICK BREAKFASTS AND SNACKS.

1 pound lean ground pork
½ cup snipped no-sugar-added dried cherries
2 tablespoons snipped fresh sage
1 tablespoon snipped fresh marjoram
1 teaspoon freshly ground black pepper
¼ teaspoon freshly ground nutmeg
⅛ teaspoon ground cloves
4 hard-cooked large eggs, cooled and peeled*
½ cup almond flour
1 teaspoon dried sage, crushed
½ teaspoon dried marjoram, crushed
2 tablespoons extra virgin olive oil
   Dijon-Style Mustard (see recipe, page 322)

1. Preheat oven to 375°F. Line a baking pan with parchment paper or foil; set aside. In a large bowl combine pork, cherries, fresh sage, fresh marjoram, pepper, nutmeg, and cloves.

2. Shape pork mixture into four equal patties. Place one egg on each patty. Shape the patty around each egg. In a shallow dish or pie plate combine almond flour, dried sage, and dried marjoram. Roll each sausage-coated egg in the almond flour mixture to coat. Place on the prepared baking sheet. Drizzle with olive oil.

3. Bake for 35 to 40 minutes or until sausage is cooked through. Serve with Dijon-Style Mustard.

***Tip:** To hard-cook eggs, place eggs in a single layer in a large saucepan. Cover with 1 to 2 inches water. Bring to boiling. Allow to boil for 1 minute. Remove from heat. Cover and let stand for 12 to 15 minutes.

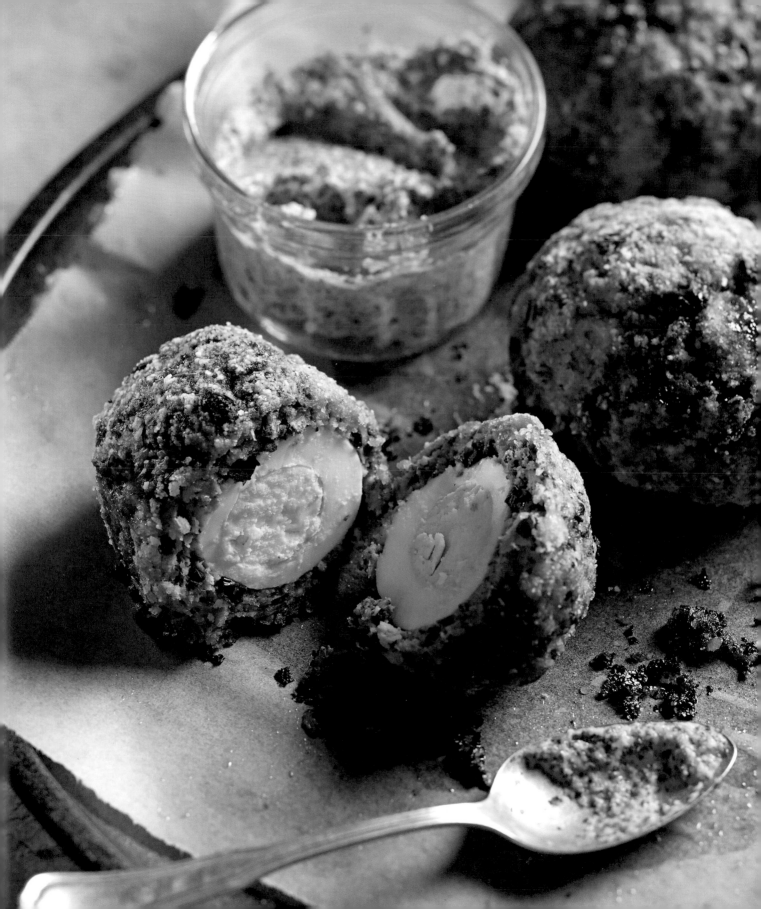

CAULIFLOWER STEAKS AND EGGS

PREP: 20 minutes   COOK: 25 minutes   MAKES: 4 servings

THICK SLICES ARE CUT FROM A HEAD OF CAULIFLOWER TO CREATE HEARTY "STEAKS" THAT ARE THEN FRIED IN OLIVE OIL UNTIL BROWNED AND CRISP, TOPPED WITH A POACHED EGG, AND SERVED ON A BED OF GARLICKY SAUTÉED KALE.

1	head cauliflower, leaves removed
1½	teaspoons Smoky Seasoning, (see recipe, page 324)
5	tablespoons extra virgin olive oil
4	large eggs
1	tablespoon white or cider vinegar
2	large cloves garlic, minced
4	cups chopped kale

1. Place stem end of cauliflower on a cutting board. Using a large sharp knife, slice cauliflower into four ½-inch steaks from the center of the cauliflower, cutting through stem end (some florets may break loose; save for another use).

2. Season steaks on both sides with 1 teaspoon of the Smoky Seasoning. In an extra-large skillet heat 2 tablespoons of the olive oil over medium-high heat. Add 2 of the cauliflower steaks. Cook for 4 minutes on each side or until golden brown and just tender. Remove from pan and cover lightly with foil. Keep warm in a 200°F oven. Repeat with remaining 2 steaks, using an additional 2 tablespoons of olive oil.

3. To poach the eggs, fill a separate skillet with about 3 inches of water. Add vinegar and bring to a simmer. Crack eggs, one at a time, into a small bowl or ramekin and gently slide into the simmering water. Let eggs cook for 30 to 45 seconds or until whites start to firm up. Turn off the heat. Cover and poach for 3 to 5 minutes, depending on how soft you like your yolks.

4. Meanwhile, in the same skillet heat the remaining 1 tablespoon olive oil. Add garlic and cook for 30 seconds to 1 minute. Add kale and cook and stir for 1 to 2 minutes or just until wilted.

5. To serve, divide kale among four plates. Top each with a cauliflower steak and a poached egg. Sprinkle eggs with the remaining ½ teaspoon Smoky Seasoning and serve immediately.

TURKEY, SPINACH, AND ASPARAGUS FRITTATA

PREP: 20 minutes   BROIL: 3 minutes   MAKES: 2 to 3 servings

THIS BEAUTIFUL FRITTATA FLECKED WITH GREEN GOES TOGETHER VERY QUICKLY AND IS A GREAT WAY TO START YOUR DAY—OR END IT. IT'S PERFECT FOR A SPEEDY DINNER WHEN YOU DON'T HAVE TIME TO COOK A MORE INVOLVED MEAL. A CAST-IRON SKILLET IS NOT NECESSARY BUT WILL GIVE YOU VERY GOOD RESULTS.

2 tablespoons extra virgin olive oil

1 clove garlic, minced

4 ounces ground turkey breast

¼ to ½ teaspoon black pepper

½ cup ½-inch-long pieces fresh asparagus

1 cup fresh baby spinach leaves, chopped

4 large eggs

1 tablespoon water

2 teaspoons snipped fresh dill

1 tablespoon snipped fresh parsley

1. Preheat broiler with the oven rack positioned 4 inches from the heating element.

2. In an oven-safe medium skillet heat 1 tablespoon of the olive oil over medium heat. Add garlic; cook and stir until golden. Add the ground turkey; sprinkle with pepper. Cook and stir for 3 to 4 minutes or until meat is browned and cooked through, stirring with a wooden spoon to break up meat. Transfer cooked turkey to a bowl; set aside.

3. Return skillet to stovetop; pour the remaining 1 tablespoon olive oil into skillet. Add asparagus; cook and stir over medium-high heat until tender. Stir in the cooked turkey and the spinach. Cook for 1 minute.

4. In a medium bowl beat eggs with the water and the dill. Pour egg mixture over turkey mixture in skillet. Cook and stir for 1 minute. Transfer skillet to oven and broil for 3 to 4 minutes or until eggs are set and top is browned. Sprinkle with snipped parsley.

5 WAYS WITH EGGS

EGGS ARE AMAZINGLY VERSATILE. THEY CAN BE FRIED, BOILED, POACHED, STEAMED, SCRAMBLED, OR BAKED AND LEND THEMSELVES TO A WORLD OF FLAVORS. EAT A BREAKFAST OF PROTEIN-RICH EGGS AND VEGETABLES AND YOU WILL STAY SATISFIED AND FREE FROM HUNGER PANGS ALL MORNING.

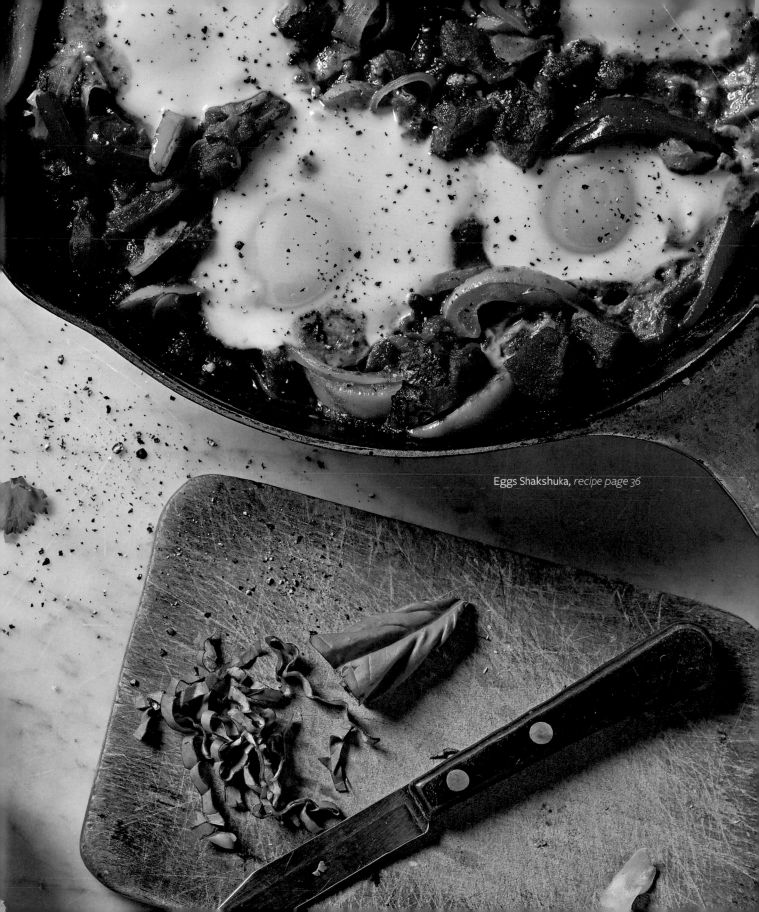

Eggs Shakshuka, *recipe page 36*

5 WAYS WITH EGGS

THE RICH BUT MILD FLAVOR OF EGGS ALLOWS THEM TO SERVE AS A BLANK CANVAS FOR AN AMAZING VARIETY OF PREPARATIONS AND FLAVOR PROFILES—FROM A NORTH AFRICAN-INSPIRED SCRAMBLE TO FRENCH OVEN-BAKED EGGS WITH SALMON AND FRESH SPINACH TO AN ASIAN-INSPIRED HOT SOUP. ONE OF THE MOST WONDERFUL AND INTERESTING THINGS ABOUT THE PALEO DIET® IS HOW IT CHANGES YOUR PARADIGMS ABOUT WHAT TO EAT AND WHEN. MEATS AND FRESH VEGETABLES BECOME PREFERRED BREAKFAST FOODS—AND SO DOES SOUP. SOUP IS EATEN FOR BREAKFAST ALL OVER THE MIDDLE EAST, ASIA, AND LATIN AMERICA— WHY SHOULDN'T WE?

1. TUNISIAN SCRAMBLED EGGS WITH ROASTED PEPPERS AND HARISSA

PREP: 30 minutes
BROIL: 8 minutes
STAND: 5 minutes
COOK: 5 minutes
MAKES: 4 servings

- 1 small red sweet pepper
- 1 small yellow sweet pepper
- 1 small poblano chile pepper (see tip, page 56)
- 1 tablespoon extra virgin olive oil
- 6 large eggs
- ¼ teaspoon ground cinnamon
- ½ teaspoon ground cumin
- ⅓ cup golden raisins
- ⅓ cup snipped fresh parsley
- 1 tablespoon Harissa (see recipe, page 322)

1. Preheat broiler with the oven rack positioned 3 to 4 inches from the heat. Halve peppers lengthwise; remove stems and seeds. Place pepper halves, cut sides down, on a foil-lined baking sheet. Broil 8 minutes or until pepper skins are black. Wrap peppers in the foil. Let cool for 5 minutes. Unwrap peppers; use a sharp knife to peel away blackened skins. Cut peppers into thin strips; set aside.

2. In a large bowl combine eggs, cinnamon, and cumin. Whisk until frothy. Add pepper strips, raisins, parsley, and Harissa.

3. In a large skillet heat olive oil over medium heat. Add the egg mixture to skillet. Cook about 5 to 7 minutes or until eggs are set but still moist and shiny, stirring frequently. Serve immediately.

2. EGGS SHAKSHUKA

START TO FINISH: 35 minutes
MAKES: 4 to 6 servings

- ¼ cup extra virgin olive oil
- 1 large onion, halved and thinly sliced
- 1 large red sweet pepper, thinly sliced
- 1 large orange sweet pepper, thinly sliced
- 1 teaspoon ground cumin
- ½ teaspoon smoked paprika
- ½ teaspoon crushed red pepper
- 4 cloves garlic, minced
- 2 14.5-ounce cans organic salt-free fire-roasted diced tomatoes
- 6 large eggs
     Freshly ground black pepper
- ¼ cup snipped fresh cilantro
- ¼ cup shredded fresh basil

1. Preheat oven to 400°F. In an oven-safe large skillet heat oil over medium heat. Add onion and sweet peppers. Cook and stir for 4 to 5 minutes or until vegetables are tender. Add cumin, paprika, crushed red pepper, and garlic; cook and stir for 2 minutes.

2. Stir in tomatoes. Bring to boiling; reduce heat. Simmer, uncovered, about 10 minutes or until thickened.

3. Crack eggs into skillet over tomato mixture. Transfer skillet to the preheated oven. Bake, uncovered, for 7 to 10 minutes or until eggs are just set (yolks should still be runny).

4. Sprinkle with black pepper. Garnish with cilantro and basil; serve immediately.

3. BAKED EGGS WITH SALMON AND SPINACH

PREP: 20 minutes
BAKE: 15 minutes
MAKES: 4 servings

- 1 tablespoon extra virgin olive oil
- 1 tablespoon fresh thyme leaves
     Freshly grated nutmeg
- 10 ounces baby spinach leaves (6 cups packed)
- 2 tablespoons water
- 8 ounces grilled or roasted salmon
- 1 teaspoon finely shredded lemon peel
- ½ teaspoon Smoky Seasoning (see recipe, page 324)
- 8 large eggs

1. Preheat oven to 375°F. Brush the insides of four 6- to 8-ounce ramekins with olive oil. Sprinkle thyme leaves evenly among the ramekins; lightly sprinkle with freshly grated nutmeg. Set aside.

2. In a covered medium saucepan combine spinach and the water.

Bring to boiling; remove from heat. Lift and turn spinach with tongs just until wilted. Place spinach in a fine-mesh sieve; press firmly to release excess liquid. Divide spinach among prepared ramekins. Flake salmon evenly among ramekins. Sprinkle salmon with lemon peel and Smoky Seasoning. Crack 2 of the eggs into each ramekin.

3. Place filled ramekins in a large baking pan. Pour hot water into the baking pan until it is halfway up the sides of the ramekins. Carefully transfer baking pan to the oven.

4. Bake for 15 to 18 minutes or until egg whites are set. Serve immediately.

4. EGG DROP SOUP WITH SCALLIONS, MUSHROOMS, AND BOK CHOY

PREP: 30 minutes
STAND: 10 minutes
COOK: 5 minutes
MAKES: 4 to 6 servings

0.5 ounce sun-dried wakame
3 tablespoons unrefined coconut oil
2 shallots, minced
1 2-inch piece fresh ginger, peeled and cut into very thin matchstick-size strips
1 star anise
1 pound shiitake mushrooms, stemmed and sliced
1 teaspoon five-spice powder
¼ teaspoon black pepper
8 cups Beef Bone Broth (see recipe, page 131) or no-salt-added beef broth
¼ cup fresh lemon juice
3 large eggs
6 scallions, thinly sliced
2 heads baby bok choy, cut into ¼-inch-thick slices

1. In a medium bowl cover wakame with hot water. Let stand for 10 minutes or until soft and pliable. Drain well; rinse well and drain again. Cut strips of wakame into 1-inch pieces; set aside.

2. In a large pot heat coconut oil over medium heat. Add shallots, ginger, and star anise. Cook and stir for about 2 minutes or until shallots are translucent. Add mushrooms; cook and stir for 2 minutes. Sprinkle five-spice powder and pepper over mushrooms; cook and stir for 1 minute. Add reserved wakame, Beef Bone Broth, and lemon juice. Bring mixture to simmering.

3. In a small bowl beat eggs. Drizzle beaten eggs into simmering broth, swirling broth in a figure-eight motion. Remove soup from heat. Stir in scallions. Divide bok choy among large warmed bowls. Ladle soup into bowls; serve immediately.

5. PERSIAN SWEET OMELET

START TO FINISH: 30 minutes
MAKES: 4 servings

6 large eggs
½ teaspoon ground cinnamon
¼ teaspoon ground cardamom
¼ teaspoon ground coriander
1 teaspoon finely shredded orange peel
½ teaspoon pure vanilla extract
1 tablespoon refined coconut oil
⅔ cup raw cashews, coarsely chopped and toasted
⅔ cup raw almonds, coarsely chopped and toasted
⅔ cup pitted and chopped Medjool dates
½ cup raw shredded coconut

1. In a medium bowl whisk together eggs, cinnamon, cardamom, coriander, orange peel, and vanilla extract until frothy; set aside.

2. In a large skillet heat coconut oil over medium-high heat until a drop of water dropped in the center of the skillet sizzles. Add egg mixture; reduce heat to medium.

3. Let eggs cook until they begin to set around the edges of the pan. Using a heatproof spatula, gently push one edge of the egg mixture toward the center of the pan while tilting the pan to allow the remaining liquid egg mixture to flow underneath. Repeat process around edges of pan until liquid is almost set but eggs are still moist and shiny. Loosen edges of omelet with the spatula; slide omelet gently out of skillet and onto a serving plate.

4. Sprinkle cashews, almonds, dates, and coconut over top of omelet. Serve immediately.

SHRIMP AND CRAB CHAWANMUSHI

PREP: 30 minutes   COOK: 30 minutes   COOL: 30 minutes   MAKES: 4 servings

"CHAWANMUSHI" TRANSLATES LITERALLY TO "TEACUP STEAMING," WHICH REFERS TO HOW THIS JAPANESE EGG CUSTARD IS TRADITIONALLY COOKED—STEAMED IN A TEACUP. THE CREAMY, SAVORY DISH CAN BE SERVED WARM OR CHILLED. A BIT OF CULINARY TRIVIA: IT'S ONE OF THE RARE JAPANESE DISHES THAT IS EATEN WITH A SPOON.

2   ounces fresh or frozen shrimp, peeled, deveined, and chopped

1½ ounces fresh or frozen Dungeness or snow crab meat*

2½ cups Chicken Bone Broth (see recipe, page 235), Beef Bone Broth (see recipe page 131), or no-salt-added chicken or beef broth, chilled

⅔   cup shiitake mushrooms, stemmed and chopped

1   1-inch piece fresh ginger, peeled and thinly sliced

⅛   teaspoon salt-free five-spice powder

3   large eggs, beaten

⅓   cup small diced zucchini

2   tablespoons snipped fresh cilantro

1. Thaw shrimp and crab, if frozen. Rinse shrimp and crab; pat dry with paper towels. Set aside. In a small saucepan bring 1½ cups broth, ⅓ cup chopped shiitake mushrooms, ginger, and five-spice powder to boiling; reduce heat. Boil gently until reduced to 1 cup, about 15 minutes. Remove saucepan from heat. Stir in the remaining 1 cup of broth; let cool to room temperature, about 20 minutes.

2. When broth is cooled completely, gently whisk in the eggs, incorporating as little air as possible. Over a bowl strain the mixture through a fine-mesh sieve; discard solids.

3. Divide the shrimp, crab, zucchini, cilantro, and the remaining ⅓ cup mushrooms among four 8- to 10-ounce ramekins or mugs. Divide the egg mixture among the ramekins filling each one-half to three-fourths full; set aside.

4. Fill an extra-large stockpot with 1½ inches of water. Cover and bring to boiling. Reduce heat to medium-low. Arrange the four ramekins inside of the stockpot. Carefully pour in enough additional boiling water to reach halfway up the sides of the ramekins. Cover ramekins loosely with foil. Cover the pot with a tight-fitting lid and steam about 15 minutes or until egg mixture is set. To test for doneness, insert a toothpick into the center of the custard. When clear broth comes out, it is done. Carefully remove the ramekins. Let cool for 10 minutes before serving. Serve warm or chilled.

Note: Before beginning the recipe, find an extra-large stockpot with a tight-fitting lid that allows four ramekins or mugs to stand upright inside of it. While the mugs are inside, find a clean 100%-cotton kitchen wash cloth or towel that will cover the tops of the mugs without obstructing the lid.

***Tip:** You will need 4 ounces crab in the shell to get 1½ ounces crabmeat.

Tip: The mushrooms and spices infuse flavor into the broth in Step 1. For a quicker version, use 2 cups broth and start with Step 2, omitting the ginger, five-spice powder, and ⅓ cup of the shiitakes. No need to strain the egg mixture.

CHICKEN SAUSAGE HASH

PREP: 20 minutes   COOK: 15 minutes   MAKES: 4 to 6 servings

ALTHOUGH THIS SAVORY HASH IS PERFCTLY DELICIOUS ON ITS OWN, CRACKING FRESH EGGS INTO INDENTATIONS IN THE HASH AND LETTING THEM COOK JUST UNTIL SLIGHTLY FIRM—SO THE YOLK RUNS INTO THE HASH—MAKES IT PARTICULARLY TASTY.

2 pounds ground chicken
1 teaspoon dried thyme
1 teaspoon dried sage
½ teaspoon dried rosemary
¼ teaspoon black pepper
2 tablespoons extra virgin olive oil
2 cups chopped onions
1 tablespoon minced garlic
1 cup chopped green sweet pepper
1 cup shredded red or golden beets
½ cup Chicken Bone Broth (see recipe, page 235) or no-salt-added chicken broth

1. In a large bowl combine ground chicken, thyme, sage, rosemary, and black pepper, working mixture together with your hands to evenly distribute seasonings through the meat.

2. In an extra-large skillet heat 1 tablespoon of the oil over medium-high heat. Add chicken; cook about 8 minutes or until lightly browned, stirring with a wooden spoon to break up meat. Using a slotted spoon, remove meat from skillet; set aside. Drain fat from skillet. Wipe skillet with a clean paper towel.

3. In the same skillet heat the remaining 1 tablespoon oil over medium heat. Add onions and garlic; cook about 3 minutes or until onions are tender. Add sweet pepper and shredded beets to onion mixture; cook about 4 to 5 minutes or until vegetables are tender, stirring occasionally. Stir in reserved chicken mixture and Chicken Bone Broth. Heat through.

Tip: If you like, make four indentations in the hash; crack an egg into each indentation. Cover and cook over medium heat until eggs are desired doneness.

ROSEMARY-PEAR BREAKFAST SAUSAGES

PREP: 20 minutes   COOK: 8 minutes per batch   MAKES: 4 (2-patty) servings

SHREDDED PEAR GIVES THESE SAVORY SAUSAGES A TOUCH OF SWEETNESS—WHICH IS A TERRIFIC COMPLEMENT TO THE SMOKY FLAVOR FROM THE PAPRIKA. ENJOY THEM ALONE OR WITH EGGS.

1 pound ground pork
1 ripe medium pear (such as Bosc, Anjou, or Bartlett), peeled, cored, and shredded
2 tablespoons finely chopped scallions
2 teaspoons snipped fresh rosemary
1 teaspoon fennel seeds, crushed
½ teaspoon smoked paprika
¼ to ½ teaspoon freshly ground black pepper
2 cloves garlic, minced
1 tablespoon olive oil

1. In a medium bowl combine ground pork, pear, scallions, rosemary, fennel seeds, smoked paprika, pepper, and garlic. Gently mix ingredients until thoroughly combined. Divide the mixture into eight equal portions. Shape into eight ½-inch-thick patties.

2. In an extra-large skillet heat olive oil over medium heat until hot. Add half of the patties; cook for 8 to 10 minutes or until well browned and cooked through, flipping sausages halfway through. Remove from skillet and place on a paper towel-lined plate to drain; tent lightly with foil to keep warm while cooking remaining sausages.

CUBAN-STYLE SHREDDED BEEF SKILLET

START TO FINISH: 30 minutes   MAKES: 4 servings

LEFTOVER BRISKET IS IDEAL FOR USE IN THIS RECIPE. TRY IT AFTER YOU'VE ENJOYED MEXICAN BRAISED BRISKET WITH MANGO, JICAMA, CHILE, AND ROASTED PUMPKIN SEED SALAD (PAGE 86) OR ROMAINE WRAPS WITH SHREDDED BEEF BRISKET AND FRESH RED CHILE HARISSA (PAGE 88) FOR DINNER.

1 bunch collard greens or 4 cups lightly packed raw spinach

2 tablespoons extra virgin olive oil

½ cup chopped onion

2 medium green sweet peppers, cut into strips

2 teaspoons dried oregano

½ teaspoon ground cumin

½ teaspoon ground coriander

½ teaspoon smoked paprika

3 cloves garlic, minced

2 ounces cooked beef, shredded

1 teaspoon finely shredded orange peel

⅓ cup fresh orange juice

1 cup halved cherry tomatoes

1 tablespoon fresh lime juice

1 ripe avocado, seeded, peeled, and sliced

1. Remove and discard thick stems from collard greens. Cut leaves into bite-size pieces; set aside.

2. In an extra-large skillet heat olive oil over medium heat. Add onion and sweet peppers; cook for 3 to 5 minutes or just until vegetables are tender. Add oregano, cumin, coriander, smoked paprika, and garlic; stir well. Add shredded beef, orange peel, and orange juice; stir to combine. Add collard greens and tomatoes. Cook, covered, for 5 minutes or just until tomatoes start to juice out and collard greens are just tender. Drizzle with lime juice. Serve with sliced avocado.

FRENCH POULET SKILLET

PREP: 40 minutes   COOK: 10 minutes   STAND: 2 minutes   MAKES: 4 to 6 servings

COOKED CHICKEN IS CONVENIENT TO HAVE IN THE REFRIGERATOR FOR MAKING PROTEIN-RICH BREAKFASTS MUCH QUICKER TO MAKE. WHETHER IT'S FROM LEFTOVER ROAST CHICKEN WITH SAFFRON AND LEMON (PAGE 186) OR SIMPLY FROM BAKED CHICKEN YOU MAKE SPECIFICALLY TO USE IN DISHES SUCH AS THIS ONE, IT'S GREAT TO HAVE ON HAND.

1 0.5-ounce package dried chanterelle mushrooms

8 ounces fresh asparagus

2 tablespoons olive oil

1 medium bulb fennel, cored and thinly sliced

⅔ cup sliced leek, white and light green parts only

1 tablespoon herbes de Provence

3 cups diced cooked chicken

1 cup chopped, seeded tomatoes

¼ cup Chicken Bone Broth (see recipe, page 235) or no-salt-added chicken broth

¼ cup dry white wine

2 teaspoons finely shredded lemon peel

4 cups roughly chopped red or rainbow Swiss chard leaves

¼ cup snipped fresh basil

2 tablespoons snipped fresh mint

1. Rehydrate dried mushrooms according to package directions; drain. Rinse and drain again; set aside.

2. Meanwhile, snap off and discard woody bases from asparagus. If desired, scrape off scales. Bias-slice asparagus into 2-inch pieces. In a large saucepan cook asparagus in boiling water for 3 minutes or until crisp-tender; drain. Immediately plunge into ice water to stop cooking; set aside.

3. In an extra-large skillet heat oil over medium heat. Add fennel, leek, and herbes de Provence; cook for 5 minutes or just until fennel begins to brown, stirring occasionally. Add the rehydrated mushrooms, asparagus, chicken, tomatoes, Chicken Bone Broth, wine, and lemon peel. Bring to a simmer. Cover and reduce heat to low. Simmer for 5 minutes or just until fennel and asparagus are tender and tomatoes are juicy. Remove from heat. Stir in Swiss chard and let stand for 2 minutes or until wilted. Sprinkle with basil and mint.

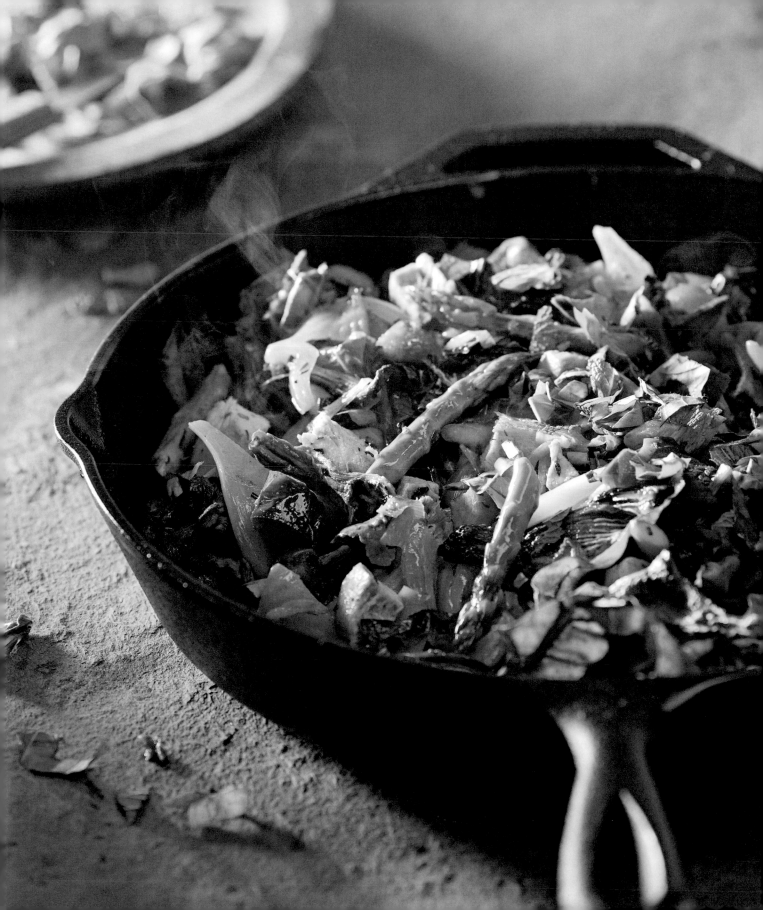

TROUT WITH SHOESTRING SWEET POTATOES

PREP: 35 minutes   BAKE: 6 minutes   COOK: 1 minute per batch of potatoes   MAKES: 4 servings

EVEN IF YOU DIDN'T CATCH THE TROUT IN A MOUNTAIN STREAM, THIS DISH WILL MAKE YOU FEEL A LITTLE BIT AS IF YOU'RE ENJOYING A "SHORE BREAKFAST" NEXT TO A CRACKLING CAMPFIRE.

4 6-ounce fresh or frozen skinless trout fillets, ¼ to ½ inch thick
1½ teaspoons Smoky Seasoning (see recipe, page, 324)
¼ to ½ teaspoon black pepper (optional)
3 tablespoons refined coconut oil
1½ pounds white or yellow sweet potatoes, peeled
Refined coconut oil for frying*
Chopped fresh parsley
Sliced scallions

1. Preheat oven to 400°F. Thaw fish, if frozen. Rinse fish; pat dry with paper towels. Sprinkle fillets with Smoky Seasoning and, if desired, pepper. In an extra-large oven-going skillet heat 2 tablespoons of the oil over medium-high heat. Place fillets in skillet and bake, uncovered, for 6 to 8 minutes or until fish begins to flake when tested with a fork. Remove from oven.

2. Meanwhile, using a julienne peeler or mandoline fitted with the julienne cutter, cut sweet potatoes lengthwise into long thin strips. Wrap potato strips in a double thickness of paper towels and absorb any excess water.

3. In a large stockpot with at least 8-inch-tall sides, heat 2 to 3 inches of refined coconut oil to 365°F. Carefully add potatoes, about one-fourth at a time, to the hot oil. (Oil will rise in the pot.) Fry about 1 to 3 minutes per batch or until just starting to brown, stirring once or twice. Quickly remove potatoes using a long slotted spoon and drain on paper towels. (Potatoes can overcook quickly, so check early and often.) Be sure to heat oil back up to 365°F before adding each batch of potatoes.

4. Sprinkle trout with parsley and scallions; serve with sweet potato shoestrings.

***Tip:** You will need two to three 29-ounce containers of coconut oil to have enough oil for frying.

SALMON PATTIES WITH TOMATILLO-MANGO SALSA, POACHED EGGS, AND ZUCCHINI RIBBONS

PREP: 25 minutes   CHILL: 30 minutes   COOK: 16 minutes   MAKES: 4 servings

THIS MAY NOT BE BREAKFAST BEFORE HEADING TO WORK ON A WEEKDAY MORNING, BUT IT MAKES AN IMPRESSIVE AND ABSOLUTELY DELICIOUS WEEKEND BRUNCH FOR FRIENDS OR FAMILY.

10 ounces cooked salmon*
 2 egg whites
 ½ cup almond flour
 ⅓ cup shredded sweet potato
 2 tablespoons thinly sliced scallions
 2 tablespoons snipped fresh cilantro
 2 tablespoons Chipotle Paleo Mayo (see recipe, page 323)
 1 tablespoon fresh lime juice
 1 teaspoon Mexican Seasoning (see recipe, page 324)
    Black pepper
 4 tablespoons olive oil
 1 recipe Zucchini Ribbons (see recipe, right)
 4 eggs, poached (see recipe for Cauliflower Steaks and Eggs, page 32)
    Tomatillo-Mango Salsa (see recipe, right)
 1 ripe avocado, peeled, seeded, and sliced

1. For salmon patties, in a large bowl use a fork to flake cooked salmon into small pieces. Add egg whites, almond flour, sweet potato, scallions, cilantro, Chipotle Paleo Mayo, lime juice, Mexican Seasoning, and pepper to taste. Mix lightly to combine. Divide mixture into eight portions; shape each portion into a patty. Place patties on a parchment-lined baking sheet. Cover and chill at least 30 minutes before frying. (Cakes may be chilled 1 day before serving.)

2. Preheat oven to 300°F. In a large nonstick skillet heat 2 tablespoons olive oil over medium-high heat. Add half of the cakes to the skillet; cook about 8 minutes or until golden brown, flipping the cakes halfway through cooking. Transfer the cakes to another parchment-lined baking sheet and keep warm in the oven. Fry the remaining cakes in the remaining 2 tablespoons oil as directed.

3. To serve, arrange Zucchini Ribbons in a nest on each of four serving plates. Top each with 2 salmon cakes, a poached egg, some of the Tomatillo-Mango Salsa, and avocado slices.

Zucchini Ribbons: Trim ends from 2 zucchini. Using a mandoline or vegetable peeler, shave long ribbons from each zucchini. (To keep ribbons intact, stop shaving once you reach the seed core in center of squash.) In a large skillet heat 1 tablespoon olive oil over medium-high heat. Add zucchini and ⅛ teaspoon ground cumin; cook for 2 to 3 minutes or until crisp-tender, using tongs to gently toss ribbons to cook evenly. Drizzle with lime juice.

Tomatillo-Mango Salsa: Preheat the oven to 450°F. Husk and halve 8 tomatillos. On a baking sheet arrange tomatillos; 1 cup chopped onion; 1 chopped, seeded fresh jalapeño; and 2 cloves peeled garlic. Drizzle with 1 tablespoon olive oil; toss to coat. Roast vegetables about 15 minutes or until they begin to soften and brown. Let cool for 10 minutes. Transfer vegetables and any juices to a food processor. Add ¾ cup chopped, peeled mango and ¼ cup fresh cilantro. Cover and pulse to coarsely chop. Transfer salsa to a bowl; stir in an additional ¾ cup chopped, peeled mango. (Salsa may be made 1 day ahead and chilled. Bring to room temperature before serving.)

*Tip: For cooked salmon, preheat oven to 425°F. Place an 8-ounce salmon fillet on a parchment paper-lined baking sheet. Bake for 6 to 8 minutes per ½ inch thickness of fish or until fish flakes easily when tested with a fork.

APPLE-FLAX JACKS

START TO FINISH: **30 minutes**   MAKES: **4 servings**

THESE FLOURLESS FLAPJACKS ARE CRISP ON THE OUTSIDE AND TENDER ON THE INSIDE. MADE WITH SHREDDED APPLE AND JUST A LITTLE BIT OF FLAXMEAL AND EGG TO BIND THEM, THEY ARE A BREAKFAST TREAT KIDS (AND GROWN-UPS TOO) WILL GOBBLE UP.

4 large eggs, lightly beaten

2 large unpeeled apples, cored and finely shredded

½ cup flaxmeal

¼ cup finely chopped walnuts or pecans

2 teaspoons finely shredded orange peel

1 teaspoon pure vanilla extract

1 teaspoon ground cardamom or cinnamon

3 tablespoons unrefined coconut oil

½ cup almond butter

2 teaspoons finely shredded orange peel

¼ teaspoon ground cardamom or cinnamon

1. In a large bowl combine eggs, shredded apples, flaxmeal, nuts, orange peel, vanilla, and 1 teaspoon cardamom. Stir until well combined. Let batter stand for 5 to 10 minutes to thicken.

2. On a griddle or skillet melt 1 tablespoon of the coconut oil over medium heat. For each Apple-Flax Jack, drop about ⅓ cup batter onto the griddle, spreading slightly. Cook over medium heat for 3 to 4 minutes on each side or until jacks are golden brown.

3. Meanwhile, in a small microwave-safe bowl heat almond butter on low until spreadable. Serve on top of Apple-Flax Jacks and sprinkle with orange peel and additional cardamom.

ORANGE-GINGER PALEO GRANOLA

PREP: 15 minutes   COOK: 5 minutes   STAND: 4 minutes
BAKE: 27 minutes   COOL: 30 minutes   MAKES: 8 (½-cup) servings

THIS CRUNCHY NUT AND DRIED FRUIT "CEREAL" IS DELICIOUS TOPPED WITH ALMOND OR COCONUT MILK AND EATEN WITH A SPOON, BUT IT ALSO MAKES A GREAT GRAB-AND-GO BREAFAST OR SNACK MUNCHED ON DRY.

⅔ cup fresh orange juice

1 ½-inch piece fresh ginger, peeled and thinly sliced

1 teaspoon green tea leaves

2 tablespoons unrefined coconut oil

1 cup coarsely chopped raw almonds

1 cup raw macadamia nuts

1 cup shelled raw pistachio nuts

½ cup unsweetened coconut chips

¼ cup chopped unsulfured, unsweetened dried apricots

2 tablespoons chopped dried unsulfured, unsweetened stemmed dried figs

2 tablespoons unsulfured, unsweetened golden raisins

Unsweetened almond milk or coconut milk

1. Preheat oven to 325°F. In a small saucepan heat orange juice just until boiling. Add ginger slices. Boil gently, uncovered, about 5 minutes or until reduced to about ⅓ cup. Remove from the heat; add green tea leaves. Cover and let steep for 4 minutes. Strain orange juice mixture through a fine-mesh sieve. Discard tea leaves and ginger slices. Add coconut oil to hot orange juice mixture and stir until melted. In a large bowl combine almonds, macadamia nuts, and pistachio nuts. Add orange juice mixture; toss to coat. Spread evenly in a large rimmed baking pan.

2. Bake, uncovered, for 15 minutes, stirring halfway through baking time. Add coconut chips; stir mixture and spread to an even layer. Bake about 12 to 15 minutes more or until nuts are toasted and golden brown, stirring once. Add apricots, figs, and raisins; stir until well combined. Spread granola onto a large piece of foil or clean rimmed baking sheet; cool completely. Serve with almond or coconut milk.

To store: Place granola in an airtight container; store at room temperature for up to 2 weeks or in the freezer for up to 3 months.

STEWED PEACHES AND BERRIES WITH TOASTED COCONUT-ALMOND CRUNCH

PREP: 20 minutes   BAKE: 1 hour   COOK: 10 minutes   MAKES: 4 to 6 servings

SAVE THIS FOR PEACH SEASON—GENERALLY LATE JULY, AUGUST, AND EARLY SEPTEMBER IN MOST PARTS OF THE COUNTRY— WHEN PEACHES ARE AT THEIR SWEETEST AND JUICIEST. THIS MAKES A WONDERFUL BREAKFAST BUT CAN ALSO BE ENJOYED AS DESSERT.

6 ripe peaches
½ cup unsweetened, unsulfored dried peaches, finely chopped*
¾ cup fresh orange juice
¼ cup unrefined coconut oil
½ teaspoon ground cinnamon
1 cup unsweetened coconut flakes
1 cup coarsely chopped raw almonds
¼ cup unsalted raw sunflower seeds
1 tablespoon fresh lemon juice
1 vanilla bean, split and seeds scraped
1 cup raspberries, blueberries, blackberries, and/or coarsely chopped strawberries

1. In a large saucepan bring 8 cups water to boiling. Using a sharp knife, cut a shallow X on the bottom of each peach. Immerse peaches, two at a time, in boiling water for 30 to 60 seconds or until skins begin to split. Using a slotted spoon, transfer peaches to a large bowl of ice water. When cool enough to handle, use a knife or your fingers to peel off skins; discard skins. Cut peaches into wedges, discarding the pits; set aside.

2. Preheat oven to 250°F. Line a large baking sheet with parchment paper. In a food processor or blender combine 1 cup of the peach wedges, the dried peaches, ¼ cup of the orange juice, the coconut oil, and cinnamon. Cover and process or blend until smooth; set aside.

3. In a large bowl combine the coconut flakes, almonds, and sunflower seeds. Add pureed peach mixture. Toss to coat. Transfer nut mixture to the prepared baking sheet, spreading evenly. Bake for 60 to 75 minutes or until dry and crisp, stirring occasionally. (Be careful not to burn; mixture will crisp up more as it cools.)

4. Meanwhile, place the remaining peach wedges into a medium heavy saucepan. Stir in the remaining ½ cup orange juice, the lemon juice, and split vanilla bean (with seeds). Bring to boiling over medium heat, stirring occasionally. Reduce heat to low; simmer, uncovered, for 10 to 15 minutes or until thickened, stirring occasionally. Remove vanilla bean pod. Stir in berries. Cook for 3 to 4 minutes or just until berries are warmed through.

5. To serve, spoon stewed peaches into bowls. Sprinkle each serving with nut mixture.

*Note: If you can't find unsulfured dried peaches, you can use ⅓ cup unsulfured dried apricots, chopped, instead.

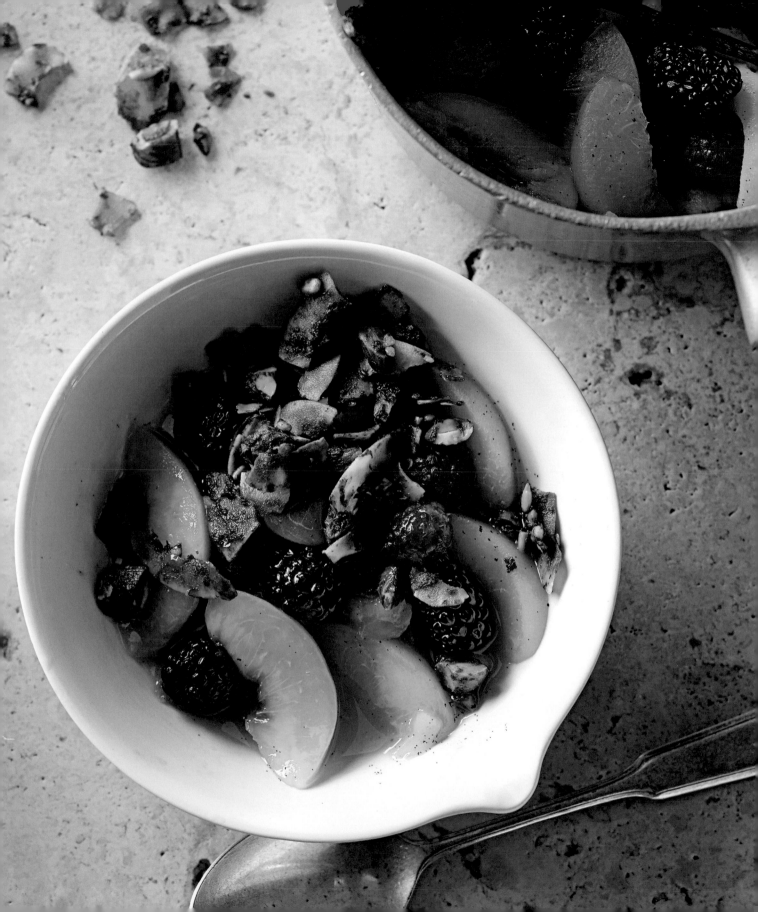

STRAWBERRY-MANGO POWER SMOOTHIES

PREP: 15 minutes   COOK: 30 minutes   MAKES: 4 (about 8-ounce) servings

THE BEET IN THIS BREAKFAST DRINK GIVES IT A VITAMIN AND MINERAL BOOST AND A GORGEOUS RED HUE. THE EGG WHITE POWDER PROVIDES PROTEIN AND GETS WHIPPED AS THE DRINK IS BLENDED, FOR A LIGHTER, FROTHIER SMOOTHIE.

1 medium red beet, peeled and quartered (about 4 ounces)

2½ cups hulled fresh strawberries

1½ cups frozen unsweetened mango chunks*

1¼ cups unsweetened coconut milk or almond milk

¼ cup unsweetened pomegranate juice

¼ cup unsalted almond butter

2 teaspoons egg white powder

1. In a medium saucepan cook beet, covered, in a small amount of boiling water for 30 to 40 minutes** or until very tender. Drain beet; run cold water over beet to cool quickly. Drain well.

2. In a blender combine beet, strawberries, mango chunks, coconut milk, pomegranate juice, and almond butter. Cover and blend until smooth, stopping to scrape sides of blender as needed. Add egg white powder. Cover and blend just until combined.

*Note: To freeze fresh mango pieces, arrange cut-up mango in a single layer in a 15×10×1-inch baking pan lined with waxed paper. Cover loosely and freeze for several hours or until very firm. Transfer frozen mango pieces to an airtight container; freeze for up to 3 months.

**Note: The beet can be cooked up to 3 days ahead. Cool beet completely. Store in a tightly sealed container in the refrigerator.

DATE SHAKES

START TO FINISH: 10 minutes   MAKES: 2 (about 8-ounce) servings

THIS IS A PALEO TAKE ON THE CREAMY DATE SHAKES USUALLY MADE WITH ICE CREAM THAT HAVE BEEN POPULAR IN SOUTHERN CALIFORNIA SINCE THE 1930S. WITH DATES, FROZEN BANANA, ALMOND BUTTER, ALMOND MILK, AND EGG WHITE POWDER, THIS VERSION IS DECIDEDLY MORE NUTRITIOUS. FOR A CHOCOLATE VERSION, ADD THE 1 TABLESPOON UNSNWEETENED COCOA POWDER.

⅓ cup chopped, pitted Medjool dates
1 cup unsweetened almond or coconut milk (with vanilla if desired)
1 ripe banana, frozen and sliced
2 tablespoons almond butter
1 tablespoon egg white powder
1 tablespoon unsweetened cocoa powder (optional)
½ teaspoon fresh lemon juice
⅛ to ¼ teaspoon ground nutmeg*

1. In a small bowl combine dates and ½ cup water. Microwave on high for 30 seconds or until dates are softened; drain off water.

2. In a blender combine the dates, almond milk, banana slices, almond butter, egg white powder, cocoa powder (if using), lemon juice, and nutmeg. Cover and blend until smooth.

*Tip: If using cocoa powder, use ¼ teaspoon ground nutmeg.

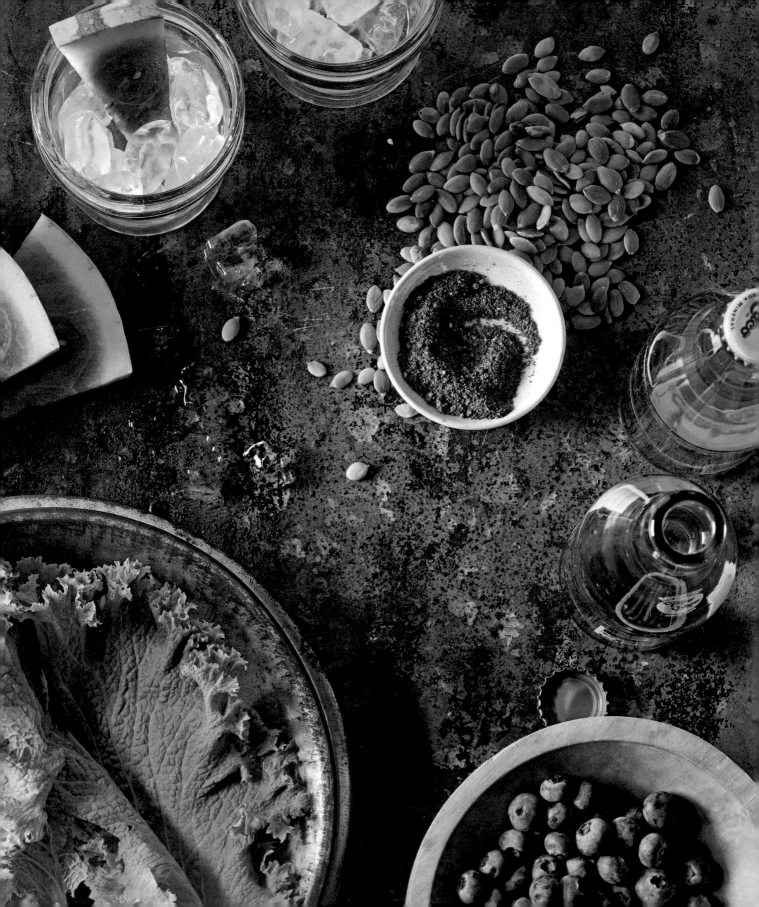

APPETIZERS, SNACKS & BEVERAGES

Snack foods, appetizers, and beverages are absolutely essential to The Paleo Diet®, and you should snack between meals whenever you feel the desire. For instance, if you haven't ever tried an *agua fresca*, you are in for a surprise. These refreshing beverages quench your thirst in a most delicious and healthful manner. They are concocted from fresh fruits, veggies, and herbs and are much healthier for you and your children than "healthy" sugar-free soft drinks.

Snacks and appetizers are social foods, festivity foods, and group foods that encourage conversation and get the party started. Along with your agua fresca, serve a bowl of Spicy Roasted Pepitas—and note how good these little seeds taste with absolutely no added salt. Try Chorizo-Stuffed Jalapeño Poppers for a real taste treat. Or how about Scallop and Avocado Endive Bites along with a good wine of your choice? Remember, wine, spirits, and gluten-free beers can be part of The Paleo Diet® when consumed in moderation, so there is no need to forgo these libations when entertaining. Unless you were to enlighten your guests, very few people would even know that the food you offer is Paleo. As a host or hostess, you will be secure in the knowledge that your snacks and appetizers not only taste good but are also good for the health of your friends, family, and visitors.

Two party-friendly recipes that stand out in this chapter are Roasted Red Pepper "Hummus" with Veggies and Spinach-Artichoke Dip. Both of these dishes are much healthier Paleo versions of their commercial counterparts—and taste a helluva lot better.

Traditional hummus is a Middle Eastern spread made from cooked, mashed chickpeas blended with tahini (sesame seed paste), olive oil, lemon juice, salt, and garlic. Unfortunately, hummus is a very non-Paleo food because it is based upon legumes (chickpeas) and contains significant amounts of salt and a seed paste (tahini) that has excessive omega-6 fatty acids. Our creative cooks have produced a Paleo version of hummus that sidesteps all of these deleterious nutritional issues and offers you a delectable appetizer without chickpeas, legumes, or salt.

Similarly, most of you are familiar with generic spinach and artichoke dip that can be purchased in supermarkets, delis, and grocery stores. This product normally contains a ridiculous jumble of artificial ingredients (trans fats, sugars, salt, vegetable oils, preservatives, chemical stabilizers, etc.) that is routinely mixed into virtually all processed food to fool our taste buds, increase shelf life, and alter food texture. The middlemen and food processors who create these unnatural products do so not because they have a campaign to ruin our health, but rather because they can produce a highly profitable and appetite-enticing product that has absolutely no redeeming nutritional qualities. So take a look at our version of Spinach-Artichoke Dip, which contains no added salts, sugars, preservatives, or unnatural ingredients. You are actually getting real spinach and artichokes in a creamy blend of spices and citrus.

With these dips, feel free to offer your guests any raw vegetables you prefer. We recommend sliced fresh vegetables or vegetable sticks such as broccoli florets, sliced broccoli stems, carrots, daikon radishes, cucumber, celery, jicama, sliced Jerusalem artichokes, green onions, red and yellow sweet peppers, radishes, turnips, zucchini—or any other fresh vegetable that strikes your fancy. And don't forget to slice up some fruits that many people consider to be veggies—avocados and tomatoes.

CHORIZO-STUFFED JALAPEÑO POPPERS

PREP: 30 minutes   BAKE: 25 minutes   MAKES: 12 appetizers

A DRIZZLE OF CILANTRO-LIME CASHEW CREAM COOLS THE FIRE OF THESE SPICY SNACKS. FOR A MILDER FLAVOR, SUBSTITUTE 6 MINIATURE SWEET PEPPERS, STEMMED, SEEDED, AND HALVED VERTICALLY, FOR THE JALAPEÑOS.

 2 teaspoons ancho chile powder*
1½ teaspoons preservative-free
       granulated garlic
1½ teaspoons ground cumin
 ¾ teaspoon dried oregano
 ¾ teaspoon ground coriander
 ½ teaspoon black pepper
 ¼ teaspoon ground cinnamon
 ⅛ teaspoon ground cloves
12 ounces ground pork
 2 tablespoons red wine vinegar
 6 large jalapeño chiles, cut in
       half horizontally and seeded**
       (leave stems intact if possible)
 ½ cup Cashew Cream (see recipe,
       page 327)
 1 tablespoon finely chopped fresh
       cilantro
 1 teaspoon finely shredded lime
       peel

1. Preheat oven to 400°F.

2. For chorizo, in a small bowl combine chile powder, garlic, cumin, oregano, coriander, black pepper, cinnamon, and cloves. Place pork in a medium bowl. Gently break it up with your hands. Sprinkle seasoning mixture over the pork; add vinegar. Gently work meat mixture until seasonings and vinegar are evenly distributed.

3. Stuff chorizo into jalapeño halves, dividing evenly and mounding slightly (chorizo will shrink as it cooks). Arrange stuffed jalapeño halves on a large rimmed baking sheet. Bake for 25 to 30 minutes or until chorizo is cooked through.

4. Meanwhile, in a small bowl combine Cashew Cream, cilantro, and lime peel. Drizzle stuffed jalapeños with Cashew Cream mixture before serving.

***Note:** If you like, substitute 2 tablespoons paprika and ¼ teaspoon ground cayenne for the ancho chile powder.

****Tip:** Chile peppers contain oils that can burn your skin, eyes, and the sensitive tissue in your nose. Avoid direct contact with cut sides and seeds of the chiles as much as possible. If your bare hands do touch either of those parts of the peppers, wash your hands thoroughly with soap and warm water.

ROASTED BEET BITES WITH ORANGE-WALNUT DRIZZLE

PREP: 20 minutes   BAKE: 40 minutes   MARINATE: 8 hours   MAKES: 12 servings

WALNUT OIL SHOULD NEVER BE USED FOR COOKING. WHEN HEATED, ITS HIGH CONCENTRATION OF POLYUNSATURATED FATS MAKES IT SUSCEPTIBLE TO OXIDATION AND DEGRADATION, BUT IT IS PERFECTLY WONDERFUL USED IN DISHES THAT ARE SERVED COLD OR AT ROOM TEMPERATURE—SUCH AS THIS ONE.

3 large beets, trimmed and peeled (about 1 pound)
1 tablespoon olive oil
¼ cup walnut oil
1½ teaspoons finely shredded orange peel
¼ cup fresh orange juice
2 teaspoons fresh lemon juice
2 tablespoons finely chopped walnuts, toasted*

1. Preheat oven to 425°F. Cut each beet into 8 wedges. (If beets are smaller, cut them into ½-inch wedges. You want about 24 wedges total.) Place beets in a 2-quart baking dish; drizzle with the olive oil and toss to coat. Cover dish with foil. Bake, covered, for 20 minutes. Stir beets and roast, uncovered, about 20 minutes more or until beets are tender. Let cool slightly.

2. Meanwhile, for marinade, in a small bowl combine walnut oil, orange peel, orange juice, and lemon juice. Pour marinade over beets; cover and refrigerate for 8 hours or overnight. Drain marinade.

3. Place beets in a serving bowl and sprinkle with the toasted walnuts. Serve with picks.

***Tip:** To toast nuts, spread them in a shallow baking pan. Bake in a 350°F oven for 5 to 10 minutes or until lightly browned, shaking pan once or twice. Watch carefully so they don't burn.

CAULIFLOWER CUPS WITH HERB PESTO AND LAMB

PREP: 45 minutes   COOK: 15 minutes   BAKE: 10 minutes   MAKES: 6 servings

THE CAULIFLOWER CUPS ARE VERY LIGHT AND TENDER. YOU MIGHT WANT TO SERVE THESE SAVORY SNACKS WITH FORKS SO THAT GUESTS CAN GET EVERY LAST NIBBLE—AND STILL KEEP THEIR MANNERS INTACT.

2 tablespoons refined coconut oil, melted

4 cups coarsely chopped fresh cauliflower

2 large eggs

½ cup almond meal

¼ teaspoon black pepper

4 scallions

12 ounces ground lamb or ground pork

3 cloves garlic, minced

12 cherry or grape tomatoes, quartered

1 teaspoon Mediterranean Seasoning (see recipe, page 324)

¾ cup firmly packed fresh cilantro

½ cup firmly packed fresh parsley

¼ cup firmly packed fresh mint

⅓ cup pine nuts, toasted (see tip, page 57)

¼ cup olive oil

1. Preheat oven to 425°F. Brush the bottoms and sides of twelve 2½-inch muffin cups with coconut oil. Set aside. Place cauliflower in a food processor. Cover and pulse until cauliflower is finely chopped but not pureed. Fill a large skillet with water to a depth of 1 inch; bring to boiling. Set a steamer basket in skillet over water. Add cauliflower to steamer basket. Cover and steam for 4 to 5 minutes or until tender. Remove steamer basket with cauliflower from skillet and set over a large plate. Let cauliflower cool slightly.

2. In a large bowl lightly beat eggs with a whisk. Stir in cooled cauliflower, almond meal, and pepper. Spoon cauliflower mixture evenly into prepared muffin cups. Using your fingers and the back of a spoon, press cauliflower onto bottoms and up the sides of the cups.

3. Bake cauliflower cups for 10 to 15 minutes or until cauliflower cups are lightly browned and centers are set. Place on wire rack but do not remove from the pan.

4. Meanwhile, thinly slice scallions, keeping white bottoms separate from the green tops. In a large skillet cook lamb, the sliced white bottoms of the scallions, and the garlic over medium-high heat until meat is cooked through, stirring with a wooden spoon to break up meat as it cooks. Drain off fat. Add green parts of scallions, tomatoes, and Mediterranean Seasoning. Cook and stir for 1 minute. Spoon lamb mixture evenly into cauliflower cups.

5. For herb pesto, in a food processor combine cilantro, parsley, mint, and pine nuts. Cover and process until mixture is finely chopped. With the processor running, slowly add oil through the feed tube until mixture is well combined.

6. Run a thin sharp knife around the edges of the cauliflower cups. Carefully remove the cups from the pan and set on a serving platter. Spoon herb pesto over cauliflower cups.

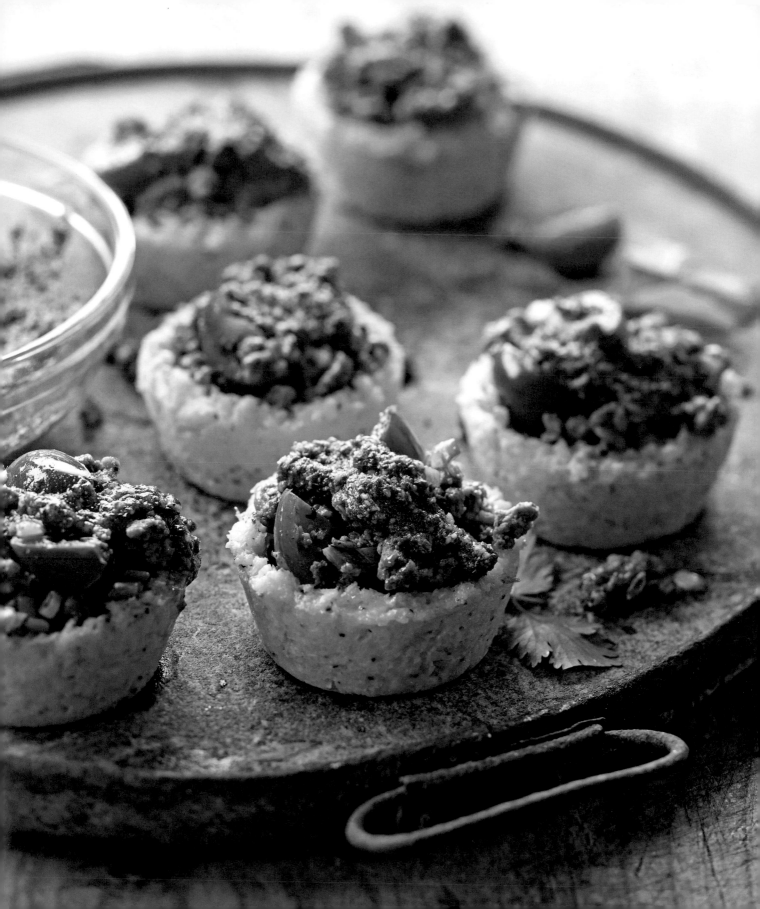

SPINACH-ARTICHOKE DIP

START TO FINISH: 20 minutes   MAKES: 6 servings

IT SEEMS THAT ALMOST EVERY PARTY INCLUDES SOME VERSION OF SPINACH-ARTICHOKE DIP ON THE TABLE—HOT OR COLD—BECAUSE PEOPLE LOVE IT. UNFORTUNATELY, THE COMMERCIALLY MADE VERSIONS—AND EVEN MOST OF THE HOMEMADE VERSIONS —DON'T LOVE YOU BACK. THIS ONE DOES.

1 tablespoon extra virgin olive oil

1 cup chopped sweet onion

3 cloves garlic, minced

1 9-ounce box frozen artichoke hearts, thawed

¾ cup Paleo Mayo (see recipe, page 323)

¾ cup Cashew Cream (see recipe, page 327)

½ teaspoon finely shredded lemon peel

2 teaspoons fresh lemon juice

2 teaspoons Smoky Seasoning (see recipe, page 324)

2 10-ounce boxes chopped frozen spinach, thawed and well drained

Assorted cut-up vegetables such as cucumbers, carrots, and red sweet peppers

1. In a large skillet heat olive oil over medium heat. Add onion; cook and stir about 5 minutes or until translucent. Add garlic; cook for 1 minute.

2. Meanwhile, place drained artichokes in a food processor fitted with the chopping/mixing blade. Cover and pulse until finely chopped; set aside.

3. In a small bowl combine Paleo Mayo and Cashew Cream. Stir in lemon peel, lemon juice, and Smoky Seasoning; set aside.

4. Add chopped artichokes and spinach to the onion mixture in skillet. Stir in mayonnaise mixture; heat through. Serve with cut-up vegetables.

ASIAN MEATBALLS WITH STAR ANISE DIPPING SAUCE

PREP: 30 minutes   COOK: 5 minutes per batch   MAKES: 8 servings

FOR THIS RECIPE, YOU NEED THE STEMS AND RIBS FROM 1 BUNCH OF MUSTARD GREENS. MAKE IT AT THE SAME TIME YOU MAKE SESAME-FLECKED MUSTARD GREEN CHIPS (PAGE 70) OR START WITH A BUNCH OF MUSTARD GREENS AND CHOP UP THE SMALLER LEAVES ALONG WTH THE STEMS AND RIBS FOR THE MEATBALLS—AND SAVE THE LARGER LEAVES TO STIR-FRY WITH GARLIC FOR A QUICK SIDE DISH.

Stems and ribs from 1 bunch of mustard greens
1 6-inch piece fresh ginger, peeled and sliced
12 ounces ground pork
12 ounces ground turkey (dark and white meat)
½ teaspoon black pepper
4 cups Beef Bone Broth (see recipe, page 131) or no-salt-added beef broth
2 star anise
½ cup finely chopped scallions
3 teaspoons finely shredded orange peel
2 tablespoons apple cider vinegar
1 teaspoon Hot Chile Oil (see recipe, right) (optional)
8 savoy cabbage leaves
1 tablespoon finely chopped scallions
2 teaspoons crushed red pepper

1. Coarsely chop the mustard greens stems and ribs; place in a food processor. Cover and process until finely chopped. (You should have 2 cups.) Place in a large bowl. Place the sliced ginger in the food processor; cover and process until minced. Add ¼ cup of the minced ginger, ground pork, ground turkey, and black pepper to the bowl. Lightly mix until well combined. Shape meat mixture into 32 mini meatballs using about 1 tablespoon meat mixture for each meatball.

2. For star anise dipping sauce, in a medium saucepan combine 2 tablespoons of the reserved minced ginger, 2 cups of the Beef Bone Broth, 1 star anise, ¼ cup of the scallions, 2 teaspoons of the orange peel, the apple cider vinegar, and, if desired, Hot Chile Oil. Bring to boiling; reduce heat. Simmer, covered, while cooking the meatballs.

3. Meanwhile, in another medium saucepan combine the remaining 2 tablespoons minced ginger, 2 cups broth, 1 star anise, ¼ cup of the scallions, and 1 teaspoon orange peel. Bring to boiling; add as many meatballs as will float in the cooking liquid without being overcrowded. Cook meatballs for 5 minutes; remove with a slotted spoon. Keep cooked meatballs warm in a serving bowl while cooking remaining meatballs. Discard cooking liquid.

4. Remove dipping sauce from heat. Strain and discard solids.

5. To serve, place a cabbage leaf on an appetizer plate and place 4 meatballs on each leaf. Drizzle with warm dipping sauce; sprinkle with scallions and crushed red pepper.

Hot Chile Oil: In a small saucepan heat 2 tablespoons sunflower oil over medium heat; add 2 teaspoons crushed red pepper and 2 whole dried ancho chiles. Cook for 1 minute or just until chile peppers begin to sizzle (do not let them brown or you need to start over). Add ¾ cup sunflower oil; heat just until warmed through. Remove from heat; let cool to room temperature. Strain oil through a fine-mesh sieve; discard chiles. Store oil in an airtight container or glass jar in the refrigerator for up to 3 weeks.

DEVILED EGGS

START TO FINISH: 25 minutes   MAKES: 12 servings

IF YOU OPT FOR THE WASABI DEVILED EGGS, BE SURE TO LOOK FOR A WASABI POWDER THAT CONTAINS ONLY NATURAL INGREDIENTS, NO SALT, AND NO ARTIFICIAL COLORING. WASABI IS A ROOT THAT IS GRATED AND USED FRESH OR DRIED AND GROUND INTO A POWDER. WHILE 100% WASABI POWDER IS HARD TO FIND OUTSIDE OF JAPAN— AND VERY EXPENSIVE—THERE ARE COMMERCIALLY AVAILABLE WASABI POWDERS THAT CONTAIN ONLY WASABI, HORSERADISH, AND DRY MUSTARD.

6   hard-cooked eggs, peeled*
¼   cup Paleo Mayo (see recipe, page 323)
1   teaspoon Dijon-Style Mustard (see recipe, page 322)
1   teaspoon cider vinegar or white wine vinegar
½   teaspoon black pepper
    Smoked paprika or fresh parsley sprigs

1. Cut eggs in half horizontally. Remove yolks and place in a medium bowl. Arrange whites on a serving platter.

2. Using a fork, mash the yolks. Stir in Paleo Mayo, Dijon-Style Mustard, vinegar, and black pepper. Mix well.

3. Spoon yolk mixture into egg white halves. Cover and chill until serving time. Garnish with paprika or parsley sprigs.

Wasabi Deviled Eggs: Prepare as directed, except omit Dijon-Style Mustard and use ¼ cup plus 1 teaspoon Paleo Mayo. In a small bowl combine 1 teaspoon wasabi powder and 1 teaspoon water to make a paste. Stir into yolk mixture, along with ¼ cup thinly sliced scallions. Garnish with sliced scallions.

Chipotle Deviled Eggs: Prepare as directed, except stir ¼ cup finely chopped cilantro, 2 tablespoons finely chopped red onion, and ½ teaspoon ground chipotle chile pepper into the yolk mixture. Sprinkle with additional ground chipotle chile pepper.

Avocado-Ranch Deviled Eggs: Reduce Paleo Mayo to 2 tablespoons and omit Dijon-Style Mustard and vinegar. Stir ¼ cup mashed avocado, 2 tablespoons chopped fresh chives, 1 tablespoon fresh lime juice, 1 tablespoon snipped parsley, 1 teaspoon snipped dill, ½ teaspoon onion powder, and ¼ teaspoon garlic powder into the yolk mixture. Garnish with finely chopped chives.

*Tip: To hard-cook eggs, place eggs in a single layer in a large saucepan. Cover with cold water by 1 inch. Bring to boiling over high heat. Remove from heat. Cover and let stand for 15 minutes; drain. Run cool water over eggs; drain again.

ROASTED EGGPLANT AND ROMESCO ROLLS

PREP: 45 minutes   BROIL: 10 minutes   BAKE: 15 minutes   MAKES: about 24 rolls

ROMESCO IS A SPANISH SAUCE TRADITIONALLY MADE FROM ROASTED RED SWEET PEPPERS PUREED WITH TOMATOES, OLIVE OIL, ALMONDS, AND GARLIC. THIS RECIPE MAKES ABOUT 2½ CUPS OF SAUCE. STORE ANY LEFTOVER SAUCE IN A TIGHTLY SEALED CONTAINER IN THE REFRIGERATOR FOR UP TO 1 WEEK. USE ON ROASTED OR GRILLED MEAT, POULTRY, FISH, OR VEGETABLES.

3 red sweet peppers, halved, stems removed, and seeded
4 roma tomatoes, cored
1 1-pound eggplant, ends trimmed
½ cup extra virgin olive oil
1 tablespoon Mediterranean Seasoning (see recipe, page 324
¼ cup almonds, toasted (see tip, page 57)
3 tablespoons Roasted Garlic Vinaigrette (see recipe, page 321)
   Extra virgin olive oil

1. For the romesco sauce, preheat broiler with the oven rack positioned 4 to 5 inches from the heating element. Line a rimmed baking sheet with foil. Place sweet peppers, cut sides down, and tomatoes on the prepared baking sheet. Broil about 10 minutes or until skins are blackened. Remove baking sheet from broiler and wrap vegetables in the foil; set aside.

2. Decrease oven temperature to 400°F. Using a mandoline or slicer, cut eggplant lengthwise into ¼-inch slices. (You should have about 12 to 14 slices.) Line two baking sheets with foil; place eggplant slices in a single layer on prepared baking sheets. Brush both sides of eggplant slices with olive oil; sprinkle with Mediterranean Seasoning. Bake about 15 minutes or until tender, turning slices once. Set baked eggplant aside to cool.

3. In a food processor combine the broiled peppers and tomatoes, the almonds, and Roasted Garlic Vinaigrette. Cover and process until smooth, adding additional olive oil as needed to make a smooth sauce.

4. Spread each slice of roasted eggplant with about 1 teaspoon of romesco sauce. Starting from the short end of roasted eggplant slices, roll each slice into a spiral and cut in half crosswise. Secure each roll with a wooden toothpick.

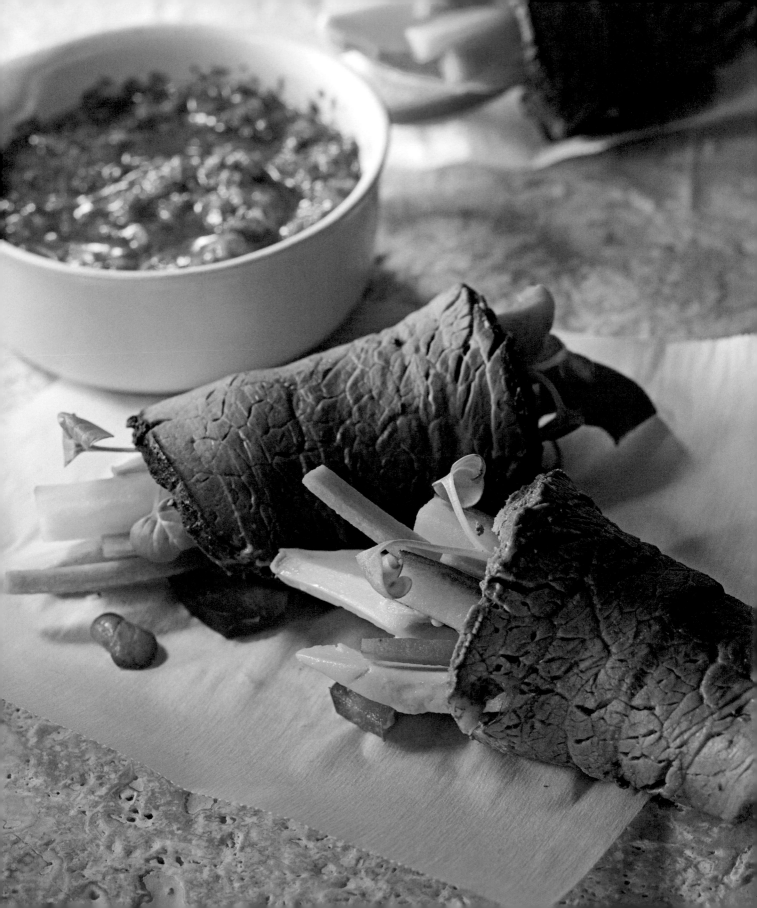

VEGGIE-BEEF WRAPS

START TO FINISH: 15 minutes   MAKES: 6 servings (12 wraps)

THESE CRUNCHY ROLLS ARE ESPECIALLY GOOD MADE WITH LEFTOVER SLOW-ROASTED BEEF TENDERLOIN (PAGE 84). CHILLING THE MEAT BEFORE SLICING HELPS IT TO CUT MORE CLEANLY, SO YOU CAN GET THE SLICES OF BEEF AS THIN AS POSSIBLE.

1 small red sweet pepper, stemmed, halved, and seeded
2 3-inch pieces English cucumber, halved lengthwise and seeded
2 3-inch pieces carrot, peeled
½ cup daikon radish sprouts
1 pound leftover roast beef tenderloin or other leftover roast beef, chilled
1 avocado, peeled, seeded, and cut into 12 slices
   Chimichurri Sauce (see recipe, page 323)

1. Cut the red pepper, cucumber, and carrot into long matchstick-size pieces.

2. Thinly slice roast beef (you will need 12 slices). If necessary, trim slices to make approximately 4×2-inch pieces. For each wrap, on a clean dry work surface place 4 beef slices in a single layer. In the center of each piece place an avocado slice, a piece of red pepper, a piece of cucumber, a piece of carrot, and some of the sprouts. Roll beef up and over the vegetables. Place wraps on a platter, seam sides down (secure wraps with toothpicks if necessary). Repeat two times to make 12 wraps total. Serve with Chimichurri Sauce for dipping.

SCALLOP AND AVOCADO ENDIVE BITES

START TO FINISH: 25 minutes   MAKES: 24 appetizers

ENDIVE LEAVES MAKE GREAT SCOOPS FOR FORK-FREE EATING OF ALL KINDS OF FILLINGS. HERE, THEY HOLD A CITRUSY AVOCADO-SWEET PEPPER RELISH TOPPED WITH QUICK-SEARED CAJUN SCALLOPS. THE RESULT IS AT ONCE CREAMY AND CRUNCHY, COOL AND HOT.

1 pound fresh or frozen bay scallops

1 to 2 teaspoons Cajun Seasoning (see recipe, page 324)

24 medium- to large-size endive leaves (from 3 to 4 heads endive)*

1 ripe avocado, peeled, seeded, and chopped

1 red or orange sweet pepper, finely chopped

2 green onions, chopped

2 tablespoons Bright Citrus Vinaigrette (see recipe, page 320) or fresh lime juice

1 tablespoon extra virgin olive oil

1. Thaw scallops, if frozen. Rinse scallops and pat dry with paper towels. In a medium bowl toss scallops with Cajun Seasoning; set aside.

2. Arrange endive leaves on a large platter. In a medium bowl gently stir together avocado, sweet pepper, green onions, and Bright Citrus Vinaigrette. Spoon onto endive leaves.

3. In a large skillet heat olive oil over medium-high heat.** Add scallops; cook for 1 to 2 minutes or until opaque, stirring frequently. Spoon scallops over avocado mixture on endive leaves. Serve immediately or cover and chill for up to 2 hours. Makes 24 appetizers.

***Note:** Reserve the smaller leaves for chopping and tossing in a salad.

****Note:** Bay scallops are delicately textured and can stick easily when cooking. A well-seasoned cast-iron pan has a nonstick surface that is an excellent choice for this job.

HERBED OYSTER MUSHROOM CHIPS WITH LEMON AÏOLI

PREP: 10 minutes   BAKE: 30 minutes   COOL: 5 minutes   MAKES: 4 to 6 servings

MAKE THESE IN SPRING AND FALL, WHEN OYSTER MUSHROOMS ARE PLENTIFUL. IN ADDITION TO BEING VERY TASTY WHEN ROASTED WITH OLIVE OIL AND FRESH HERBS, OYSTER MUSHROOMS ARE A GREAT SOURCE OF PROTEIN—UP TO 30% PROTEIN BY DRY WEIGHT—AND CONTAIN A COMPOUND CALLED LOVASTATIN, WHICH CAN HELP LOWER CHOLESTEROL LEVELS IN THE BLOOD.

1 pound oyster mushrooms, stemmed

2 tablespoons extra virgin olive oil

3 tablespoons snipped fresh rosemary, thyme, sage, and/or oregano

½ cup Paleo Aïoli (Garlic Mayo) (see recipe, page 323)

½ teaspoon finely shredded lemon peel

1 tablespoon fresh lemon juice

1. Preheat oven to 400°F. Place a metal rack on a large baking sheet; set aside. In a large bowl combine mushrooms, olive oil, and fresh herbs. Toss to coat mushrooms evenly. Spread mushrooms in a single layer on rack in baking sheet.

2. Bake for 30 to 35 minutes or until mushrooms are browned, sizzling, and slightly crisp. Cool for 5 to 10 minutes before serving (the mushrooms will crisp up as they cool).

3. For the lemon aïoli, in a small bowl combine Paleo Aïoli, lemon peel, and lemon juice. Serve with mushroom chips.

ROOT VEGETABLE CHIPS

START TO FINISH: **30 minutes**

THESE CRUNCHY CHIPS ARE EVERY BIT AS DELICIOUS AS THE ONES YOU BUY IN THE BAG—WITHOUT BEING FRIED IN A POTENTIALLY UNHEALTHY OIL (SUCH AS CANOLA OR SAFFLOWER) AND SEASONED WITH ADDED SALT. START WITH VERY THIN SLICES TO GET THEM AS CRISP AS POSSIBLE.

Sweet potato, beet, parsnip, carrot, turnip, parsnip, or rutabaga, scrubbed and peeled
Extra virgin olive oil
Seasoning blend of choice (see recipes, page 324)

1. Using a mandoline or a sharp chef's knife, thinly the slice the vegetable(s) into $\frac{1}{16}$- to $\frac{1}{32}$-inch slices. Transfer the slices to a bowl of ice water as you work to remove starch from the surface of the slices.

2. Using a salad spinner, spin the slices dry (or pat dry between paper towels or clean cotton towels). Line a microwave-safe plate with a paper towel. Arrange as many vegetables slices as you can without touching on the plate. Brush with olive oil and sprinkle lightly with seasoning.

3. Microwave on high for 3 minutes. Turn slices over and microwave on medium for 2 to 3 minutes, removing any slices that begin to brown quickly. Continue cooking on medium in 1-minute intervals until chips are crisp and lightly browned, taking care that the spices don't burn. Allow cooked chips to cool on plate until completely crisp, then transfer to a serving bowl. Repeat with remaining vegetable slices.

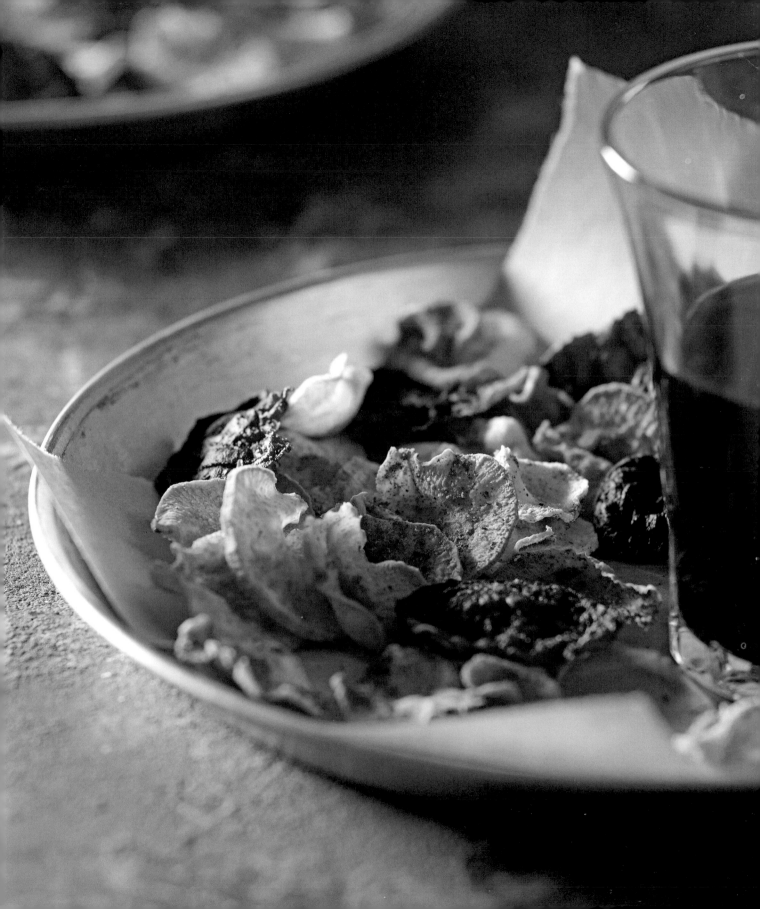

SESAME-FLECKED MUSTARD GREEN CHIPS

PREP: 10 minutes   BAKE: 20 minutes   MAKES: 4 to 6 servings

THESE ARE SIMILAR TO CRISP KALE CHIPS BUT MORE DELICATE. TO KEEP THEM CRISP, STORE THEM IN A ROLLED-DOWN PAPER BAG AND NOT A TIGHTLY SEALED CONTAINER—WHICH WILL MAKE THEM WILT.

1 bunch mustard greens, stems and ribs removed*
2 tablespoons extra virgin olive oil
2 teaspoons white sesame seeds
1 teaspoon black sesame seeds

1. Preheat oven to 300°F. Line two 15×10×1-inch baking pans with parchment paper.

2. Tear mustard greens into bite-size pieces. In a large bowl combine greens and olive oil. Toss to coat, gently rubbing the oil over the surface of the leaves. Sprinkle with sesame seeds; toss lightly to coat.

3. Arrange mustard leaves in a single layer on the prepared baking pans. Bake about 20 minutes or until darkened and crisp, turning once. Serve immediately or store cooled chips in a paper bag for up to 3 days.

*Note: The stems and ribs can be used to make the Asian Meatballs with Star Anise Dipping Sauce (see recipe, page 61).

SPICY ROASTED PEPITAS

PREP: 5 minutes   BAKE: 20 minutes   MAKES: 2 cups

THESE ARE JUST THE THING TO MUNCH ON WHEN YOU'RE HUNGRY AND IN THE MIDDLE OF MAKING DINNER. PEPITAS ARE SHELLED PUMPKIN SEEDS, BUT YOU COULD SUBSTITUTE A NUT SUCH AS ALMONDS OR PECANS IF YOU PREFER.

1 egg white
2 teaspoons fresh lime juice
1 teaspoon ground cumin
½ teaspoon no-salt-added chili powder
½ teaspoon smoked paprika
½ teaspoon black pepper
¼ teaspoon cayenne pepper
¼ teaspoon ground cinnamon
2 cups raw pepitas (shelled pumpkin seeds)

1. Preheat oven to 350°F. Line a baking sheet with parchment paper; set aside.

2. In a medium bowl whisk egg white until frothy. Add lime juice, cumin, chili powder, paprika, black pepper, cayenne pepper, and cinnamon. Whisk until well combined. Add pepitas. Stir until all pepitas are well coated. Spread pepitas evenly on prepared baking sheet.

3. Bake about 20 minutes or until golden brown and crisp, stirring frequently. While pepitas are still warm, separate any clumps.

4. Cool completely. Store in an airtight container at room temperature for up to 1 week.

HERB-CHIPOTLE NUTS

PREP: 10 minutes   BAKE: 12 minutes   MAKES: 4 to 6 serving (2 cups)

CHIPOTLE CHILES ARE DRIED, SMOKED JALAPEÑOS. ALTHOUGH THEY'VE BECOME VERY POPULAR COMMERCIALLY CANNED IN ADOBO SAUCE—WHICH CONTAINS SUGAR, SALT, AND SOYBEAN OIL—IN THEIR PUREST FORM, THERE ARE NO INGREDIENTS OTHER THAN THE CHILES THEMSELVES. THEY PROVIDE WONDERFUL, SMOKY-HOT FLAVOR TO FOODS.

1 egg white
2 tablespoons extra virgin olive oil
2 teaspoons snipped fresh thyme
1 teaspoon snipped fresh rosemary
1 teaspoon ground chipotle chile pepper
1 teaspoon finely shredded orange peel
2 cups unsalted whole nuts (almonds, pecans, walnuts, and/or cashews)

1. Preheat oven to 350°F. Line a 15×10×1-inch baking pan with foil; set pan aside.

2. In a medium bowl whisk egg white until frothy. Add olive oil, thyme, rosemary, ground chipotle pepper, and orange peel. Whisk until combined. Add nuts and stir to coat. Spread nuts in a single layer in the prepared baking pan.

3. Bake for 20 minutes or until nuts are golden brown and crisp, stirring frequently. While still warm, separate any clumps. Cool completely.

4. Store in an airtight container at room temperature for up to 1 week.

ROASTED RED PEPPER "HUMMUS" WITH VEGGIES

PREP: 20 minutes   ROAST: 20 minutes   STAND: 15 minutes   MAKES: 4 servings

IF YOU LIKE, YOU CAN MAKE THIS SAVORY DIP UP TO 3 DAYS AHEAD. PREPARE IT AS DIRECTED THROUGH STEP 2, THEN TRANSFER TO A SERVING BOWL. COVER AND CHILL FOR UP TO 2 DAYS. STIR IN THE PARSLEY JUST BEFORE SERVING.

1 medium red sweet pepper, seeded and quartered

3 cloves garlic, peeled

¼ teaspoon extra virgin olive oil

½ cup slivered almonds

3 tablespoons pine nuts

2 tablespoons Pine Nut Butter (see recipe, page 327)

1 teaspoon finely shredded lemon peel

2 to 3 tablespoons fresh lemon juice

¼ cup snipped fresh parsley
Fresh vegetable sticks (carrots, sweet peppers, cucumber, celery, and/or zucchini)

1. Preheat oven to 425°F. Line a small baking pan with foil; place pepper quarters, cut sides down, on the foil. Place garlic cloves on a small piece of foil; drizzle with olive oil. Wrap foil up around the garlic cloves. Place packet of garlic in the pan with the pepper quarters. Roast pepper and garlic for 20 to 25 minutes or until peppers are charred and very tender. Set garlic packet on a wire rack to cool. Bring the foil up around pepper quarters and fold edges together to enclose. Let stand about 15 minutes or until cool enough to handle. Use a sharp knife to loosen edges of the pepper skins; gently pull off the skins in strips and discard.

2. Meanwhile, in a small skillet toast pine nuts over medium heat for 3 to 5 minutes or until lightly toasted. Cool slightly.

3. Transfer toasted nuts to a food processor. Cover and process until finely chopped. Add pepper quarters, garlic cloves, Pine Nut Butter, lemon peel, and lemon juice. Cover and process until very smooth, stopping to scrape sides of the bowl occasionally.

4. Transfer nut mixture to a serving bowl; stir in parsley. Serve with fresh vegetables for dipping.

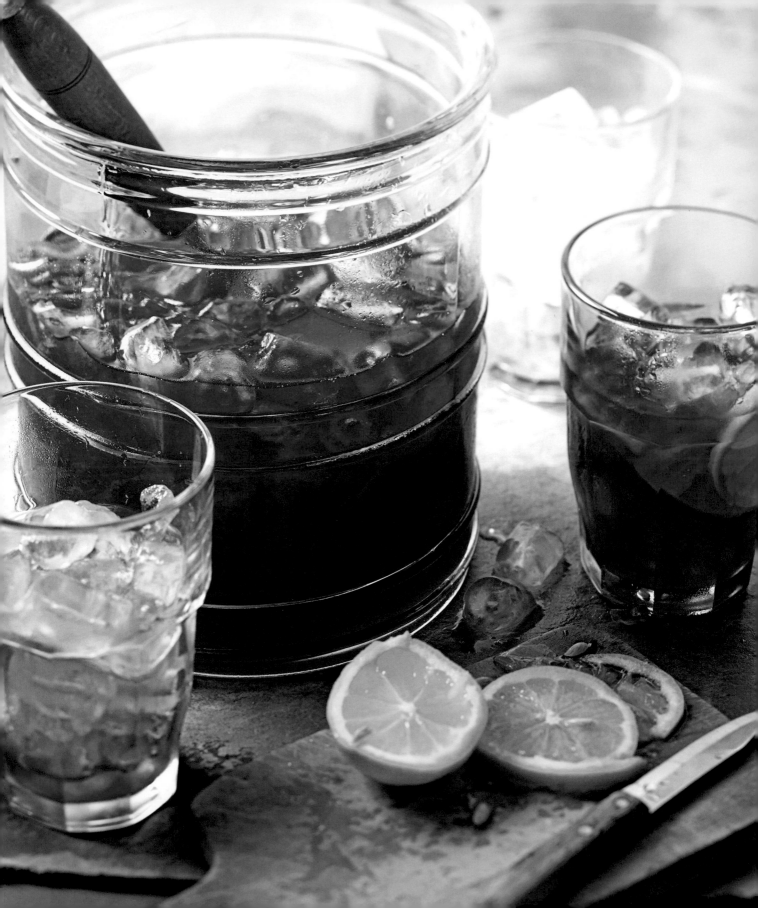

ICED GINGER-HIBISCUS TEA

PREP: **10 minutes**   STAND: **20 minutes**   MAKES: **6 (8-ounce) servings**

DRIED HIBISCUS FLOWERS MAKE A VERY REFRESHING, TARTLY FLAVORED TEA POPULAR IN MEXICO AND OTHER PARTS OF THE WORLD. STEEPING WITH GINGER GIVES IT SOME ZING. STUDIES HAVE SUGGESTED THAT HIBISCUS IS BENEFICIAL IN MAINTAINING HEALTHY BLOOD PRESSURE AND CHOLESTEROL—AND IT IS VERY HIGH IN VITAMIN C.

6 cups cold water
1 cup uncut, dried hibiscus
   flowers (flor de jamaica)
2 tablespoons coarsely grated,
   peeled fresh ginger
   Ice cubes
   Orange and lime slices

1. Bring 2 cups of the water to boiling. Combine hibiscus flowers and ginger in a large container. Pour boiling water over hibiscus mixture; cover and let stand for 20 minutes.

2. Strain mixture through a fine-mesh sieve into a large pitcher. Discard solids. Add the remaining 4 cups cold water; mix well.

3. Serve tea in tall glasses over ice. Garnish with orange and lime slices.

STRAWBERRY-MELON-MINT AGUA FRESCA

START TO FINISH: 20 minutes   MAKES: about 8 servings (10 cups)

AGUA FRESCA MEANS "FRESH WATER" IN SPANISH, AND IF YOU CAN IMPROVE ON WATER FOR REFRESHMENT, THIS IS IT. MOST AGUA FRESCAS CONTAIN ADDED SUGAR ALONG WITH FRUIT, BUT THESE RELY ONLY ON THE NATURAL SUGAR IN THE FRUITS. ON A HOT DAY, NOTHING TASTES BETTER—AND THEY MAKE A GREAT ALCOHOL-FREE PARTY DRINK.

2   pounds fresh strawberries, hulled and halved
3   cups cubed honeydew melon
6   cups cold water
1   cup fresh mint leaves, torn
     Juice of 2 limes, plus wedges for serving
     Ice cubes
     Mint sprigs
     Lime wedges

1. In a blender combine strawberries, melon, and 2 cups of the water. Cover and blend until smooth. Strain mixture through a fine-mesh sieve into a pitcher or large glass jar. Discard solids.

2. In the blender combine the 1 cup mint leaves, lime juice, and 1 cup water. Strain the mixture through the fine-mesh sieve into the strawberry-melon mixture.

3. Stir in 3 cups water. Serve immediately or chill until ready to serve. Serve in tall glasses over ice. Garnish with mint sprigs and lime wedges.

WATERMELON AND BLUEBERRY AGUA FRESCA

PREP: 20 minutes   CHILL: 2 to 24 hours   MAKES: 6 servings

THE FRUIT PUREE FOR THIS DRINK CAN BE CHILLED BETWEEN 2 AND 24 HOURS. IT'S A LITTLE DIFFERENT THAN SOME AGUA FRESCAS IN THAT IT HAS CARBONATED WATER BLENDED WITH THE FRUIT FOR A BUBBLY DRINK. BE SURE YOU BUY NATURALLY CARBONATED MINERAL WATER—NOT "SPARKLING" WATER OR SODA WATER, WHICH IS HIGH IN SODIUM.

 6 cups cubed, seeded watermelon
 1 cup fresh blueberries
¼ cup loosely packed fresh mint leaves
¼ cup fresh lime juice
12 ounces naturally carbonated mineral water, chilled
    Ice cubes
    Mint leaves
    Lime slices

1. In a blender or food processor combine the watermelon cubes, blueberries, ¼ cup mint, and lime juice, working in batches if necessary. Puree until smooth. Chill pureed fruit for 2 to to 24 hours.

2. To serve, stir chilled carbonated water into pureed fruit mixture. Pour into tall glasses over ice. Garnish with additional mint leaves and lime slices.

CUCUMBER AGUA FRESCA

PREP: 15 minutes   CHILL: 1 hour   MAKES: 6 servings

FRESH BASIL HAS A LICORICE FLAVOR THAT PAIRS WONDERFULLY WITH FRUIT OF ALL KINDS—STRAWBERRIES, PEACHES, APRICOTS, AND CANTALOUPE, IN PARTICULAR.

1 large seedless (English) cucumber, peeled and sliced (about 2 cups)
1 cup raspberries
2 ripe apricots, pitted and quartered
¼ cup fresh lime juice
1 tablespoon snipped fresh basil
½ teaspoon snipped fresh thyme
2 to 3 cups water
Ice cubes

1. In a blender or food processor combine cucumber, raspberries, apricots, lime juice, basil, and thyme. Add 2 cups water. Cover and blend or process until smooth. Add additional water, if you like, until desired consistency.

2. Chill for at least 1 hour or up to 1 week. Serve in tall glasses over ice.

COCONUT CHAI

START TO FINISH: 25 minutes   MAKES: 5 to 6 servings (about 5½ cups)

THIS CHAI CONTAINS NO TEA—JUST WELL-SPICED COCONUT MILK AND A SPLASH OF FRESH ORANGE JUICE. FOR A FROTHY TOPPING, ADDITIONAL COCONUT MILK CAN BE WHIPPED AND SPOONED ON TOP OF EACH SERVING.

12 whole cardamom pods
10 whole star anise
10 whole cloves
 2 teaspoons black peppercorns
 1 teaspoon whole dried allspice
 4 cups water
 3 2½-inch cinnamon sticks
 2 2-inch-long by 1-inch-wide
    strips orange peel
 1 3-inch piece fresh ginger, cut
    into thin rounds
½ teaspoon ground nutmeg
 1 15-ounce can whole coconut
    milk
½ cup fresh orange juice
 2 teaspoons pure vanilla extract

1. In an electric spice grinder combine cardamom pods, star anise, cloves, peppercorns, and allspice. Pulse until very coarsely ground. (Or in a large resealable plastic bag combine the cardamom pods, star anise, cloves, peppercorns, and allspice. Use a meat mallet or the bottom of a heavy-duty skillet to coarsely crush the spices.) Transfer spices to a medium saucepan.

2. Lightly toast the crushed spices in the saucepan over medium-low heat about 2 minutes or until fragrant, stirring frequently. Do not burn. Add the water, cinnamon sticks, orange peel, ginger, and nutmeg. Bring to boiling; reduce heat. Simmer, uncovered, for 15 minutes.

3. Stir in coconut milk, orange juice, and vanilla extract. Cook until heated through. Strain through a cheesecloth-lined fine-mesh strainer and serve immediately.

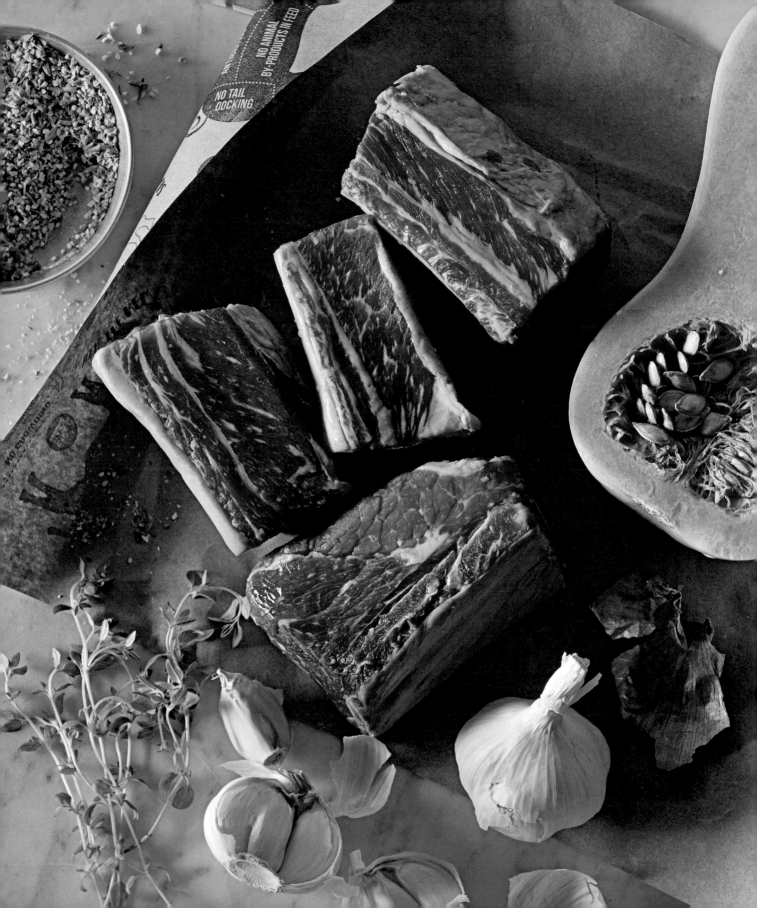

BEEF & BISON

One of my mother's famous clichés during my childhood was "What a difference a day makes." Fifty years later, as a retired college professor, I now fully "get" my mother's wisdom in this saying. The "difference a day makes" actually symbolizes not just a day but also a week, a month, a year, a decade, or a lifetime that it takes for our perceptions to change as we obtain more and more information about any issue—including food and diet.

Just a few short years ago, many people were under the misguided impression that all red meats were harmful and should be avoided. I am here to inform you unequivocally that you should enjoy these nutritious and delicious foods and eat them whenever possible. Red meat, particularly beef, represents the major source of highly absorbable iron and zinc in the U.S. food supply. If they are grass-produced or free-ranging, both beef and bison are good sources of healthful omega-3 fatty acids. Red meats, including beef and bison, are also excellent sources of vitamins B1, B6, and B12 and niacin. Numerous human experiments now confirm that high-protein diets based upon red meats reduce total blood cholesterol and triglycerides and increase HDL cholesterol (the good cholesterol) while lowering high blood pressure. All of these therapeutic effects will reduce your risk for heart disease.

As I mentioned in Paleo Principles, grass-produced meats are generally nutritionally superior to feedlot-produced meats, but they are frequently more expensive as well. If you can afford it, then go for grass-fed meats. Regardless, you should include red meat in your diet on a regular basis. High-quality cuts of beef and bison are available in the supermarket at reasonable prices—particularly if you buy in bulk or on sale. Simply put, red meat represents a delicious addition to our daily menus and can be incorporated into a plethora of dishes, along with fruits and veggies that you may have never considered. Look no further than the appealing recipes in this chapter.

One of my favorites is the Vietnamese-Style Rare Beef Salad. To my palate, one of the best food combinations ever is thinly sliced beef combined with fresh salad veggies and dressed exquisitely. You are going to experience some incredible flavors and textures with this creative and delectable salad that deftly mixes together iceberg lettuce; red and white onion and scallions; cilantro; mint; basil; sesame seeds; and an appetizing dressing comprised of lime juice, pineapple juice, crushed red peppers, and macadamia nut oil.

SLOW-ROASTED BEEF TENDERLOIN

PREP: 10 minutes   STAND: 50 minutes   ROAST: 1 hour 45 minutes   MAKES: 8 to 10 servings

THIS IS A SPECIAL-OCCASION ROAST, TO BE SURE. LETTING IT STAND AT ROOM TEMPERATURE ACCOMPLISHES TWO THINGS—IT ALLOWS THE SEASONING TO FLAVOR THE MEAT BEFORE ROASTING AND ALSO SHORTENS THE COOKING TIME SO THAT THE ROAST STAYS AS TENDER AND JUICY AS POSSIBLE. MEAT OF THIS QUALITY SHOULD BE EATEN NO MORE THAN MEDIUM RARE. USE LEFTOVERS IN VEGGIE-BEEF WRAPS (PAGE 65).

1   3½- to 4-pound center-cut beef tenderloin, trimmed and tied with 100%-cotton kitchen string
Extra virgin olive oil
½   cup Mediterranean Seasoning (see recipe, page 324)
½   teaspoon black pepper
Truffle-infused olive oil (optional)

1. Rub all sides of tenderloin with olive oil and coat with Mediterranean Seasoning and pepper. Let stand at room temperature for 30 to 60 minutes.

2. Preheat oven to 450°F with the rack in the lower third of the oven. Line a rimmed baking sheet with foil; place a roasting rack on the baking sheet.

3. Place meat on rack on baking sheet. Roast for 15 minutes. Decrease oven to 250°F. Roast for 1¾ to 2½ hours more or until internal temperature reaches 135°F for medium rare. Remove from oven; tent with foil. Let meat stand for 20 to 30 minutes. Remove string. Cut meat into ⅓-inch slices. If desired, lightly drizzle meat with truffle oil.

VIETNAMESE-STYLE RARE BEEF SALAD

PREP: 40 minutes   FREEZE: 45 minutes   CHILL: 15 minutes   STAND: 5 minutes   MAKES: 4 servings

ALTHOUGH THE COOKING PROCESS FOR THE MEAT STARTS IN THE BOILING PINEAPPLE JUICE, IT FINISHES IN THE MIXTURE OF LIME AND COLD PINEAPPLE JUICE. THE ACID IN THESE JUICES CONTINUES TO "COOK" THE MEAT WITHOUT HEAT—TOO MUCH OF WHICH CAN DESTROY FLAVOR AND TENDERNESS.

BEEF

- 1 pound beef tenderloin
- 4½ cups 100% pineapple juice
- 1 cup fresh lime juice
- ¼ of a red onion, very thinly sliced
- ¼ of a white onion, very thinly sliced
- ½ cup thinly sliced scallions
- ½ cup coarsely chopped fresh cilantro
- ½ cup coarsely chopped fresh mint
- ½ cup coarsely chopped fresh Thai basil (see page 99)
  Macadamia Dressing (see recipe, right)

SALAD

- 8 iceberg lettuce leaves
- 2 tablespoons chopped cashews, toasted (see tip, page 57)
- 1 Thai bird chile, very thinly sliced (see tip, page 56) (optional)
- 1 tablespoon sesame seeds
  Black pepper
  Fresh cilantro sprigs (optional)
  Lime wedges (optional)

1. Freeze beef about 45 minutes or until partially frozen. Using a very sharp knife, cut meat into paper-thin slices. In a large saucepan heat 4 cups of the pineapple juice to a boiling. Reduce heat to keep juice at a simmer. Blanch the beef in small batches in simmering juice for just a few seconds (the meat should be quite rare). Shake off excess liquid and place meat in a medium bowl. Chill meat in the refrigerator for 15 to 20 minutes to cool slightly.

2. Add the 1 cup lime juice and the remaining ½ cup pineapple juice to meat in bowl. Allow the beef to "cook" in juices at room temperature for 5 to 10 minutes or until desired doneness. Drain and squeeze excess liquid from meat and transfer to a large bowl. Add red onion, white onion, scallions, cilantro, mint, and basil; toss to combine. Pour Macadamia Dressing over beef mixture; toss to coat.

3. To assemble salads, line each serving plate with 2 lettuce leaves. Divide beef mixture among lettuce-lined plates. Sprinkle with cashews, Thai chile (if desired), sesame seeds, and black pepper to taste. If desired, garnish with cilantro sprigs and serve with lime wedges.

Macadamia Dressing: In a small jar with a tight-fitting lid combine ¼ cup macadamia oil, 1 tablespoon fresh lime juice, 1 tablespoon pineapple juice, and ¼ to ½ teaspoon crushed red pepper. Cover and shake well.

MEXICAN BRAISED BRISKET WITH MANGO, JICAMA, CHILE, AND ROASTED PUMPKIN SEED SALAD

PREP: **20 minutes**   MARINATE: **overnight**   COOK: **3 hours**   STAND: **15 minutes**   MAKES: **6 servings**

MARINATING THE BRISKET OVERNIGHT IN THE MIXTURE OF TOMATOES, CHIPOTLE CHILE, AND MEXICAN SEASONING GIVES IT INCREDIBLE FLAVOR AND FALL-APART TENDERNESS. BE SURE TO MARINATE IT IN A NONREACTIVE POT, SUCH STAINLESS STEEL OR ENAMELED CAST IRON. ALUMINUM REACTS WITH ACIDIC INGREDIENTS SUCH AS TOMATO AND CAN CREATE OFF FLAVORS—AND IT'S A BAD IDEA FOR HEALTH REASONS AS WELL (SEE PAGE 22).

BRISKET

- 1 3-pound beef brisket
- 2 cups Beef Bone Broth (see recipe, page 131) or no-salt-added beef broth
- 1 15-ounce can no-salt-added crushed tomatoes
- 1 cup water
- 1 dried chipotle or ancho chile pepper, snipped
- 2 teaspoons Mexican Seasoning (see recipe, page 324)

SALAD

- 1 ripe mango, peeled and pitted
- 1 jicama, peeled and cut into julienne strips
- 3 tablespoons green pumpkin seeds, toasted*
- ½ of a jalapeño, seeded and finely chopped (see tip, page 56)
- 1 to 2 tablespoons snipped fresh cilantro
- 3 tablespoons fresh lime juice
- 1 tablespoon extra virgin olive oil
   Lime wedges

1. Trim excess fat from brisket. Place in a stainless-steel or enamel Dutch oven. Add Beef Bone Broth, undrained tomatoes, the water, chipotle pepper, and Mexican Seasoning. Cover and refrigerate overnight.

2. Place Dutch oven over high heat; bring to boiling. Reduce heat and simmer, covered, for 3 to 3½ hours or until tender. Remove from oven, uncover, and let stand for 15 minutes.

3. Meanwhile, for the salad, cut peeled mango into ¼-inch-thick slices. Cut each slice into 3 strips. In a medium bowl combine mango, jicama, pumpkin seeds, jalapeño, and cilantro. In a small bowl stir together lime juice and olive oil; add to the salad and toss; set aside.

4. Transfer meat to a cutting board; slice the meat across the grain. If desired, drizzle meat with a little bit of the cooking juices. Serve meat with the salad. Garnish with lime wedges.

*Tip: To toast seeds and finely chopped nuts, scatter them in a small dry skillet and heat over medium heat just until golden. Stir frequently so they don't burn.

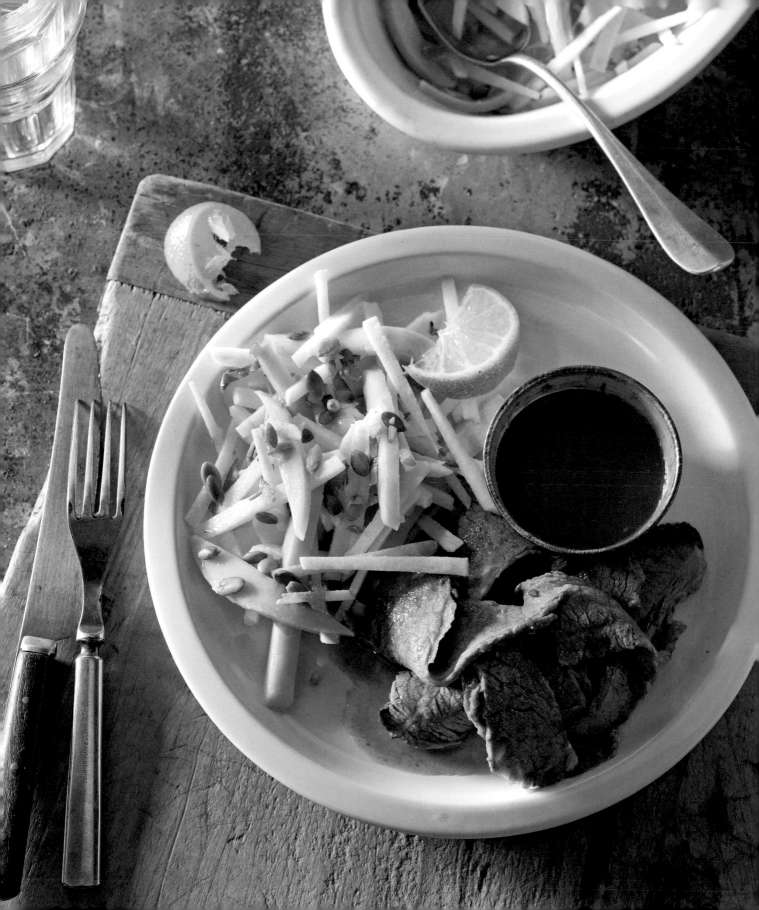

ROMAINE WRAPS WITH SHREDDED BEEF BRISKET AND FRESH RED CHILE HARISSA

PREP: 20 minutes   ROAST: 4 hours   STAND: 15 minutes   MAKES: 6 to 8 servings

HARISSA IS A FIERY-HOT SAUCE FROM TUNISIA THAT IS USED AS A CONDIMENT FOR ROASTED MEATS AND FISH AND IN STEWS AS A FLAVORING. EACH COOK HAS HIS OR HER OWN VERSION OF IT, BUT—IN ADDITION TO CHILES—IT ALMOST ALWAYS CONTAINS CARAWAY, CUMIN, GARLIC, CORIANDER, AND OLIVE OIL.

BRISKET

1 3- to 3 ½-pound beef brisket
2 teaspoons ground ancho chile pepper
1 teaspoon garlic powder
1 teaspoon onion powder
1 teaspoon ground cumin
¼ cup extra virgin olive oil
1 cup Beef Bone Broth (see recipe, page 131) or no-salt-added beef broth

HARISSA

1 teaspoon coriander seeds
1 teaspoon caraway seeds
½ teaspoon cumin seeds
8 to 10 red Fresno chile peppers, red Anaheim chile peppers, or red jalapenos, stemmed, seeded (if desired), and chopped (see tip, page 56)
3 cloves garlic, minced
   Romaine lettuce leaves

1. Preheat oven to 300°F. Trim any excess fat from brisket. In a small bowl combine ground ancho chile pepper, garlic powder, onion powder, and cumin. Sprinkle spice mixture over meat; rub into meat.

2. In a 5- to 6-quart Dutch oven heat 1 tablespoon of the olive oil over medium-high heat. Brown the brisket on both sides in the hot oil; remove Dutch oven from heat. Add the Beef Bone Broth. Cover and roast for 4 to 4½ hours or until meat is tender.

3. Meanwhile, for the harissa, in a small skillet combine coriander seeds, caraway seeds, and cumin seeds. Place skillet over medium heat. Toast seeds about 5 minutes or until fragrant, shaking skillet frequently; let cool. Use a spice grinder or mortar and pestle to grind the toasted seeds. In a food processor combine the ground seed mixture, fresh chiles, garlic, and the remaining 3 tablespoons olive oil. Process until smooth. Transfer to a bowl; cover and chill for at least 1 hour.

4. Remove Dutch oven from oven. Let stand for 15 minutes. Transfer meat to a cutting board; slice meat across the grain. Place on a serving platter and drizzle with some of the cooking liquid. To serve, fill romaine leaves with sliced brisket; top with harissa.

HERB-CRUSTED ROAST EYE OF ROUND WITH MASHED ROOT VEGETABLES AND PAN SAUCE

PREP: 25 minutes   COOK: 25 minutes   ROAST: 40 minutes   STAND: 10 minutes   MAKES: 6 servings

BE SURE TO SAVE ALL OF THE COOKING WATER WHEN YOU DRAIN THE VEGETABLES. THE RESERVED WATER IS USED IN BOTH THE MASHED ROOT VEGETABLES AND IN THE SAUCE FOR THE MEAT.

ROAST
- ½ cup tightly packed fresh parsley leaves
- ¼ cup snipped fresh thyme
- 1 tablespoon cracked black pepper
- 2 teaspoons finely shredded lemon peel
- 4 cloves garlic, peeled
- 4 tablespoons extra virgin olive oil
- 1 3-pound eye of round roast
- 2 tablespoons Dijon-Style Mustard (see recipe, page 322)

PAN SAUCE
- 1 cup chopped onion
- 1 cup sliced button mushrooms
- 1 bay leaf
- ¼ cup dry red wine
- 1 cup Beef Bone Broth (see recipe, page 131) or no-salt-added beef broth
- 1 tablespoon extra virgin olive oil
- 2 teaspoons sherry or balsamic vinegar
- 1 recipe Mashed Root Vegetables (see recipe, right)

1. Position oven rack in lower third of oven. Preheat oven to 400°F. In a food processor combine parsley, thyme, pepper, lemon peel, garlic cloves, and 2 tablespoons of the olive oil. Pulse until garlic is coarsely chopped. Set garlic mixture aside.

2. In a medium roasting pan or extra-large ovenproof sauté pan heat the remaining 2 tablespoons olive oil over medium-high heat. Add the roast and sear until browned on all sides, about 4 minutes per side. Remove roast from pan; remove pan from the burner. Spread the Dijon-Style Mustard over the roast. Sprinkle garlic mixture on the roast, pressing to adhere. Return roast to the pan. Roast, uncovered, for 40 to 45 minutes or until a meat thermometer inserted in center of roast registers 130°F to 135°F. Transfer the meat to a cutting board; loosely tent with foil. Let stand for 10 minutes before slicing.

3. Meanwhile, for sauce, place the roasting or sauté pan on the stovetop. Heat over medium-high heat. Add the onion, mushrooms, and bay leaf; cook and stir about 5 minutes or until onion is translucent. Stir in wine; simmer about 2 minutes or until wine is nearly evaporated, scraping up any browned bits from bottom of the pan. Add 1 cup of the reserved vegetable cooking water and Beef Bone Broth. Bring to boiling; reduce heat. Simmer, uncovered, until sauce reduces to about 1 cup, about 4 minutes, stirring occasionally.

4. Strain sauce through a fine-mesh sieve into a large measuring cup; discard solids. Whisk olive oil and vinegar into the sauce. Serve roast beef with Mashed Root Vegetables; drizzle with sauce.

Mashed Root Vegetables: In a large saucepan combine 3 medium carrots, peeled and cut into large chunks; 3 medium parsnips, peeled and cut into large chunks; 2 medium turnips, peeled and cut into large chunks; 1 large sweet potato, peeled and cut into large chunks; and 2 sprigs fresh rosemary. Add enough water to cover vegetables. Bring to boiling; reduce heat. Simmer, covered, for 15 to 20 minutes or until vegetables are very tender. Drain the vegetables, reserving the cooking water. Discard rosemary. Return vegetables to the pan. Mash with a potato masher or electric mixer, drizzling in some of the reserved cooking water until desired consistency (reserve remaining vegetable water for pan sauce). Season with cayenne. Cover and keep warm until ready to serve.

BEEF-VEGETABLE SOUP WITH ROASTED RED PEPPER PESTO

PREP: 40 minutes   COOK: 1 hour 25 minutes   STAND: 20 minutes   MAKES: 8 servings

SMOKED PAPRIKA—ALSO CALLED PIMENTON—IS A SPANISH PAPRIKA MADE BY DRYING PEPPERS OVER A SMOKY OAK-WOOD FIRE, WHICH IMPARTS INCREDIBLE FLAVOR. IT COMES IN THREE VARIETIES—SWEET AND MILD (*DULCE*), MEDIUM-HOT (*AGRIDULCE*), AND HOT (*PICANTE*). CHOOSE BASED ON YOUR TASTE.

1 tablespoon extra virgin olive oil
2 pounds boneless beef chuck roast, trimmed of excess fat and cut into 1-inch cubes
1 cup chopped onion
1 cup sliced carrots
1 cup sliced celery
1 cup sliced parsnips
1 cup sliced fresh mushrooms
½ cup diced turnip
½ teaspoon smoked paprika
½ teaspoon dried rosemary, crushed
½ teaspoon crushed red pepper
½ cup dry red wine
8 cups Beef Bone Broth (see recipe, page 131) or no-salt-added beef broth
2 cups diced fresh tomatoes
1 bay leaf
1 cup cubed, peeled sweet potato or butternut squash
2 cups shredded kale leaves or green cabbage
¾ cup diced zucchini or yellow summer squash
¾ cup chopped asparagus
¾ cup very small cauliflower florets
  Red Pepper Pesto (see recipe, right)

1. In a 6- to 8-quart Dutch oven heat the olive oil over medium-high heat. Add half of the beef to hot oil in pan; cook for 5 to 6 minutes or until well browned on all sides. Remove beef from pan. Repeat with remaining beef. Adjust heat as necessary to prevent the browned bits on the bottom of the pot from scorching.

2. Add the onion, carrots, celery, parsnips, mushrooms, and turnip to the Dutch oven. Reduce heat to medium. Cook and stir for 7 to 8 minutes or until vegetables are crisp-tender, scraping up any browned bits with a wooden spoon. Add the paprika, rosemary, and crushed red pepper; cook and stir for 1 minute. Stir in the wine; simmer until nearly evaporated. Add the Beef Bone Broth, tomatoes, bay leaf, and browned beef and accumulated juices. Bring to boiling; reduce heat. Simmer, covered, about 1 hour or until beef and vegetables are tender. Stir in the sweet potato and kale; simmer for 20 minutes. Add the zucchini, asparagus, and cauliflower; cook about 5 minutes or just until crisp-tender. Remove and discard bay leaf.

3. To serve, ladle soup into serving bowls and top with some of the Red Pepper Pesto.

Red Pepper Pesto: Preheat broiler with oven rack positioned in the upper third of the oven. Place 3 red sweet peppers on a foil-lined baking sheet. Rub surfaces of peppers with 1 tablespoon extra virgin olive oil. Broil peppers for 10 to 15 minutes or until skin darkens and blisters and peppers soften, turning halfway during roasting. Transfer peppers to a large bowl. Cover bowl with plastic wrap. Let stand about 20 minutes or until cool. Remove seeds, stems, and skins from the peppers and discard. Cut peppers into pieces. In a food processor pulse ½ cup fresh parsley leaves, ¼ cup slivered almonds, and 3 cloves garlic until finely chopped. Add roasted peppers, 2 tablespoons extra virgin olive oil, 1 tablespoon finely shredded orange peel, 2 teaspoons balsamic or sherry vinegar, and paprika and cayenne to taste. Pulse until finely chopped but not runny. If necessary, add an additional 1 tablespoon olive oil to reach desired consistency. Transfer to an airtight container. Cover and chill until ready to serve.

SLOW-COOKED SWEET AND SAVORY BEEF STEW

PREP: 25 minutes   COOK: 6 minutes   STAND: 10 minutes
SLOW COOK: 9 hours (low) or 4½ hours (high) + 15 minutes (high)   MAKES: 4 servings

THE SWEETNESS IN THIS HEARTY STEW COMES FROM A SMALL AMOUNT OF DRIED APRICOTS AND DRIED CHERRIES. LOOK FOR UNSULFURED, UNSWEETENED DRIED FRUITS AT ANY MARKET THAT CARRIES WHOLE FOODS.

1½ pounds boneless beef arm pot roast or boneless beef chuck roast

2 tablespoons refined coconut oil

1 cup boiling water

½ cup dried shiitake mushrooms

1 cup fresh peeled or frozen pearl onions, halved if large

3 medium parsnips, halved lengthwise and cut crosswise into 2-inch pieces

3 medium carrots, halved lengthwise and cut crosswise into 2-inch pieces

6 cloves garlic, thinly sliced

1 bay leaf

1 teaspoon dried sage or thyme or 1 tablespoon snipped fresh sage or thyme

2½ cups Beef Bone Broth (see page 131) or no-salt-added beef broth

4 cups coarsely chopped, trimmed fresh Swiss chard or kale

½ cup dry red wine

2 tablespoons chopped unsulfured, unsweetened dried apricots

2 tablespoons unsulfured, unsweetened dried cherries

1. Trim fat from beef. Cut beef into 1½-inch pieces. In a large skillet heat 1 tablespoon of the coconut oil over medium-high heat. Add beef; cook for 5 to 7 minutes or until browned, stirring occasionally. Using a slotted spoon transfer beef to a 3½- or 4-quart slow cooker. Repeat with remaining coconut oil and beef. If desired, scrape the drippings from the skillet into cooker with beef.

2. Meanwhile, in a small bowl combine the boiling water and dried mushrooms. Cover; let stand for 10 minutes. Drain mushrooms, reserving the soaking liquid. Rinse the mushrooms; coarsely chop mushrooms and add to cooker with beef. Pour the soaking liquid through a fine-mesh sieve into the slow cooker.

3. Add onions, parsnips, carrots, garlic, bay leaf, and dried sage or thyme (if using). Pour Beef Bone Broth over all. Cover; cook on low-heat setting for 9 to 10 hours or on high-heat setting for 4½ to 5 hours.

4. Remove and discard the bay leaf. Add Swiss chard, wine, apricots, cherries, and fresh sage or thyme (if using) to stew in cooker. If using low-heat setting, turn to high-heat setting. Cover; cook for 15 minutes more. To serve, ladle into warm serving bowls.

5 WAYS WITH FLANK STEAK

FLANK STEAK IS A LONG, LEAN AND FLAVORFUL CUT FROM THE ABDOMINAL MUSCLES OF THE ANIMAL. IT IS VERY VERSATILE—IT CAN BE GRILLED, BROILED, SLICED THIN AND STIR-FRIED, STUFFED AND ROLLED AND ROASTED, AND COOKED IN A SOUP TO MAKE IT MORE TENDER. IT ALSO TAKES TO A WIDE VARIETY OF FLAVOR PROFILES AND IS OFTEN USED AS A SUBSTITUTE IN FAJITAS FOR THE MORE TRADITIONAL SKIRT STEAK.

Asian Flank Steak Soup,
recipe page 94

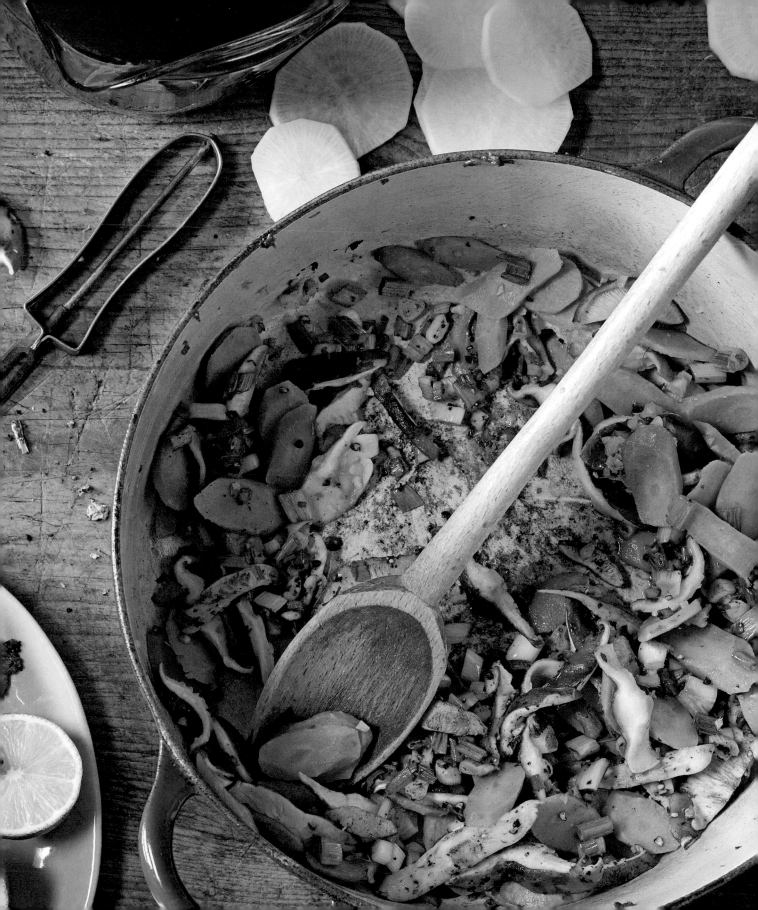

5 WAYS WITH FLANK STEAK

BECAUSE FLANK STEAK COMES FROM A WELL-EXERCISED AREA OF THE COW, IT HAS A STRONG GRAIN—THE MUSCLE FIBERS IN THE MEAT. WHEN SLICING IT, BE SURE TO CUT IT ACROSS THE GRAIN TO MAXIMIZE ITS TENDERNESS. THESE RECIPES SHOW OFF ITS VERSATILITY IN FLAVORS THAT RUN THE GAMUT FROM ASIAN TO LATIN AMERICAN TO NEW AMERICAN. LOOK FOR FLANK STEAK THAT IS BRIGHT RED IN COLOR TO GET THE FRESHEST MEAT.

1. PAN-SEARED FLANK STEAK WITH BRUSSELS SPROUTS AND CHERRIES

PREP: 20 minutes
COOK: 20 minutes
MAKES: 4 servings

- 3 tablespoons refined coconut oil
- 1½ pounds Brussels sprouts, trimmed and quartered
- ½ cup sliced shallots
- 1½ cups pitted fresh cherries
- 1 teaspoon snipped fresh thyme
- 1 tablespoon balsamic vinegar
- 1½ pounds beef flank steak
- 1 tablespoon snipped fresh rosemary
- 2 tablespoons snipped fresh thyme
- ½ teaspoon black pepper

1. In a large skillet heat 2 tablespoons of the coconut oil over medium heat. Add Brussels sprouts and shallots. Cook, covered, for 15 minutes, stirring occasionally. Add cherries and thyme, stirring to scrape up any browned bits from bottom of skillet. Cook, uncovered, about 5 minutes or until Brussels sprouts are browned and tender. Add vinegar; remove skillet from heat.

2. Cut flank steak into four portions; sprinkle both sides of each steak with rosemary, thyme, and pepper. In an extra-large skillet heat 1 tablespoon of the coconut oil over medium-high heat. Add steaks to skillet; cook for 8 to 10 minutes or until an instant-read thermometer registers 145°F for medium, turning once halfway through cooking.

3. Thinly slice steaks across the grain and serve with Brussels sprouts and cherries.

2. ASIAN FLANK STEAK SOUP

PREP: 35 minutes
COOK: 20 minutes
MAKES: 6 to 8 servings

- 1½ pounds beef flank steak
- 2 tablespoons extra virgin olive oil
- 1 pound shiitake mushrooms, stemmed and sliced
- 1 bunch scallions, thinly sliced
- 2 cups chopped bok choy
- 1 cup thinly sliced carrots
- 6 large cloves garlic, minced (1 tablespoon)
- 1 tablespoon minced fresh ginger
- 1 teaspoon black pepper
- 8 cups Beef Bone Broth (see recipe, page 131) or no-salt-added beef broth
- 1 sheet nori seaweed, crumbled
- 1 cup thinly sliced daikon radish
- ⅓ cup fresh lime juice
- 4 hard-cooked eggs, peeled and halved
  Lime wedges

1. If desired, partially freeze beef for easier slicing (about 20 minutes). Cut flank steak in half lengthwise and then thinly slice each half across the grain into strips. Cut strips in half. In a 6-quart Dutch oven heat 1 tablespoon of the olive oil over medium-high heat. Add half of the flank steak; cook about 3 minutes or until nicely browned, stirring occasionally. Remove meat from pan; repeat with remaining olive oil and flank steak. Remove steak from Dutch oven and set aside.

2. Reduce heat to medium; add shiitake mushrooms, scallions, bok choy, carrots, garlic, and pepper to the Dutch oven. Cook for 5 minutes, stirring frequently. Add the flank steak, Beef Bone Broth, and crumbled seaweed to Dutch oven. Bring to boiling; reduce heat. Simmer, covered, about 5 minutes or until carrots are tender.

3. Add daikon radish, lime juice, and hard-cooked eggs to soup. Return soup to a simmer. Immediately turn off heat. Ladle soup into warmed serving bowls. Garnish with lime wedges.

3. FLANK STEAK STIR-FRY WITH SESAME-CAULIFLOWER RICE

START TO FINISH: 1 hour
MAKES: 4 servings

- 1½ pounds beef flank steak
- 4 cups chopped cauliflower
- 2 tablespoons sesame seeds
- 2 teaspoons refined coconut oil
- ¾ teaspoon crushed red pepper
- ¼ cup snipped fresh cilantro
- 3 tablespoons coconut oil
- ½ cup thinly sliced scallions
- 1 tablespoon grated fresh ginger
- 6 cloves garlic, minced (1 tablespoon)
- 1 tablespoon thinly sliced fresh lemongrass

2 red, green, and/or yellow sweet peppers, seeded and cut into strips
2 cups small broccoli florets
½ cup Beef Bone Broth (see recipe, page 131) or no-salt-added beef broth
¼ cup fresh lime juice
  Sliced scallions (optional)
  Crushed red pepper (optional)

1. If desired, partially freeze flank steak for easier slicing (about 20 minutes). Cut flank steak in half lengthwise; thinly slice each half across the grain into strips. Set meat strips aside.

2. For the cauliflower rice, in a food processor pulse 2 cups of the cauliflower until the pieces are the size of rice; transfer to a medium bowl. Repeat with remaining 2 cups cauliflower. In a large skillet toast the sesame seeds over medium heat about 2 minutes or until golden. Add the 2 teaspoons coconut oil and ¼ teaspoon of the crushed red pepper; cook for 30 seconds. Add cauliflower rice and cilantro to skillet; stir. Reduce heat; cook, covered, for 6 to 8 minutes or until cauliflower is just tender. Keep warm.

3. In an extra-large skillet heat 1 tablespoon of the coconut oil over medium-high heat. Add half of the meat strips; cook and stir until desired doneness. Remove meat from skillet. Repeat with 1 tablespoon of the remaining coconut oil and remaining meat strips; set meat aside. Drain skillet.

4. In the same skillet heat the remaining 1 tablespoon coconut oil over medium-high heat. Add scallions, ginger, garlic, lemongrass, and the remaining ½ teaspoon crushed red pepper to the skillet; cook and stir for 30 seconds. Add sweet peppers, broccoli, and Beef Bone Broth to skillet. Cook about 5 minutes or until broccoli is tender,

stirring occasionally. Stir in meat and the lime juice; cook for 1 minute more. Serve over cauliflower rice. If desired, top with additional scallions and/or crushed red pepper.

4. STUFFED FLANK STEAK WITH CHIMICHURRI SAUCE

PREP: 30 minutes
ROAST: 35 minutes
STAND: 10 minutes
MAKES: 4 servings

1 medium sweet potato, peeled (about 12 ounces)
1 tablespoon extra virgin olive oil
6 cloves garlic, minced (1 tablespoon)
2 teaspoons extra virgin olive oil
1 5-ounce package fresh baby spinach
1½ pounds flank steak
2 teaspoons cracked black pepper
2 tablespoons extra virgin olive oil
½ cup Chimichurri Sauce (see recipe, page 323)

1. Preheat oven to 400°F. Line a large baking sheet with parchment paper. Using a mandoline, slice sweet potato lengthwise into approximately ⅛-inch thick slices. In a medium bowl toss sweet potato slices with the 1 tablespoon oil. Arrange slices in an even layer on the prepared baking sheet. Roast about 15 minutes or until tender. Set aside to cool.

2. Meanwhile, in an ovenproof extra-large skillet combine the garlic and 2 teaspoons olive oil. Cook over medium heat about 2 minutes or until garlic is slightly cooked but not brown, stirring occasionally. Add spinach to skillet; cook until wilted.

Transfer spinach to a plate to cool; set skillet aside.

3. Score both sides of the flank steak by making shallow, diagonal cuts approximately 1 inch apart in a diamond pattern. Place the flank steak between two pieces of plastic wrap. Using the flat side of a meat mallet, pound steak until it is approximately ½ inch thick. Squeeze excess liquid from the cooked spinach and arrange evenly over steak. Top with sweet potatoes, overlapping slices as necessary. Starting from a long side, roll up flank steak. Tie rolled steak at 1-inch intervals using 100%-cotton kitchen string. Sprinkle with cracked black pepper.

4. Add 2 tablespoons oil to the skillet used to cook spinach. Add meat to skillet; cook until browned on all sides, turning meat as necessary to brown evenly. Place skillet with meat in oven. Roast, uncovered, for 20 to 25 minutes or until an instant-read meat thermometer inserted in center registers 145°F.

5. Remove meat from skillet and cover with foil. Let stand for 10 minutes. Remove kitchen string; slice meat crosswise into ½-inch thick slices. Serve with Chimichurri Sauce.

5. GRILLED FLANK STEAK KABOBS WITH HORSERADISH MAYO

PREP: 30 minutes
MARINATE: 2 to 4 hours
GRILL: 48 minutes
MAKES: 4 servings

1½ pounds beef flank steak
 1 cup dry red wine
 ½ cup olive oil
 ¼ cup minced shallots
 9 cloves garlic, minced
    (1 tablespoon)
 2 tablespoons snipped fresh
    rosemary
 2 medium sweet potatoes,
    peeled and cut into 1-inch
    cubes
 2 medium turnips, peeled and
    cut into 1-inch cubes
 ½ teaspoon black pepper
 ¾ cup Paleo Mayo (see recipe,
    page 323)
 2 to 3 tablespoons grated fresh
    horseradish
 1 tablespoon snipped fresh
    chives

1. Slice flank steak against the grain into ¼-inch-thick slices. Place meat in a 1-gallon resealable plastic bag set in a shallow dish; set aside.

2. For marinade, in a small bowl combine red wine, ¼ cup of the oil, shallots, 6 cloves of minced garlic, and 1 tablespoon of the rosemary. Pour marinade over meat in bag. Seal bag and turn to coat meat. Marinate in the refrigerator for 2 to 4 hours, turning bag occasionally.

3. Meanwhile, for vegetables, combine sweet potatoes and turnips in a large bowl. In a small bowl combine remaining ¼ cup olive oil, 3 cloves minced garlic, remaining rosemary, and pepper. Drizzle over vegetables; toss to coat. Fold a 36×18-inch piece of heavy foil in half to make a double thickness of foil that measures 18×18 inches. Place coated vegetables in the center of the foil; bring up opposite edges of foil and seal with a double fold. Fold remaining edges to completely enclose the vegetables, leaving space for steam to build.

4. For a charcoal or gas grill, place foil vegetable packet on a grill rack directly over medium heat. Cover and grill for 40 minutes or until vegetables are tender, turning once halfway through grilling. Remove from grill. Let stand enclosed while grilling steak kabobs.

5. In a small bowl stir together Paleo Mayo, horseradish, and chives. Set aside. Drain flank steak; discard marinade. On twelve 12- to 14-inch metal or bamboo skewers* thread the steak accordion style. Place steak kabobs on a grill rack directly over medium heat. Cover and grill for 8 to 9 minutes, turning kabobs halfway through grilling.

6. Carefully open vegetable packet and empty into a large serving bowl. Serve steak kabobs and vegetables with horseradish mayo.

*Note: If using bamboo skewers, soak in water for 30 minutes prior to adding meat to prevent burning.

WINE-BRAISED CHUCK STEAKS WITH MUSHROOMS

PREP: 10 minutes   COOK: 30 minutes   BAKE: 1 hour 45 minutes   MAKES: 2 servings

CHUCK STEAKS ARE AN ECONOMICAL CHOICE BECAUSE THEY'RE NOT THE TENDEREST CUT. HOWEVER, AFTER AN HOUR OR SO SIMMERING IN A MIXTURE OF RED WINE, BEEF BROTH, MUSHROOMS, GARLIC, AND BLACK PEPPER, THEY CAN BE CUT WITH A BUTTER KNIFE.

2   6-ounce boneless cross rib beef chuck steaks, cut about ¾ inch thick

½   teaspoon preservative-free granulated garlic
    Black pepper

4   teaspoons extra virgin olive oil

10 ounces button mushrooms, sliced

½   cup dry red wine (such as Zinfandel)

½   cup Beef Bone Broth (see recipe, page 131), Chicken Bone Broth (see recipe, page 235), or no-salt-added beef or chicken broth

2   teaspoons snipped fresh parsley

½   teaspoon snipped fresh thyme

½   teaspoon finely shredded lemon peel

1   small garlic clove, minced
    Grated fresh horseradish (optional)

1. Preheat oven to 300°F.

2. If desired, trim fat from steaks. Pat steaks dry with paper towels. Sprinkle both sides with granulated garlic and pepper. In a ovenproof medium skillet heat 2 teaspoons of the olive oil over medium-high heat. Add steaks to skillet; cook for 3 to 4 minutes per side or until well browned. Transfer steaks to a plate; set aside.

3. Add mushrooms and the remaining 2 teaspoons olive oil to the pan. Cook for 4 minutes, stirring occasionally. Stir in the wine and Beef Bone Broth, scraping up the browned bits from the bottom of the pan. Bring to a simmer. Add steaks to the skillet, spooning mushroom mixture over steaks. Cover skillet with lid. Transfer skillet to the oven. Bake about 1¼ hours or until meat is tender.

4. For parsley topping, in a small bowl stir together the parsley, thyme, lemon peel, and garlic; set aside.

5. Transfer steaks to a plate; cover to keep warm. For sauce, heat mushrooms and liquid in skillet over medium-high heat until simmering. Cook about 4 minutes or until reduced slightly. Serve mushroom sauce over steaks. Sprinkle with the parsley topping and, if desired, grated horseradish.

STRIP STEAKS WITH
AVOCADO-HORSERADISH SAUCE

PREP: 15 minutes   STAND: 10 minutes   GRILL: 16 minutes   MAKES: 4 servings

THE HORSERADISH SAUCE MAKES A GREAT ACCOMPANIMENT TO THE SLOW-ROASTED BEEF TENDERLOIN ON PAGE 84. HERE, IT'S BLENDED WITH GRILLED AVOCADOS TO MAKE A RICH-TASTING SAUCE SPIKED WITH A LITTLE BIT OF HEAT FROM DIJON MUSTARD AND FRESHLY GRATED HORSERADISH. GRILLING THE AVOCADOS MAKES THEM EXTRA CREAMY AND NICELY SMOKY.

STEAK

1 tablespoon Smoky Seasoning
   (see recipe, page 324)
½ teaspoon dry mustard
1 teaspoon ground cumin
4 strip (top loin) steaks, cut
   1 inch thick (about 2 pounds
   total)
2 avocados, halved and seeded
   (peel on)
1 teaspoon lime juice

SAUCE

2 tablespoons Horseradish Sauce
2 tablespoons fresh lime juice
2 cloves garlic, minced

1. In a small bowl combine Smoky Seasoning, dry mustard, and cumin. Sprinkle over steaks and rub in with your fingers. Let stand for 10 minutes.

2. For a charcoal grill, arrange medium-hot coals around a drip pan. Test for medium heat above the pan. Place steaks on the grill rack over the drip pan. Cover and grill for 16 to 20 minutes for medium rare (145°F) or 20 to 24 minutes for medium (160°F), turning steaks once halfway through grilling. Brush the cut sides of the avocados with lime juice. Add to the grill rack over the drip pan, cut sides up, for the last 8 to 10 minutes of grilling or until softened. (For a gas grill, preheat grill. Reduce heat to medium. Adjust for indirect cooking. Grill as directed above.)

3. For the sauce, scoop the avocado flesh into a medium bowl. Add Horseradish Sauce, the 2 tablespoons lime juice, and garlic; mash with a fork until nearly smooth. Serve steaks with sauce.

Horseradish Sauce: In a medium bowl combine ¼ cup grated fresh horseradish, 1 cup Cashew Cream (see recipe, page 327), 1 tablespoon Dijon-Style Mustard (see recipe, page 322), 1 teaspoon white wine vinegar, and 2 teaspoons Lemon-Herb Seasoning (see recipe, page 324). Cover and refrigerate for at least 4 hours or overnight.

LEMONGRASS-MARINATED SIRLOIN STEAKS

PREP: 30 minutes   MARINATE: 2 to 10 hours   GRILL: 10 minutes   STAND: 35 minutes   MAKES: 4 servings

THAI BASIL IS DIFFERENT THAN THE SWEET BASIL USED IN MEDITERRANEAN COOKING IN BOTH APPEARANCE AND TASTE. SWEET BASIL HAS WIDE LEAVES ON GREEN STEMS; THAI BASIL HAS NARROW GREEN LEAVES ON PURPLE STEMS. BOTH HAVE AN ANISE FLAVOR, BUT IN THAI BASIL IT IS MORE PRONOUNCED. THAI BASIL ALSO HOLDS UP BETTER UNDER HEAT THAN SWEET BASIL. LOOK FOR IT AT ASIAN MARKETS AND FARMER'S MARKETS. IF YOU CAN'T FIND IT, YOU CAN CERTAINLY USE SWEET BASIL.

2 stalks lemongrass, yellow and pale green parts only
1 2-inch piece ginger, peeled and thinly sliced
½ cup chopped fresh pineapple
¼ cup fresh lime juice
1 jalapeño, seeded and chopped (see tip, page 56)
2 tablespoons extra virgin olive oil
4 6-ounce beef sirloin steaks, cut ¾ inch thick
½ cup Thai basil leaves
½ cup cilantro leaves
½ cup mint leaves
½ cup scallions, thinly sliced
2 teaspoons extra virgin olive oil
1 lime, quartered

1. For marinade, remove and discard any bruised outer layers from the lemongrass stalks. Slice into thin rounds. In a food processor combine lemongrass and ginger; pulse until very finely chopped. Add the pineapple, lime juice, jalapeño, and 2 tablespoons olive oil; puree as much as possible.

2. Place steaks in a large resealable plastic bag set in a shallow dish. Pour marinade over steaks. Seal bag; turn bag to coat. Marinate in the refrigerator for 2 to 10 hours, turning bag occasionally. Remove steaks from the marinade; discard marinade. Let steaks stand at room temperature for 30 minutes before grilling.

3. For a charcoal or gas grill, place steaks on the grill rack directly over medium heat. Cover and grill for 10 to 12 minutes for medium rare (145°F) or 12 to 15 minutes for medium (160°F), turning once halfway through grilling. Remove steaks from grill; let stand for 5 minutes before serving.

4. For herb topping, in a small bowl toss together basil, cilantro, mint, and scallions; drizzle with the 2 teaspoons olive oil; toss to coat. Top each steak with herb topping and serve with lime wedges.

BALSAMIC-DIJON SIRLOIN WITH GARLICKY SPINACH

PREP: 12 minutes   MARINATE: 4 hours   BROIL: 10 minutes   MAKES: 4 servings

BOILING THE MARINADE MAKES IT SAFE TO EAT AS A SAUCE—AND REDUCES IT SLIGHTLY TO MAKE IT THICKER AS WELL. SAUTÉ THE SPINACH WHILE THE STEAK IS BROILING—AND JUST BARELY. FOR THE BEST FLAVOR AND NUTRITION, COOK THE SPINACH ONLY UNTIL IT JUST WILTS AND IS STILL BRIGHT GREEN.

STEAK

- 4 tablespoons balsamic vinegar
- 3 tablespoons extra virgin olive oil
- 3 tablespoons fresh lemon juice
- 3 tablespoons fresh orange juice
- 1 tablespoon Dijon-Style Mustard (see recipe, page 322)
- 2 teaspoons snipped fresh rosemary
- ½ teaspoon black pepper
- 3 cloves garlic, minced
- 1 1½-pound sirloin steak, cut 1½ inches thick

SPINACH

- 1 tablespoon extra virgin olive oil
- 4 cloves garlic, thinly sliced
- 8 cups baby spinach
- ¼ teaspoon black pepper

1. For marinade, in a medium bowl whisk together vinegar, olive oil, lemon juice, orange juice, Dijon-Style Mustard, rosemary, pepper, and garlic. Place steak in a resealable plastic bag set in a shallow dish. Pour marinade over steak. Seal bag; turn to coat steak. Marinate in the refrigerator for 4 hours, turning bag occasionally.

2. Preheat broiler. Remove steak from marinade; transfer marinade to a small saucepan. For balsamic sauce, heat marinade over medium-high heat until boiling. Reduce heat; simmer for 2 to 3 minutes or until slightly thickened; set aside.

3. Place steak on unheated rack of a broiler pan. Broil 4 to 5 inches from heat about 10 minutes for medium rare (145°F) or 14 minutes for medium (160°), turning once. Transfer steak to a cutting board. Cover loosely with foil; let stand for 10 minutes.

4. Meanwhile, for spinach, in a extra-large skillet heat olive oil over medium heat. Add sliced garlic; cook for 1 minute or until light golden. Add spinach; sprinkle with pepper. Cook and stir for 1 to 2 minutes or just until spinach wilts.

5. Cut steak into four portions and drizzle with the balsamic sauce. Serve with spinach.

GRILLED STRIP STEAKS WITH GRATED ROOT VEGETABLE HASH

PREP: 20 minutes   STAND: 20 minutes   GRILL: 10 minutes   STAND: 5 minutes   MAKES: 4 servings

STRIP STEAKS HAVE A VERY TENDER TEXTURE, AND THE SMALL STRIP OF FAT ON ONE SIDE OF THE STEAK GETS CRISP AND SMOKY ON THE GRILL. MY THINKING ABOUT ANIMAL FAT HAS CHANGED SINCE MY FIRST BOOK. IF YOU ARE FAITHFUL TO THE BASIC PRINCIPLES OF THE PALEO DIET® AND KEEP SATURATED FATS WITHIN 10 TO 15 PERCENT OF YOUR DAILY CALORIES, IT WILL NOT INCREASE YOUR RISK OF HEART DISEASE—AND IN FACT, THE OPPOSITE MAY BE TRUE. NEW INFORMATION SUGGESTS THAT ELEVATIONS IN LDL CHOLESTEROL MAY ACTUALLY REDUCE SYSTEMIC INFLAMMATION, WHICH IS A RISK FACTOR FOR HEART DISEASE.

3 tablespoons extra virgin olive oil

2 tablespoons grated fresh horseradish

1 teaspoon finely shredded orange peel

½ teaspoon ground cumin

½ teaspoon black pepper

4 strip steaks (also called top loin), cut about 1 inch thick

2 medium parsnips, peeled

1 large sweet potato, peeled

1 medium turnip, peeled

1 or 2 shallots, finely chopped

2 cloves garlic, minced

1 tablespoon snipped fresh thyme

1. In a small bowl stir together 1 tablespoon of the oil, horseradish, orange peel, cumin, and ¼ teaspoon of the pepper. Spread the mixture over steaks; cover and let stand at room temperature for 15 minutes.

2. Meanwhile for hash, using a box grater or a food processor fitted with the shredding blade, shred the parsnips, sweet potato, and turnip. Place shredded vegetables in a large bowl; add shallot(s). In a small bowl combine the remaining 2 tablespoons oil, the remaining ¼ teaspoon pepper, garlic, and thyme. Drizzle over vegetables; toss to mix thoroughly. Fold a 36×18-inch piece of heavy foil in half to make a double thickness of foil that measures 18×18 inches. Place vegetable mixture in the center of the foil; bring up opposite edges of foil and seal with a double fold. Fold remaining edges to completely enclose the vegetables, leaving space for steam to build.

3. For a charcoal or gas grill, place steaks and foil packet on the grill rack directly over medium heat. Cover and grill steaks for 10 to 12 minutes for medium rare (145°F) or 12 to 15 minutes for medium (160°F), turning once halfway through grilling. Grill packet for 10 to 15 minutes or until vegetables are tender. Let steaks stand for 5 minutes while vegetables finish cooking. Divide vegetable hash among four serving plates; top with steaks.

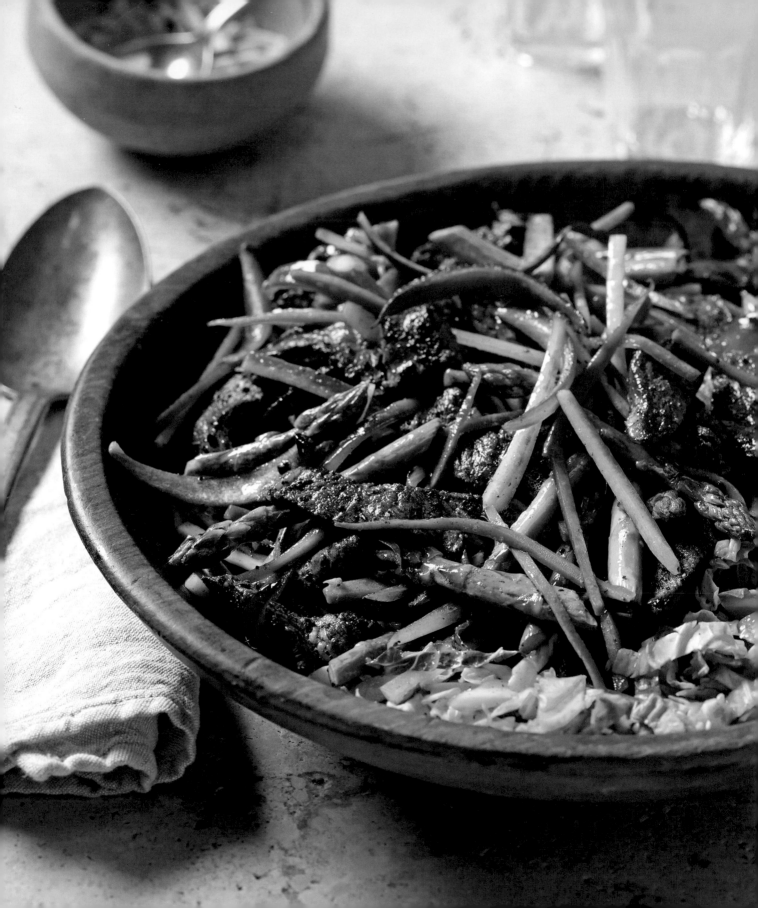

ASIAN BEEF AND VEGETABLE STIR-FRY

FIVE-SPICE POWDER IS A SALT-FREE SPICE BLEND USED WIDELY IN CHINESE COOKING. IT CONSISTS OF EQUAL PARTS GROUND CINNAMON, CLOVES, FENNEL SEEDS, STAR ANISE, AND SZECHWAN PEPPERCORNS.

1½   pounds boneless beef top sirloin steak or boneless beef round steak, cut 1 inch thick
1½   teaspoons five-spice powder
3   tablespoons refined coconut oil
1   small red onion, cut into thin wedges
1   small bunch asparagus (about 12 ounces), trimmed and cut into 3-inch pieces
1½   cups julienne-cut orange and/or yellow carrots
4   cloves garlic, minced
1   teaspoon finely shredded orange peel
¼   cup fresh orange juice
¼   cup Beef Bone Broth (see recipe, page 131) or no-salt-added beef broth
¼   cup white wine vinegar
¼   to ½ teaspoon crushed red pepper
8   cups coarsely shredded napa cabbage
½   cup unsalted slivered almonds or unsalted coarsely chopped cashews, toasted (see tip, page 57)

1. If desired, partially freeze beef for easier slicing (about 20 minutes). Cut beef into very thin slices. In a large bowl toss together beef and five-spice powder. In a large wok or extra-large skillet heat 1 tablespoon of the coconut oil over medium-high heat. Add half the beef; cook and stir for 3 to 5 minutes or until browned. Transfer beef to a bowl. Repeat with the remaining beef and another 1 tablespoon oil. Transfer beef to the bowl with the other cooked beef.

2. In the same wok add the remaining 1 tablespoon oil. Add onion; cook and stir for 3 minutes. Add asparagus and carrots; cook and stir for 2 to 3 minutes or until vegetables are crisp-tender. Add garlic; cook and stir for 1 minute more.

3. For sauce, in a small bowl combine orange peel, orange juice, Beef Bone Broth, vinegar, and crushed red pepper. Add sauce and all the beef with juices in bowl to vegetables in wok. Cook and stir for 1 to 2 minutes or until heated through. Using a slotted spoon, transfer beef vegetables to a large bowl. Cover to keep warm.

4. Cook the sauce, uncovered, over medium heat for 2 minutes. Add cabbage; cook and stir for 1 to 2 minutes or until cabbage is just wilted. Divide cabbage and any cooking juices among four serving plates. Top evenly with beef mixture. Sprinkle with nuts.

CEDAR-PLANKED FILETS WITH ASIAN SLATHER AND SLAW

SOAK: 1 hour   PREP: 40 minutes   GRILL: 13 minutes   STAND: 10 minutes   MAKES: 4 servings.

NAPA CABBAGE IS SOMETIMES CALLED CHINESE CABBAGE. IT HAS BEAUTIFUL, CRINKLY CREAM-COLOR LEAVES WITH BRIGHT YELLOW-GREEN TIPS. IT HAS A DELICATE, MILD FLAVOR AND TEXTURE—QUITE DIFFERENT THAN THE WAXY LEAVES OF ROUND-HEADED CABBAGE—AND NOT SURPRISINGLY, IS A NATURAL IN ASIAN-STYLE DISHES.

1 large cedar plank
¼ ounce dried shiitake mushrooms
¼ cup walnut oil
2 teaspoons minced fresh ginger
2 teaspoons crushed red pepper
1 teaspoon crushed Szechwan peppercorns
¼ teaspoon five-spice powder
4 cloves garlic, minced
4 4- to 5-ounce beef tenderloin steaks, cut ¾ to 1 inch thick
Asian Slaw (see recipe, right)

1. Place grill plank in water; weight down and soak for at least 1 hour.

2. Meanwhile, for Asian slather, in a small bowl pour boiling water over dried shiitake mushrooms; let stand for 20 minutes to rehydrate. Drain mushrooms and place in a food processor. Add walnut oil, ginger, crushed red pepper, Szechuan peppercorns, five-spice powder, and garlic. Cover and process until mushrooms are minced and ingredients are combined; set aside.

3. Drain grill plank. For a charcoal grill, arrange medium-hot coals around perimeter of grill. Place plank on grill rack directly over coals. Cover and grill for 3 to 5 minutes or until plank begins to crackle and smoke. Place steaks on grill rack directly over coals; grill for 3 to 4 minutes or until seared. Transfer steaks to the plank, seared sides up. Place plank in center of grill. Divide Asian Slather among steaks. Cover and grill for 10 to 12 minutes or until an instant-read thermometer inserted horizontally into the steaks reads 130°F. (For a gas grill, preheat grill. Reduce heat to medium. Place drained plank on grill rack; cover and grill for 3 to 5 minutes or until plank begins to crackle and smoke. Place steaks on grill rack for 3 to 4 minutes or until seared. Transfer steaks to the plank, seared sides up. Adjust grill for indirect cooking; place plank with steaks over the burner that is turned off. Divide slather among steaks. Cover and grill for 10 to 12 minutes or until an instant-read thermometer inserted horizontally into the steaks reads 130°F.)

4. Remove steaks from the grill. Cover steaks loosely with foil; let stand for 10 minutes. Cut steaks into ¼-inch-thick slices. Serve steak over Asian Slaw.

Asian Slaw: In a large bowl combine 1 medium head napa cabbage, thinly sliced; 1 cup finely shredded red cabbage; 2 carrots, peeled and cut into julienne strips; 1 red or yellow sweet pepper, seeded and very thinly sliced; 4 scallions, thinly bias-sliced; 1 to 2 serrano chiles, seeded and minced (see tip, page 56); 2 tablespoons chopped cilantro; and 2 tablespoons chopped mint. For dressing, in a food processor or blender combine 3 tablespoons fresh lime juice, 1 tablespoon grated fresh ginger, 1 cloves minced garlic, and ⅛ teaspoon five-spice powder. Cover and process until smooth. With the processor running, gradually add ½ cup walnut oil and process until smooth. Add 1 scallion, thinly bias-sliced, to the dressing. Drizzle over slaw and toss to coat.

PAN-SEARED TRI-TIP STEAKS WITH CAULIFLOWER PEPERONATA

PREP: 25 minutes   COOK: 25 minutes   MAKES: 2 servings

PEPERONATA IS TRADITIONALLY A SLOW-ROASTED RAGU OF SWEET PEPPERS WITH ONION, GARLIC, AND HERBS. THIS QUICK SAUTÉED VERSION—MADE HEARTIER WITH CAULIFLOWER—ACTS AS BOTH RELISH AND SIDE DISH.

2   4- to 6-ounce tri-tip steaks, cut
      ¾ to 1 inch thick
¾   teaspoon black pepper
2   tablespoons extra virgin olive
      oil
2   red and/or yellow sweet
      peppers, seeded and sliced
1   shallot, thinly sliced
1   teaspoon Mediterranean
      Seasoning (see recipe, page
      324)
2   cups small cauliflower florets
2   tablespoons balsamic vinegar
2   teaspoons snipped fresh thyme

1. Pat steaks dry with paper towels. Sprinkle steaks with ¼ teaspoon of the black pepper. In a large skillet heat 1 tablespoon of the oil over medium-high heat. Add steaks to skillet; reduce heat to medium. Cook steaks for 6 to 9 minutes for medium rare (145°F), turning occasionally. (If meat browns too quickly, reduce heat.) Remove steaks from skillet; cover loosely with foil to keep warm.

2. For the peperonata, add the remaining 1 tablespoon oil to the skillet. Add the sweet peppers and shallot. Sprinkle with Mediterranean Seasoning. Cook over medium heat about 5 minutes or until peppers are softened, stirring occasionally. Add cauliflower, balsamic vinegar, thyme, and the remaining ½ teaspoon black pepper. Cover and cook for 10 to 15 minutes or until cauliflower is tender, stirring occasionally. Return steaks to skillet. Spoon peperonata mixture over steaks. Serve immediately.

FLAT-IRON STEAKS AU POIVRE WITH MUSHROOM-DIJON SAUCE

PREP: 15 minutes   COOK: 20 minutes   MAKES: 4 servings

THIS FRENCH-INSPIRED STEAK WITH MUSHROOM SAUCE CAN BE ON THE TABLE IN JUST OVER 30 MINUTES—WHICH MAKES IT A GREAT CHOICE FOR A QUICK WEEKNIGHT MEAL.

STEAKS

- 3 tablespoons extra virgin olive oil
- 1 pound small asparagus spears, trimmed
- 4 6-ounce flat-iron (boneless beef shoulder top blade) steaks*
- 2 tablespoons snipped fresh rosemary
- 1½ teaspoons cracked black pepper

SAUCE

- 8 ounces sliced fresh mushrooms
- 2 cloves garlic, minced
- ½ cup Beef Bone Broth (see recipe, page 131)
- ¼ cup dry white wine
- 1 tablespoon Dijon-Style Mustard (see recipe, page 322)

1. In a large skillet heat 1 tablespoon of the oil over medium-high heat. Add asparagus; cook for 8 to 10 minutes or until crisp-tender, turning spears occasionally so they don't burn. Transfer asparagus to a plate; cover with foil to keep warm.

2. Sprinkle steaks with rosemary and pepper; rub in with your fingers. In the same skillet heat the remaining 2 tablespoons oil over medium-high heat. Add steaks; reduce heat to medium. Cook for 8 to 12 minutes for medium rare (145°F), turning meat occasionally. (If meat browns too quickly, reduce heat.) Remove meat from skillet, reserving drippings. Cover steaks loosely with foil to keep warm.

3. For sauce, add mushrooms and garlic to drippings in skillet; cook until tender, stirring occasionally. Add broth, wine, and Dijon-Style Mustard. Cook over medium heat, scraping up the browned bits in bottom of skillet. Bring to boiling; cook for 1 minute more.

4. Divide the asparagus among four dinner plates. Top with steaks; spoon sauce over the steaks.

*Note: If you can't find 6-ounce flat-iron steaks, purchase two 8- to 12-ounce steaks and cut them in half to make four steaks.

GRILLED FLAT-IRON STEAKS WITH CHIPOTLE-CARAMELIZED ONIONS AND SALSA SALAD

PREP: 30 minutes   MARINATE: 2 hours   BAKE: 20 minutes   COOL: 20 minutes
GRILL: 45 minutes   MAKES: 4 servings

FLAT-IRON STEAK IS A RELATIVELY NEW CUT DEVELOPED JUST A FEW YEARS AGO. CUT FROM THE FLAVORFUL CHUCK SECTION NEAR THE SHOULDER BLADE, IT IS SURPRISINGLY TENDER AND TASTES MUCH MORE EXPENSIVE THAN IT IS—WHICH LIKELY ACCOUNTS FOR ITS QUICK RISE IN POPULARITY.

STEAKS
- ⅓ cup fresh lime juice
- ¼ cup extra virgin olive oil
- ¼ cup coarsely chopped cilantro
- 5 cloves garlic, minced
- 4 6-ounce flat-iron (boneless beef shoulder top blade) steaks

SALSA SALAD
- 1 seedless (English) cucumber (peeled if desired), diced
- 1 cup quartered grape tomatoes
- ½ cup diced red onion
- ½ cup coarsely chopped cilantro
- 1 poblano chile, seeded and diced (see tip, page 56)
- 1 jalapeño, seeded and minced (see tip, page 56)
- 3 tablespoons fresh lime juice
- 2 tablespoons extra virgin olive oil

CARAMELIZED ONIONS
- 2 tablespoons extra virgin olive oil
- 2 large sweet onions (such as Maui, Vidalia, Texas Sweet, or Walla Walla)
- ½ teaspoon ground chipotle chile pepper

1. For steaks, place steaks in a resealable plastic bag set in a shallow dish; set aside. In a small bowl combine lime juice, oil, cilantro, and garlic; pour over steaks in bag. Seal bag; turn to coat. Marinate in the refrigerator for 2 hours.

2. For salad, in a large bowl combine cucumber, tomatoes, onion, cilantro, poblano, and jalapeño. Toss to combine. For dressing, in a small bowl whisk together lime juice and olive oil together. Drizzle dressing over vegetables; toss to coat. Cover and refrigerate until serving time.

3. For onions, preheat oven to 400°F. Brush the inside of a Dutch oven with some of the olive oil; set aside. Cut onions in half lengthwise, remove skins, and then slice crosswise ¼ inch thick. In the Dutch oven combine the remaining olive oil, the onions, and the chipotle chile pepper. Cover and bake for 20 minutes. Uncover and let cool about 20 minutes.

4. Transfer cooled onions to a foil grilling bag or wrap onions in a double thickness of foil. Puncture the top of the foil in several places with a skewer.

5. For a charcoal grill, arrange medium-hot coals around perimeter of grill. Test for medium heat above center of grill. Place packet in center of grill rack. Cover and grill about 45 minutes or until onions are soft and amber color. (For a gas grill, preheat grill. Reduce heat to medium. Adjust for indirect cooking. Place packet over the burner that is turned off. Cover and grill as directed.)

6. Remove steaks from marinade; discard marinade. For a charcoal or gas grill, place steaks on the grill rack directly over medium-high heat. Cover and grill for 8 to 10 minutes or until an instant-read thermometer inserted horizontally into the steaks reads 135°F, turning once. Transfer steaks to a platter, cover loosely with foil and let stand for 10 minutes.

7. To serve, divide salsa salad among four serving plates. Place a steak on each plate and top with a mound of caramelized onions. Serve immediately.

Make-Ahead Directions: Salsa salad may be made and refrigerated up to 4 hours before serving.

Grilled Ribeyes with Herbed Onion and Garlic "Butter,"
recipe page 110

Grilled Romaine Hearts
with Basil Green Goddess
Dressing, *recipe page 304*

GRILLED RIBEYES WITH HERBED ONION AND GARLIC "BUTTER"

pictured on page 108

PREP: 10 minutes   COOK: 12 minutes   CHILL: 30 minutes   GRILL: 11 minutes   MAKES: 4 servings

THE HEAT FROM JUST-OFF-THE-GRILL STEAKS MELTS THE MOUNDS OF CARAMELIZED ONIONS, GARLIC, AND HERBS SUSPENDED IN A RICH-TASTING BLEND OF COCONUT OIL AND OLIVE OIL.

2 tablespoons unrefined coconut oil

1 small onion, halved and cut into very thin slivers (about ¾ cup)

1 clove garlic, very thinly sliced

2 tablespoons extra virgin olive oil

1 tablespoon snipped fresh parsley

2 teaspoons snipped fresh thyme, rosemary, and/or oregano

4 8- to 10-ounce beef ribeye steaks, cut 1 inch thick

½ teaspoon freshly ground black pepper

1. In a medium skillet melt coconut oil over low heat. Add onion; cook for 10 to 15 minutes or until lightly browned, stirring occasionally. Add garlic; cook for 2 to 3 minutes more or until onion is golden brown, stirring occasionally.

2. Transfer onion mixture to a small bowl. Stir in olive oil, parsley, and thyme. Refrigerate, uncovered, for 30 minutes or until mixture is firm enough to mound when scooped, stirring occasionally.

3. Meanwhile, sprinkle steaks with pepper. For a charcoal or gas grill, place steaks on the grill rack directly over medium heat. Cover and grill for 11 to 15 minutes for medium rare (145°F) or 14 to 18 minutes for medium (160°F), turning once halfway through grilling.

4. To serve, place each steak on a serving plate. Immediately scoop onion mixture evenly onto steaks.

RIBEYE SALAD WITH GRILLED BEETS

PREP: 20 minutes   GRILL: 55 minutes   STAND: 5 minutes   MAKES: 4 servings

THE EARTHY FLAVOR OF BEETS PAIRS BEAUTIFULLY WITH THE SWEETNESS OF THE ORANGES—AND THE TOASTED PECANS ADD A BIT OF CRUNCH TO THIS MAIN-DISH SALAD THAT'S PERFECT FOR EATING OUTDOORS ON A WARM SUMMER NIGHT.

1 pound medium golden and/or red beets, scrubbed, trimmed, and cut into wedges

1 small onion, cut into thin wedges

2 sprigs fresh thyme

1 tablespoon extra virgin olive oil
   Cracked black pepper

2 8-ounce boneless beef ribeye steaks, cut ¾ inch thick

2 cloves garlic, halved

2 tablespoons Mediterranean Seasoning (see recipe, page 324)

6 cups mixed greens

2 oranges, peeled, sectioned, and coarsely chopped

½ cup chopped pecans, toasted (see tip, page 57)

½ cup Bright Citrus Vinaigrette (see recipe, page 320)

1. Place beets, onion, and thyme sprigs in a foil pan. Drizzle with oil and toss to combine; sprinkle lightly with cracked black pepper. For a charcoal or gas grill, place pan on the center of the grill rack. Cover and grill 55 to 60 minutes or until tender when pierced with a knife, stirring occasionally.

2. Meanwhile, rub both sides of the steaks with cut sides of garlic; sprinkle with Mediterranean Seasoning.

3. Move beets from center of grill to make room for steaks. Add steaks to grill directly over medium heat. Cover and grill for 11 to 15 minutes for medium rare (145°F) or 14 to 18 minutes for medium (160°F), turning once halfway through grilling. Remove foil pan and steaks from grill. Let steaks stand for 5 minutes. Discard thyme sprigs from foil pan.

4. Thinly slice steak diagonally into bite-size pieces. Divide greens among four serving plates. Top with sliced steak, beets, onion wedges, chopped oranges, and pecans. Drizzle with Bright Citrus Vinaigrette.

KOREAN-STYLE SHORT RIBS WITH SAUTÉED GINGER CABBAGE

PREP: 50 minutes   COOK: 25 minutes   BAKE: 10 hours   CHILL: overnight   MAKES: 4 servings

MAKE SURE THE LID OF YOUR DUTCH OVEN FITS VERY TIGHTLY SO THAT DURING THE VERY LONG BRAISING TIME, THE COOKING LIQUID DOESN'T ALL EVAPORATE THROUGH A GAP BETWEEN THE LID AND POT.

1 ounce dried shiitake mushrooms
1½ cups sliced scallions
1 Asian pear, peeled, cored, and chopped
1 3-inch piece fresh ginger, peeled and chopped
1 serrano chile pepper, finely chopped (seeded if desired) (see tip, page 56)
5 cloves garlic
1 tablespoon refined coconut oil
5 pounds bone-in beef short ribs
Freshly ground black pepper
4 cups Beef Bone Broth (see recipe, page 131) or no-salt-added beef broth
2 cups sliced fresh shiitake mushrooms
1 tablespoon finely shredded orange peel
⅓ cup fresh juice
Sautéed Ginger Cabbage (see recipe, right)
Finely shredded orange peel (optional)

1. Preheat oven to 325°F. Place dried shiitake mushrooms in a small bowl; add enough boiling water to cover. Let stand about 30 minutes or until rehydrated and soft. Drain, reserving the soaking liquid. Finely chop the mushrooms. Place mushrooms in a small bowl; cover and refrigerate until needed in Step 4. Set mushrooms and liquid aside.

2. For sauce, in a food processor combine scallions, Asian pear, ginger, serrano, garlic, and the reserved mushroom soaking liquid. Cover and process until smooth. Set sauce aside.

3. In a 6-quart Dutch oven heat the coconut oil over medium-high heat. Sprinkle short ribs with freshly ground black pepper. Cook ribs, in batches, in hot coconut oil about 10 minutes or until well browned on all sides, turning halfway through cooking. Return all the ribs to the pot; add sauce and Beef Bone broth. Cover the Dutch oven with a tight-fitting lid. Bake about 10 hours or until meat is very tender and falls off the bones.

4. Carefully remove the ribs from sauce. Place ribs and sauce in separate containers. Cover and refrigerate overnight. When cold, remove fat from surface of the sauce and discard. Bring the sauce to boiling over high heat; add hydrated mushrooms from Step 1 and the fresh mushrooms. Boil gently for 10 minutes to reduce sauce and intensify flavors. Return ribs to the sauce; simmer until heated through. Stir in 1 tablespoon orange peel and the orange juice. Serve with Sautéed Ginger Cabbage. If desired, sprinkle with additional orange peel.

Sautéed Ginger Cabbage: In a large skillet heat 1 tablespoon refined coconut oil over medium-high heat. Add 2 tablespoons minced fresh ginger; 2 cloves garlic, minced; and crushed red pepper to taste. Cook and stir until fragrant, about 30 seconds. Add 6 cups shredded napa, savoy, or green cabbage and 1 Asian pear, peeled, cored, and thinly sliced. Cook and stir for 3 minutes or until cabbage wilts slightly and pear softens. Stir in ½ cup unsweetened apple juice. Cover and cook about 2 minutes until cabbage is tender. Stir in ½ cup sliced scallions and 1 tablespoon sesame seeds.

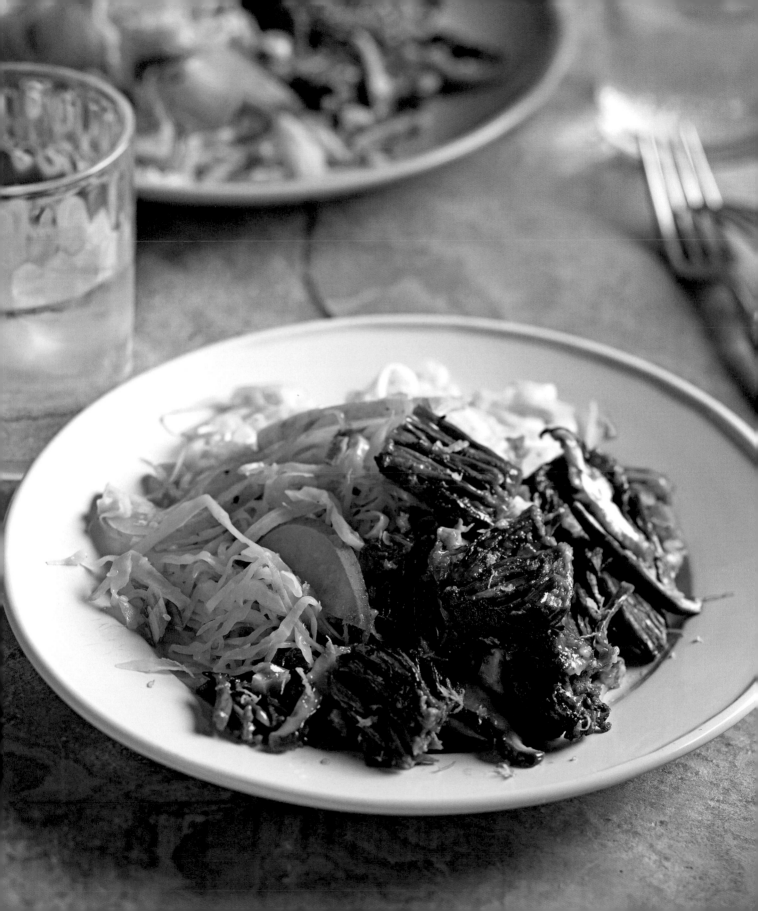

BEEF SHORT RIBS WITH CITRUS-FENNEL GREMOLATA

PREP: 40 minutes   GRILL: 8 minutes   SLOW COOK: 9 hours (low) or 4½ hours (high)   MAKES: 4 servings

GREMOLATA IS A FLAVORFUL BLEND OF PARSLEY, GARLIC, AND LEMON PEEL THAT IS SPRINKLED ON OSSO BUCCO— THE CLASSIC ITALIAN DISH OF BRAISED VEAL SHANKS—TO BRIGHTEN ITS RICH, UNCTUOUS FLAVOR. WITH THE ADDITION OF ORANGE PEEL AND FRESH FEATHERY FENNEL FRONDS, IT DOES THE SAME FOR THESE TENDER BEEF SHORT RIBS.

RIBS
2½ to 3 pounds bone-in beef short ribs

3 tablespoons Lemon-Herb Seasoning (see recipe, page 324)

1 medium fennel bulb

1 large onion, cut into large wedges

2 cups Beef Bone Broth (see recipe, page 131) or no-salt-added beef broth

2 cloves garlic, halved

PAN-ROASTED SQUASH
3 tablespoons extra virgin olive oil

1 pound butternut squash, peeled, seeded, and cut into ½-inch pieces (about 2 cups)

4 teaspoons snipped fresh thyme
Extra virgin olive oil

GREMOLATA
¼ cup snipped fresh parsley

2 tablespoons minced garlic

1½ teaspoons finely shredded lemon peel

1½ teaspoons finely shredded orange peel

1. Sprinkle short ribs with Lemon-Herb Seasoning; lightly rub into meat with your fingers; set aside. Remove fronds from fennel; set aside for Citrus-Fennel Gremolata. Trim and quarter fennel bulb.

2. For a charcoal grill, arrange medium-hot coals on one side of the grill. Test for medium heat above the side of grill without coals. Place short ribs on grill rack on side without coals; place fennel quarters and onion wedges on the rack directly over coals. Cover and grill for 8 to 10 minutes or until vegetables and ribs are just browned, turning once halfway through grilling. (For a gas grill, preheat grill, reduce heat to medium. Adjust for indirect cooking. Place ribs on grill rack over burner that is turned off; place fennel and onion on rack over burner that is turned on. Cover and grill as directed.) When cool enough to handle, coarsely chop the fennel and onion.

3. In a 5- to 6-quart slow cooker combine chopped fennel and onion, Beef Bone Broth, and garlic. Add ribs. Cover and cook on low-heat setting for 9 to 10 hours or 4½ to 5 hours on high-heat setting. Using a slotted spoon, transfer ribs to a platter; cover with foil to keep warm.

4. Meanwhile, for the squash, in a large skillet heat the 3 tablespoons oil over medium-high heat. Add squash and 3 teaspoons of the thyme, stirring to coat the squash. Arrange squash in a single layer in skillet and cook without stirring about 3 minutes or until browned on bottom sides. Turn squash pieces over; cook about 3 minutes more or until second sides are browned. Reduce heat to low; cover and cook for 10 to 15 minutes or until tender. Sprinkle with remaining 1 teaspoon fresh thyme; drizzle with additional extra virgin olive oil.

5. For the gremolata, finely chop enough reserved fennel fronds to make ¼ cup. In a small bowl stir together the chopped fennel fronds, parsley, garlic, lemon peel, and orange peel.

6. Sprinkle gremolata over ribs. Serve with squash.

SWEDISH-STYLE BEEF PATTIES WITH MUSTARD-DILL CUCUMBER SALAD

PREP: 30 minutes   COOK: 15 minutes   MAKES: 4 servings

BEEF À LA LINDSTROM IS A SWEDISH HAMBURGER THAT IS TRADITIONALLY STUDDED WITH ONIONS, CAPERS, AND PICKLED BEETS SERVED WITH GRAVY AND WITHOUT A BUN. THIS ALLSPICE-INFUSED VERSION SUBSTITUTES ROASTED BEETS FOR THE SALT-LADEN PICKLED BEETS AND CAPERS AND IS TOPPED WITH A FRIED EGG.

CUCUMBER SALAD
- 2 teaspoons fresh orange juice
- 2 teaspoons white wine vinegar
- 1 teaspoon Dijon-Style Mustard (see recipe, page 322)
- 1 tablespoon extra virgin olive oil
- 1 large seedless (English) cucumber, peeled and sliced
- 2 tablespoons sliced scallions
- 1 tablespoon chopped fresh dill

BEEF PATTIES
- 1 pound ground beef
- ¼ cup finely chopped onion
- 1 tablespoon Dijon-Style Mustard (see recipe, page 322)
- ¾ teaspoon black pepper
- ½ teaspoon ground allspice
- ½ of a small beet, roasted, peeled, and finely diced*
- 2 tablespoons extra virgin olive oil
- ½ cup Beef Bone Broth (see recipe, page 131) or no-salt-added beef broth
- 4 large eggs
- 1 tablespoon finely chopped chives

1. For cucumber salad, in a large bowl whisk together orange juice, vinegar, and Dijon-Style Mustard. Slowly add olive oil in a thin stream, whisking until dressing thickens slightly. Add cucumber, scallions, and dill; toss until combined. Cover and refrigerate until serving time.

2. For beef patties, in a large bowl combine ground beef, onion, Dijon-Style Mustard, pepper, and allspice. Add roasted beet and gently mix until evenly incorporated into the meat. Shape mixture into four ½-inch-thick patties.

3. In a large skillet heat 1 tablespoon olive oil over medium-high heat. Fry patties about 8 minutes or until browned on the exterior and cooked through (160°), turning once. Transfer patties to a plate and cover loosely with foil to keep warm. Add Beef Bone Broth, stirring to scrape up browned bits from bottom of skillet. Cook about 4 minutes or until reduced by half. Drizzle patties with reduced pan juices and re-cover loosely.

4. Rinse and wipe out skillet with a paper towel. Heat the remaining 1 tablespoon olive oil over medium heat. Fry eggs in hot oil for 3 to 4 minutes or until whites are cooked but yolks remain soft and runny.

5. Place an egg on each beef patty. Sprinkle with chives and serve with cucumber salad.

*Tip: To roast beet, scrub well and place on a piece of aluminum foil. Drizzle with a little olive oil. Wrap in foil and seal tightly. Roast in a 375°F oven about 30 minutes or until a fork easily pierces beet. Let cool; slip skin off. (Beet can be roasted up to 3 days ahead. Tightly wrap peeled roasted beets and store in the refrigerator.)

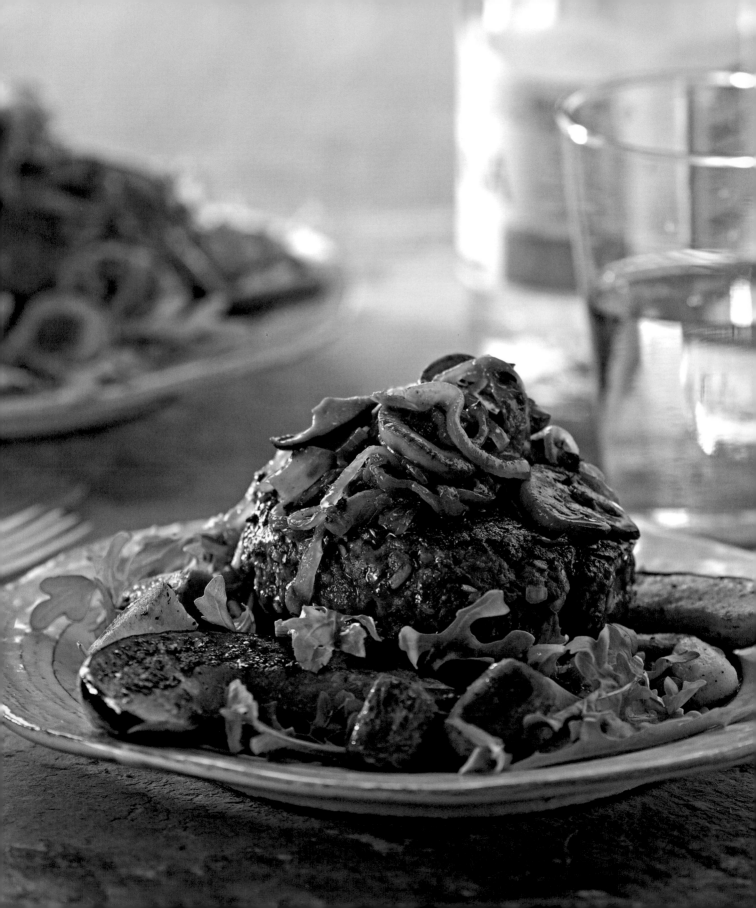

SMOTHERED BEEFBURGERS ON ARUGULA WITH ROASTED ROOT VEGETABLES

PREP: 40 minutes   COOK: 35 minutes   ROAST: 20 minutes   MAKES: 4 servings

THERE ARE A LOT OF ELEMENTS TO THESE HEARTY BURGERS—AND THEY DO TAKE A BIT OF TIME TO PUT TOGETHER—BUT THE INCREDIBLE COMBINATION OF FLAVORS MAKES IT WELL WORTH THE EFFORT: A MEATY BURGER IS TOPPED WITH CARAMELIZED ONION AND MUSHROOM PAN SAUCE AND SERVED WITH SWEET ROASTED VEGETABLES AND PEPPERY ARUGULA.

5 tablespoons extra virgin olive oil

2 cups sliced fresh button, cremini, and/or shiitake mushrooms

3 yellow onions, thinly sliced*

2 teaspoons caraway seeds

3 carrots, peeled and cut into 1-inch chunks

2 parsnips, peeled and cut into 1-inch chunks

1 acorn squash, halved, seeded, and cut into wedges
Freshly ground black pepper

2 pounds ground beef

½ cup finely chopped onion

1 tablespoon salt-free all-purpose seasoning blend

2 cups Beef Bone Broth (see recipe, page 131) or no-salt-added beef broth

¼ cup unsweetened apple juice

1 to 2 tablespoons dry sherry or white wine vinegar

1 tablespoon Dijon-Style Mustard (see recipe, page 322)

1 tablespoon snipped fresh thyme leaves

1 tablespoon snipped fresh parsley leaves

8 cups arugula leaves

1. Preheat oven to 425°F. For sauce, in a large skillet heat 1 tablespoon of the olive oil over medium-high heat. Add mushrooms; cook and stir about 8 minutes or until well browned and tender. Using a slotted spoon, transfer the mushrooms to a plate. Return the skillet to the burner; reduce heat to medium. Add the remaining 1 tablespoon olive oil, sliced onions, and the caraway seeds. Cover and cook for 20 to 25 minutes or until onions are very soft and richly browned, stirring occasionally. (Adjust heat as needed to prevent the onions from burning.)

2. Meanwhile, for roasted root vegetables, on a large baking sheet arrange carrots, parsnips, and squash. Drizzle with 2 tablespoons olive oil and sprinkle with pepper to taste; toss to coat vegetables. Roast for 20 to 25 minutes or until tender and beginning to brown, turning once halfway through roasting. Keep vegetables warm until ready to serve.

3. For burgers, in a large bowl combine the ground beef, finely chopped onion, and seasoning blend. Divide meat mixture into four equal portions and shape into patties, about ¾ inch thick. In an extra-large skillet heat the remaining 1 tablespoon olive oil over medium-high heat. Add burgers to skillet; cook about 8 minutes or until seared on both sides, turning once. Transfer burgers to a plate.

4. Add caramelized onions, reserved mushrooms, Beef Bone Broth, apple juice, sherry, and Dijon-Style Mustard to the skillet, stirring to combine. Return burgers to skillet. Bring to simmering. Cook until burgers are done (160°F), about 7 to 8 minutes. Stir in fresh thyme, parsley, and pepper to taste.

5. To serve, arrange 2 cups of arugula on each of four serving plates. Divide the roasted vegetables among the salads, then top with burgers. Generously spoon the onion mixture on the burgers.

***Tip:** A mandoline slicer is a great help in thinly slicing onions.

GRILLED BEEFBURGERS WITH SESAME-CRUSTED TOMATOES

PREP: 30 minutes   STAND: 20 minutes   GRILL: 10 minutes   MAKES: 4 servings

CRISP, GOLDEN-BROWN SESAME-CRUSTED SLICES OF TOMATO STAND IN FOR THE TRADITIONAL SESAME SEED BUN IN THESE SMOKY BURGERS. SERVE THEM WITH A KNIFE AND FORK.

4   ½-inch-thick red or green tomato slices*
1¼ pounds lean ground beef
1   tablespoon Smoky Seasoning (see recipe, page 324)
1   large egg
¾   cup almond meal
¼   cup sesame seeds
¼   teaspoon black pepper
1   small red onion, halved and sliced
1   tablespoon extra virgin olive oil
¼   cup refined coconut oil
1   small head Bibb lettuce
    Paleo Ketchup (see recipe, page 322)
    Dijon-Style Mustard (see recipe, page 322)

1. Place tomato slices on a double layer of paper towels. Top tomatoes with another double layer of paper towels. Press down lightly on paper towels so they stick to the tomatoes. Let stand at room temperature for 20 to 30 minutes so some of the tomato juice is absorbed.

2. Meanwhile, in a large bowl combine ground beef and Smoky Seasoning. Shape into four ½-inch-thick patties.

3. In a shallow bowl lightly beat egg with a fork. In another shallow bowl combine almond meal, sesame seeds, and pepper. Dip each tomato slice into the egg, turning to coat. Allow excess egg to drip off. Dip each tomato slice into almond meal mixture, turning to coat. Place coated tomatoes on a flat plate; set aside. Toss onion slices with olive oil; place onion slices in a grill basket.

4. For a charcoal or gas grill, place onions in basket and beef patties on grill rack over medium heat. Cover and grill for 10 to 12 minutes or onions are golden brown and lightly charred and patties are done (160°), stirring onions occasionally and turning patties once.

5. Meanwhile, in a large skillet heat oil over medium heat. Add tomato slices; cook for 8 to 10 minutes or until golden brown, turning once. (If tomatoes brown too quickly, reduce heat to medium-low. If necessary, add additional oil.) Drain on a paper towel-lined plate.

6. To serve, divide lettuce among four serving plates. Top with patties, onions, Paleo Ketchup, Dijon-Style Mustard, and sesame-crusted tomatoes.

*Note: You'll probably need 2 large tomatoes. If using red tomatoes, choose tomatoes that are just ripe but still slightly firm.

BURGERS ON A STICK WITH BABA GHANOUSH DIPPING SAUCE

SOAK: 15 minutes   PREP: 20 minutes   GRILL: 35 minutes   MAKES: 4 servings

BABA GHANOUSH IS A MIDDLE EASTERN SPREAD MADE FROM SMOKY GRILLED EGGPLANT PUREED WITH OLIVE OIL, LEMON, GARLIC, AND TAHINI, A PASTE MADE FROM GROUND SESAME SEEDS. A SPRINKLING OF SESAME SEEDS IS FINE, BUT WHEN THEY ARE MADE INTO OIL OR PASTE, THEY BECOME A CONCENTRATED SOURCE OF LINOLEIC ACID, WHICH CAN CONTRIBUTE TO INFLAMMATION. THE PINE NUT BUTTER USED HERE MAKES A FINE SUBSTITUTE.

4 dried tomatoes
1½ pounds lean ground beef
3 to 4 tablespoons finely chopped onion
1 tablespoon finely snipped fresh oregano and/or finely snipped fresh mint or ½ teaspoon dried oregano, crushed
¼ teaspoon cayenne pepper
Baba Ghanoush Dipping Sauce (see recipe, right)

1. Soak eight 10-inch wooden skewers in water for 30 minutes. Meanwhile, in a small bowl pour boiling water over tomatoes; let stand for 5 minutes to rehydrate. Drain tomatoes and pat dry with paper towels.

2. In large bowl combine chopped tomatoes, ground beef, onion, oregano, and cayenne pepper. Divide meat mixture into eight portions; roll each portion into a ball. Remove skewers from water; pat dry. Thread one ball onto a skewer and shape into a long oval around the skewer, starting just below the pointed tip and leaving enough room on the other end to be able to hold the stick. Repeat with remaining skewers and balls.

3. For a charcoal or gas grill, place beef skewers on a grill rack directly over medium heat. Cover and grill about 6 minutes or until done (160°F), turning once halfway through grilling. Serve with Baba Ghanoush Dipping Sauce.

Baba Ghanoush Dipping Sauce: Poke 2 medium eggplants in several places with a fork. For a charcoal or gas grill, place eggplants on a grill rack directly over medium heat. Cover and grill for 10 minutes or until charred on all sides, turning several times during grilling. Remove eggplants and carefully wrap in foil. Place wrapped eggplants back on the grill rack but not directly over the coals. Cover and grill for 25 to 35 minutes more or until collapsed and very tender. Cool. Halve eggplants and scrape out the flesh; place flesh in a food processor. Add ¼ cup Pine Nut Butter (see recipe, page 327); ¼ cup fresh lemon juice; 2 cloves garlic, minced; 1 tablespoon extra virgin olive oil; 2 to 3 tablespoons snipped fresh parsley; and ½ teaspoon ground cumin. Cover and process just until almost smooth. If sauce is too thick for dipping, stir in enough water to make desired consistency.

SMOKY STUFFED SWEET PEPPERS

PREP: 20 minutes   COOK: 8 minutes   BAKE: 30 minutes   MAKES: 4 servings

MAKE THIS FAMILY FAVORITE WITH A MIX OF COLORED SWEET PEPPERS FOR AN EYE-CATCHING DISH. THE FIRE-ROASTED TOMATOES ARE A FINE EXAMPLE OF HOW TO ADD GREAT TASTE TO FOOD IN A HEALTHY WAY. THE SIMPLE ACT OF SLIGHTLY CHARRING THE TOMATOES BEFORE THEY ARE CANNED (WITHOUT SALT) BUMPS UP THEIR FLAVOR.

4 large green, red, yellow, and/or orange sweet peppers
1 pound ground beef
1 tablespoon Smoky Seasoning (see recipe, page 324)
1 tablespoon extra virgin olive oil
1 small yellow onion, chopped
3 cloves garlic, minced
1 small head cauliflower, cored and broken into florets
1 15-ounce can no-salt-added diced fire-roasted tomatoes, drained
¼ cup finely chopped fresh parsley
½ teaspoon black pepper
⅛ teaspoon cayenne pepper
½ cup Walnut Crumb Topping (see recipe, right)

1. Preheat oven to 375°F. Cut sweet peppers in half vertically. Remove stems, seeds, and membranes; discard. Set pepper halves aside.

2. Place ground beef in a medium bowl; sprinkle with Smoky Seasoning. Use your hands to gently mix seasoning into meat.

3. In a large skillet heat olive oil over medium heat. Add meat, onion, and garlic; cook until meat is browned and onion is tender, stirring with a wooden spoon to break up meat. Remove skillet from heat.

4. In a food processor process cauliflower florets until very finely chopped. (If you don't have a food processor, grate the cauliflower on a box grater.) Measure 3 cups of the cauliflower. Add to ground beef mixture in skillet. (If there is any remaining cauliflower, save it for another use.) Stir in drained tomatoes, parsley, black pepper, and cayenne pepper.

5. Fill pepper halves with ground beef mixture, packing it lightly and mounding slightly. Arrange filled pepper halves in a baking dish. Bake for 30 to 35 minutes or until peppers are crisp-tender.* Top with Walnut Crumb Topping. If desired, return to oven for 5 minutes to crisp topping before serving.

Walnut Crumb Topping: In a medium skillet heat 1 tablespoon extra virgin olive oil over medium low heat. Stir in 1 teaspoon dried thyme, 1 teaspoon smoked paprika, and ¼ teaspoon garlic powder. Add 1 cup very finely chopped walnuts. Cook and stir about 5 minutes or until walnuts are golden brown and lightly toasted. Stir in a dash or two of cayenne pepper. Let cool completely. Store leftover topping in a tightly sealed container in the refrigerator until ready to use. Makes 1 cup.

***Note:** If using green peppers, bake for an additional 10 minutes.

BISON BURGERS WITH CABERNET ONIONS AND ARUGULA

PREP: 30 minutes   COOK: 18 minutes   GRILL: 10 minutes   MAKES: 4 servings

BISON HAS A VERY LOW FAT CONTENT AND WILL COOK 30% TO 50% FASTER THAN BEEF. THE MEAT RETAINS ITS RED COLOR AFTER COOKING, SO COLOR IS NOT AN INDICATOR OF DONENESS. BECAUSE BISON IS SO LEAN, DO NOT COOK IT BEYOND AN INTERNAL TEMPERATURE OF 155°F.

2 tablespoons extra virgin olive oil

2 large sweet onions, thinly sliced

¾ cup Cabernet Sauvignon or other dry red wine

1 teaspoon Mediterranean Seasoning (see recipe, page 324)

¼ cup extra virgin olive oil

¼ cup balsamic vinegar

1 tablespoon finely chopped shallot

1 tablespoon snipped fresh basil

1 small clove garlic, minced

1 pound ground bison

¼ cup Basil Pesto (see recipe, page 320)

5 cups arugula

Raw unsalted pistachios, toasted (see tip, page 57)

1. In a large skillet heat the 2 tablespoons oil over medium-low heat. Add onions. Cook, covered, for 10 to 15 minutes or until onions are tender, stirring occasionally. Uncover; cook and stir over medium-high heat for 3 to 5 minutes or until onions are golden. Add wine; cook about 5 minutes or until most of the wine evaporates. Sprinkle with Mediterranean Seasoning; keep warm.

2. Meanwhile, for vinaigrette, in a screw-top jar combine the ¼ cup olive oil, vinegar, shallot, basil, and garlic. Cover and shake well.

3. In a large bowl lightly mix ground bison and Basil Pesto. Lightly shape meat mixture into four ¾-inch-thick patties.

4. For a charcoal or gas grill, place patties on a lightly greased grill rack directly over medium heat. Cover and grill about 10 minutes to desired doneness (145°F for medium rare or 155°F for medium), turning once halfway through grilling.

5. Place arugula in a large bowl. Drizzle vinaigrette over arugula; toss to coat. To serve, divide onions among four serving plates; top each with a bison burger. Top burgers with arugula and sprinkle with pistachios.

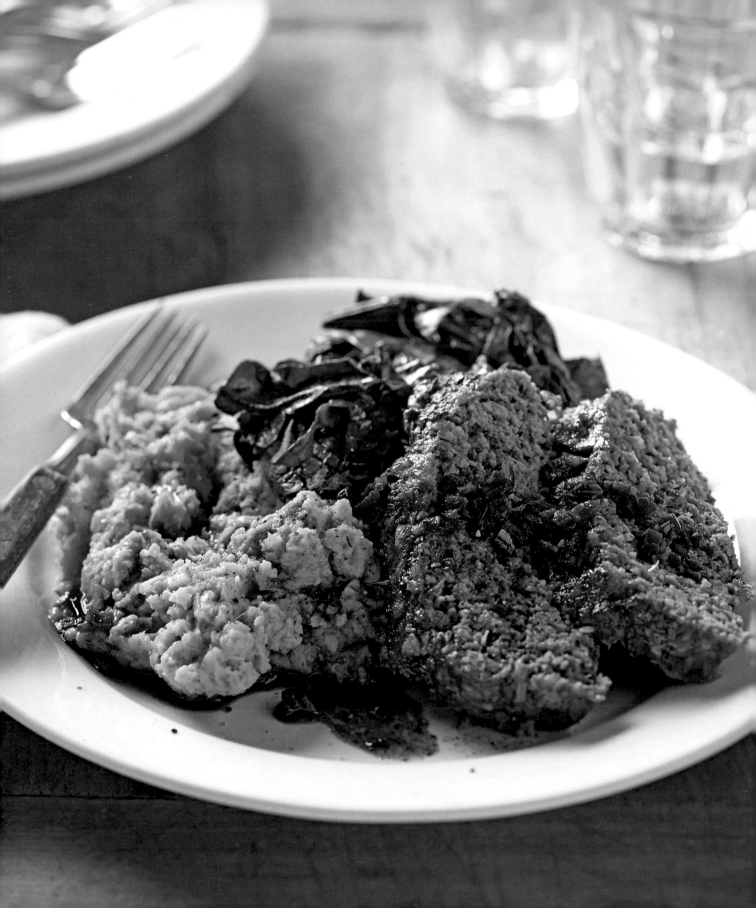

BISON AND LAMB MEAT LOAF ON CHARD AND SWEET POTATOES

PREP: 1 hour   COOK: 20 minutes   BAKE: 1 hour   STAND: 10 minutes   MAKES: 4 servings

THIS IS OLD-FASHIONED COMFORT FOOD WITH A MODERN TWIST. A RED-WINE PAN SAUCE GIVES THE MEAT LOAF A FLAVOR BOOST, AND THE GARLICKY CHARD AND SWEET POTATOES MASHED WITH CASHEW CREAM AND COCONUT OIL OFFER INCREDIBLE NUTRITIONAL CONTENT.

2 tablespoons olive oil
1 cup finely chopped cremini mushrooms
½ cup finely chopped red onion (1 medium)
½ cup finely chopped celery (1 stalk)
⅓ cup finely chopped carrot (1 small)
½ of a small apple, cored, peeled, and shredded
2 cloves garlic, minced
½ teaspoon Mediterranean Seasoning (see recipe, page 324)
1 large egg, lightly beaten
1 tablespoon snipped fresh sage
1 tablespoon snipped fresh thyme
8 ounces ground bison
8 ounces ground lamb or beef
¾ cup dry red wine
1 medium shallot, finely chopped
¾ cup Beef Bone Broth (see recipe, page 131) or no-salt-added beef broth
  Mashed Sweet Potatoes (see recipe, right)
  Garlicky Swiss Chard (see recipe, right)

1. Preheat oven to 350°F. In a large skillet heat oil over medium heat. Add mushrooms, onion, celery, and carrot; cook and stir about 5 minutes or until vegetables are softened. Reduce heat to low; add shredded apple and garlic. Cook, covered, about 5 minutes or until vegetables are very tender. Remove from heat; stir in Mediterranean Seasoning.

2. Using a slotted spoon, transfer mushroom mixture to a large bowl, reserving drippings in skillet. Stir in egg, sage, and thyme. Add ground bison and ground lamb; lightly mix. Spoon meat mixture into a 2-quart rectangular baking dish; shape into a 7×4-inch rectangle. Bake about 1 hour or until an instant-read thermometer registers 155°F. Let stand for 10 minutes. Carefully remove meat loaf to a serving platter. Cover and keep warm.

3. For the pan sauce, scrape drippings and crusty browned bits from the baking dish into reserved drippings in the skillet. Add wine and shallot. Bring to boiling over medium heat; cook until reduced by half. Add Beef Bone Broth; cook and stir until reduced by half. Remove skillet from heat.

4. To serve, divide Mashed Sweet Potatoes among four serving plates; top with some of the Garlicky Swiss Chard. Slice meat loaf; place slices on Garlicky Swiss Chard and drizzle with the pan sauce.

Mashed Sweet Potatoes: Peel and coarsely chop 4 medium sweet potatoes. In a large saucepan cook potatoes in enough boiling water to cover for 15 minutes or until tender; drain. Mash with a potato masher. Add ½ cup Cashew Cream (see recipe, page 327) and 2 tablespoons unrefined coconut oil; mash until smooth. Keep warm.

Garlicky Swiss Chard: Remove stems from 2 bunches Swiss chard and discard. Coarsely chop leaves. In a large skillet heat 2 tablespoons olive oil over medium heat. Add Swiss chard and 2 cloves garlic, minced; cook until chard is wilted, tossing occasionally with tongs.

APPLE-CURRANT-SAUCED BISON MEATBALLS WITH ZUCCHINI PAPPARDELLE

PREP: 25 minutes   BAKE: 15 minutes   COOK: 18 minutes   MAKES: 4 servings

THE MEATBALLS WILL BE VERY WET AS YOU FORM THEM. TO KEEP THE MEAT MIXTURE FROM STICKING TO YOUR HANDS, KEEP A BOWL OF COOL WATER HANDY AND WET YOUR HANDS OCCASIONALLY AS YOU WORK. CHANGE THE WATER A COUPLE OF TIMES AS YOU MAKE THE MEATBALLS.

MEATBALLS
Olive oil
½ cup coarsely chopped red onion
2 cloves garlic, minced
1 egg, lightly beaten
½ cup finely chopped button mushrooms and stems
2 tablespoon snipped fresh Italian (flat-leaf) parsley
2 teaspoons olive oil
1 pound ground bison (coarse ground if available)

APPLE-CURRANT SAUCE
2 tablespoons olive oil
2 large Granny Smith apples, peeled, cored, and finely chopped
2 shallots, minced
2 tablespoons fresh lemon juice
½ cup Chicken Bone Broth (see page 235) or no-salt-added chicken broth
2 to 3 tablespoons dried currants

ZUCCHINI PAPPARDELLE
6 zucchini
2 tablespoons olive oil
¼ cup finely chopped scallions
½ teaspoon crushed red pepper
2 cloves garlic, minced

1. For meatballs, preheat oven to 375°F. Lightly brush a rimmed baking sheet with olive oil; set aside. In a food processor or blender combine onion and garlic. Pulse until smooth. Transfer onion mixture to a medium bowl. Add egg, mushrooms, parsley, and 2 teaspoons oil; stir to combine. Add ground bison; mix lightly but well. Divide meat mixture into 16 portions; shape into meatballs. Place meatballs, evenly spaced, on the prepared baking sheet. Bake for 15 minutes; set aside.

2. For sauce, in a skillet heat 2 tablespoons oil over medium heat. Add apples and shallots; cook and stir for 6 to 8 minutes or until very tender. Stir in lemon juice. Transfer mixture to a food processor or blender. Cover and process or blend until smooth; return to the skillet. Stir in Chicken Bone Broth and currants. Bring to boiling; reduce heat. Simmer, uncovered, for 8 to 10 minutes, stirring frequently. Add meatballs; cook and stir over low heat until heated through.

3. Meanwhile, for pappardelle, trim ends of zucchini. Using a mandoline or very sharp vegetable peeler, shave zucchini into thin ribbons. (To keep the ribbons intact, stop shaving once you reach the seeds in the center of the squash.) In a extra-large skillet heat 2 tablespoons oil over medium heat. Stir in scallions, crushed red pepper, and garlic; cook and stir for 30 seconds. Add zucchini ribbons. Cook and gently stir about 3 minutes or just until wilted.

4. To serve, divide pappardelle among four serving plates; top with meatballs and apple-currant sauce.

BISON-PORCINI BOLOGNESE WITH ROASTED GARLIC SPAGHETTI SQUASH

PREP: 30 minutes   COOK: 1 hour 30 minutes   BAKE: 35 minutes   MAKES: 6 servings

IF YOU THOUGHT YOU'D EATEN YOUR LAST DISH OF SPAGHETTI WITH MEAT SAUCE WHEN YOU ADOPTED THE PALEO DIET®, THINK AGAIN. THIS RICH BOLOGNESE FLAVORED WITH GARLIC, RED WINE, AND EARTHY PORCINI MUSHROOMS IS LADELED OVER SWEET, TOOTHSOME STRANDS OF SPAGHETTI SQUASH. YOU WON'T MISS THE PASTA ONE BIT.

1 ounce dried porcini mushrooms
1 cup boiling water
3 tablespoons extra virgin olive oil
1 pound ground bison
1 cup finely chopped carrots (2)
½ cup chopped onion (1 medium)
½ cup finely chopped celery (1 stalk)
4 cloves garlic, minced
3 tablespoons salt-free tomato paste
½ cup red wine
2 15-ounce cans no-salt-added crushed tomatoes
1 teaspoon dried oregano, crushed
1 teaspoon dried thyme, crushed
½ teaspoon black pepper
1 medium spaghetti squash (2½ to 3 pounds)
1 bulb garlic

1. In a small bowl combine the porcini mushrooms and boiling water; let stand for 15 minutes. Strain through a sieve lined with 100%-cotton cheesecloth, reserving the soaking liquid. Chop the mushrooms; set side.

2. In a 4- to 5-quart Dutch oven heat 1 tablespoon of the olive oil over medium heat. Add ground bison, carrots, onion, celery, and garlic. Cook until meat is browned and vegetables are tender, stirring with a wooden spoon to break up meat. Add tomato paste; cook and stir for 1 minute. Add red wine; cook and stir for 1 minute. Stir in porcini mushrooms, tomatoes, oregano, thyme, and pepper. Add reserved mushroom liquid, being careful to avoid adding any sand or grit that may be present in the bottom of the bowl. Bring to boiling, stirring occasionally; reduce heat to low. Simmer, covered, for 1½ to 2 hours or until desired consistency.

3. Meanwhile, preheat oven to 375°F. Halve squash lengthwise; scrape out seeds. Place squash halves, cut sides down, in a large baking dish. Using a fork, prick the skin all over. Cut off the top ½ inch of the head of garlic. Place the garlic, cut end up, in the baking dish with the squash. Drizzle with the remaining 1 tablespoon olive oil. Bake for 35 to 45 minutes or until squash and garlic are tender.

4. Using a spoon and fork, remove and shred the squash flesh from each squash half; transfer to a bowl and cover to keep warm. When the garlic is cool enough to handle, squeeze the bulb from the bottom to pop out the cloves. Use a fork to mash the garlic cloves. Stir mashed garlic into the squash, distributing garlic evenly. To serve, spoon sauce over squash mixture.

BISON CHILI CON CARNE

PREP: 25 minutes   COOK: 1 hour 10 minutes   MAKES: 4 servings

UNSWEETENED CHOCOLATE, COFFEE, AND CINNAMON ADD INTEREST TO THIS HEARTY FAVORITE. IF YOU'D LIKE EVEN MORE SMOKY FLAVOR, SUBSTITUTE 1 TABLESPOON OF SWEET SMOKED PAPRIKA FOR THE REGULAR PAPRIKA.

3 tablespoons extra virgin olive oil
1 pound ground bison
½ cup chopped onion (1 medium)
2 cloves garlic, minced
2 14.5-ounce cans diced no-salt-added tomatoes, undrained
1 6-ounce can salt-free tomato paste
1 cup Beef Bone Broth (page 131) or no-salt-added beef broth
½ cup strong coffee
2 ounces 99% cacao baking bar, chopped
1 tablespoon paprika
1 teaspoon ground cumin
1 teaspoon dried oregano
1½ teaspoons Smoky Seasoning (see recipe, page 324)
½ teaspoon ground cinnamon
⅓ cup pepitas
1 teaspoon olive oil
½ cup Cashew Cream (see recipe, page 327)
1 teaspoon fresh lime juice
½ cup fresh cilantro leaves
4 lime wedges

1. In a Dutch oven heat the 3 tablespoons olive oil over medium heat. Add ground bison, onion, and garlic; cook about 5 minutes or until meat is browned, stirring with a wooden spoon to break up meat. Stir in undrained tomatoes, tomato paste, Beef Bone Broth, coffee, baking chocolate, paprika, cumin, oregano, 1 teaspoon of the Smoky Seasoning, and cinnamon. Bring to boiling; reduce heat. Simmer, covered, for 1 hour, stirring occasionally.

2. Meanwhile, in a small skillet toast pepitas in the 1 teaspoon olive oil over medium heat until they start to pop and turn golden. Place pepitas in a small bowl; add the remaining ½ teaspoon Smoky Seasoning; toss to coat.

3. In a small bowl combine Cashew Cream and lime juice.

4. To serve, ladle chili into bowls. Top servings with Cashew Cream, pepitas, and cilantro. Serve with lime wedges.

MOROCCAN-SPICED BISON STEAKS WITH GRILLED LEMONS

SERVE THESE QUICK-TO-FIX STEAKS WITH COOL AND CRISP SPICED CARROT SLAW (PAGE 315). IF YOU'RE CRAVING A TREAT, GRILLED PINEAPPLE WITH COCONUT CREAM (PAGE 340) WOULD BE A GREAT WAY TO END THE MEAL.

2 tablespoons ground cinnamon
2 tablespoons paprika
1 tablespoon garlic powder
¼ teaspoon cayenne pepper
4 6-ounce bison filet mignon
    steaks, cut ¾ to 1 inch thick
2 lemons, halved horizontally

1. In a small bowl stir together the cinnamon, paprika, garlic powder, and cayenne pepper. Pat steaks dry with paper towels. Rub both sides of steaks with the spice mixture.

2. For a charcoal or gas grill, place steaks on the grill rack directly over medium heat. Cover and grill for 10 to 12 minutes for medium rare (145°F) or 12 to 15 minutes for medium (155°F), turning once halfway through grilling. Meanwhile, place lemon halves, cut sides down, on grill rack. Grill for 2 to 3 minutes or until slightly charred and juicy.

3. Serve with grilled lemon halves to squeeze over steaks.

HERBES DE PROVENCE-RUBBED BISON SIRLOIN ROAST

PREP: 15 minutes   COOK: 15 minutes   ROAST: 1 hour 15 minutes   STAND: 15 minutes   MAKES: 4 servings

HERBES DE PROVENCE IS A BLEND OF DRIED HERBS THAT GROW IN PROFUSION IN THE SOUTH OF FRANCE. THE MIX USUALLY CONTAINS SOME COMBINATION OF BASIL, FENNEL SEEDS, LAVENDER, MARJORAM, ROSEMARY, SAGE, SUMMER SAVORY, AND THYME. IT FLAVORS THIS VERY AMERICAN ROAST BEAUTIFULLY.

1 3-pound bison sirloin roast
3 tablespoons herbes de Provence
4 tablespoons extra virgin olive oil
3 cloves garlic, minced
4 small parsnips, peeled and chopped
2 ripe pears, cored and chopped
½ cup unsweetened pear nectar
1 to 2 teaspoons fresh thyme

1. Preheat oven to 375°F. Trim fat from roast. In a small bowl combine Herbes de Provence, 2 tablespoons of the olive oil, and garlic; rub over the entire roast.

2. Place the roast on a rack in a shallow roasting pan. Insert an oven-going thermometer into the center of the roast.* Roast, uncovered, for 15 minutes. Reduce oven temperature to 300°F. Roast for 60 to 65 minutes more or until meat thermometer registers 140°F (medium rare). Cover with foil and let stand for 15 minutes.

3. Meanwhile, in a large skillet heat the remaining 2 tablespoons olive oil over medium heat. Add parsnips and pears; cook for 10 minutes or until parsnips are crisp-tender, stirring occasionally. Add pear nectar; cook about 5 minutes or until sauce is slightly thickened. Sprinkle with thyme.

4. Thinly slice roast across the grain. Serve meat with parsnips and pears.

***Tip:** Bison is very lean and cooks faster than beef. Additionally, the color of the meat is redder than beef, so you can't rely on a visual cue to determine doneness. You will need a meat thermometer to let you know when the meat is done. An oven-going thermometer is ideal, though not a necessity.

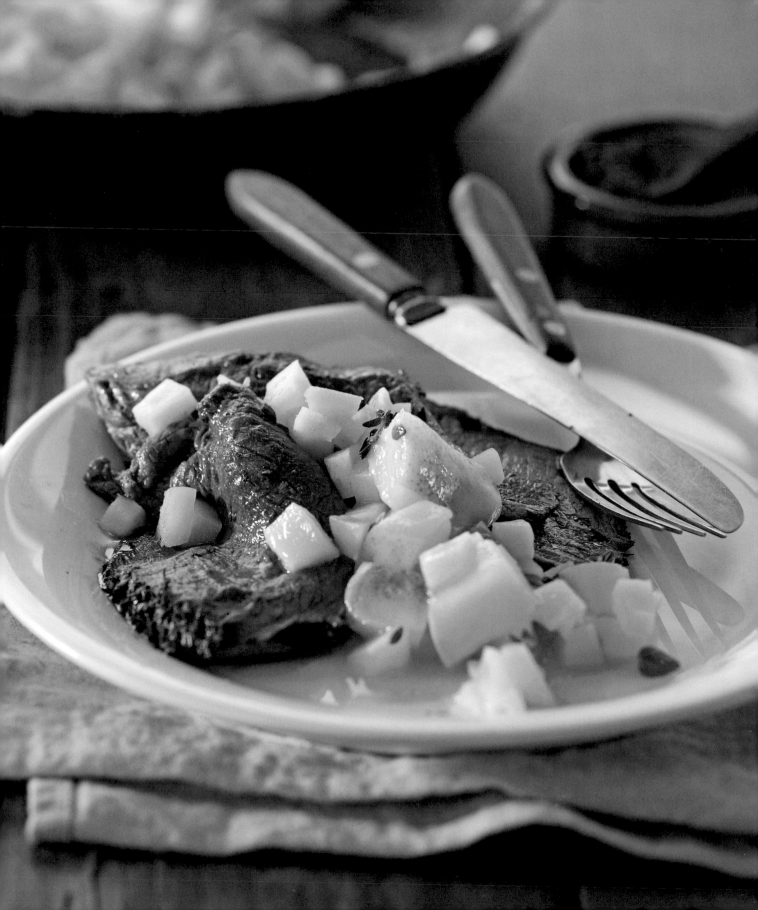

COFFEE-BRAISED BISON SHORT RIBS WITH TANGERINE GREMOLATA AND CELERY ROOT MASH

PREP: 15 minutes   COOK: 2 hours 45 minutes   MAKES: 6 servings

BISON SHORT RIBS ARE BIG AND MEATY. THEY REQUIRE A GOOD LONG COOK IN LIQUID TO GET TENDER. GREMOLATA MADE WITH TANGERINE PEEL BRIGHTENS UP THE FLAVOR OF THIS HEARTY DISH.

MARINADE

- 2 cups water
- 3 cups strong coffee, chilled
- 2 cups fresh tangerine juice
- 2 tablespoons snipped fresh rosemary
- 1 teaspoon coarsely ground black pepper
- 4 pounds bison short ribs, cut between ribs to separate

BRAISE

- 2 tablespoons olive oil
- 1 teaspoon black pepper
- 2 cups chopped onions
- ½ cup chopped shallots
- 6 garlic cloves, chopped
- 1 jalapeño chile, seeded and chopped (see tip, page 56)
- 1 cup strong coffee
- 1 cup Beef Bone Broth (see recipe, page 131) or no-salt-added beef broth
- ¼ cup Paleo Ketchup (see recipe, page 322)
- 2 tablespoons Dijon-Style Mustard (see recipe, page 322)
- 3 tablespoons cider vinegar

  Celery Root Mash (see recipe, right)
  Tangerine Gremolata (see recipe, right)

1. For the marinade, in a large nonreactive container (glass or stainless steel) combine water, chilled coffee, tangerine juice, rosemary, and black pepper. Add ribs. Place a plate on top of ribs if necessary to keep them submerged. Cover and chill 4 to 6 hours, rearranging and stirring once.

2. For the braise, preheat oven to 325°F. Drain ribs, discarding marinade. Pat ribs dry with paper towels. In a large Dutch oven heat olive oil over medium-high heat. Season ribs with black pepper. Brown ribs in batches until browned on all sides, about 5 minutes per batch. Transfer to a large plate.

3. Add onions, shallots, garlic, and jalapeño to pot. Reduce heat to medium, cover, and cook until vegetables are soft, stirring occasionally, about 10 minutes. Add coffee and broth; stir, scraping up browned bits. Add Paleo Ketchup, Dijon-Style Mustard, and vinegar. Bring to boiling. Add ribs. Cover and transfer to oven. Cook until meat is tender, about 2 hours 15 minutes, stirring gently and rearranging ribs once or twice.

4. Transfer ribs to a plate; tent with foil to keep warm. Spoon fat from surface of sauce. Boil sauce until reduced to 2 cups, about 5 minutes. Divide Celery Root Mash among 6 plates; top with ribs and sauce. Sprinkle with Tangerine Gremolata.

Celery Root Mash: In a large saucepan combine 3 pounds celery root, peeled and cut into 1-inch pieces and 4 cups Chicken Bone Broth (see recipe, page 235) or unsalted chicken broth. Bring to boiling; reduce heat. Drain celery root, reserving broth. Return celery root to saucepan. Add 1 tablespoon olive oil and 2 teaspoons snipped fresh thyme. Using a potato masher, mash the celery root, adding reserved broth, a few tablespoons at a time, as needed to achieve desired consistency.

Tangerine Gremolata: In a small bowl combine ½ cup snipped fresh parsley, 2 tablespoons finely shredded tangerine peel, and 2 cloves minced garlic.

BEEF BONE BROTH

PREP: 25 minutes   ROAST: 1 hour   COOK: 8 hours   MAKES: 8 to 10 cups

BONY OXTAILS MAKE AN EXTREMELY RICH-TASTING BROTH THAT CAN BE USED IN ANY RECIPE THAT CALLS FOR BEEF BROTH—OR SIMPLY ENJOYED AS A PICK-ME-UP IN A MUG ANY TIME OF DAY. THOUGH THEY ACTUALLY USED TO COME FROM AN OX, OXTAILS NOW COME FROM A BEEF ANIMAL.

5 carrots, roughly chopped
5 stalks celery, roughly chopped
2 yellow onions, unpeeled, halved
8 ounces white mushrooms
1 bulb garlic, unpeeled, halved
2 pounds oxtail bones or beef
   bones
2 tomatoes
12 cups cold water
3 bay leaves

1. Preheat oven to 400°F. In a large rimmed baking sheet or shallow baking pan arrange the carrots, celery, onions, mushrooms, and garlic; place the bones on top of the vegetables. In a food processor pulse tomatoes until smooth. Spread tomatoes over the bones to coat (it's okay if some of the puree drips onto the pan and the vegetables). Roast for 1 to 1½ hours or until bones are deep brown and the vegetables are caramelized. Transfer bones and vegetables to a 10- to 12-quart Dutch oven or stockpot. (If some of the tomato mixture caramelizes on the bottom of the pan, add 1 cup of hot water to the pan and scrape up any bits. Pour the liquid over the bones and vegetables and reduce water amount by 1 cup.) Add the cold water and bay leaves.

2. Slowly bring the mixture to a simmer over medium-high to high heat. Reduce heat; cover and simmer broth for 8 to 10 hours, stirring occasionally.

3. Strain broth; discard bones and vegetables. Cool broth; transfer broth to storage containers and refrigerate for up to 5 days; freeze for up to 3 months.*

Slow Cooker Directions: For a 6- to 8-quart slow cooker, use 1 pound beef bones, 3 carrots, 3 stalks celery, 1 yellow onion, and 1 bulb garlic. Puree 1 tomato and rub onto the bones. Roast as directed, then transfer the bones and vegetables to the slow cooker. Scrape off any caramelized tomato as directed and add to the slow cooker. Add enough water to cover. Cover and cook on high-heat setting until broth comes to boiling, about 4 hours. Reduce to low-heat setting; cook for 12 to 24 hours. Strain broth; discard bones and vegetables. Store as directed.

***Tip:** To easily skim fat off broth, store broth in a covered container in the refrigerator overnight. Fat will rise to the top and form a firm layer that can easily be scraped off. Broth may thicken after chilling.

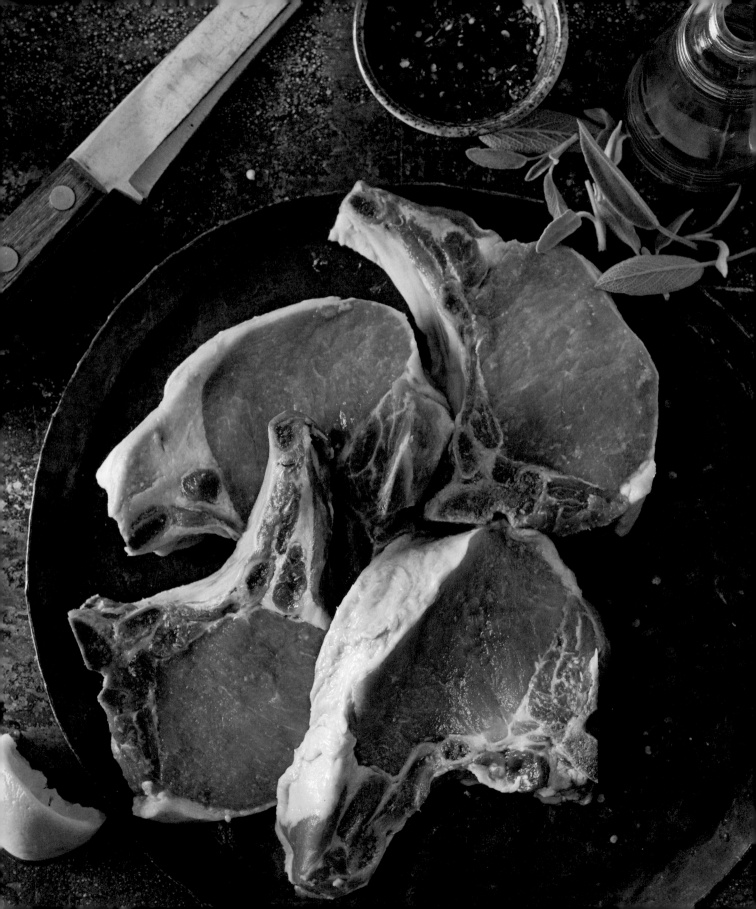

PORK & LAMB

Many people new to The Paleo Diet® have avoided eating pork and/or lamb for years—or even decades—because they assumed that these meats were decadently fatty and would make them fat and cause heart disease and other health problems. Nothing could be further from the truth. Let's clear up these myths first and then move on to the incredibly delicious recipes for lamb and pork in this chapter.

As is the case with beef and bison, fresh pork and lamb are highly nutritious, "real" living foods that should become a regular part of your daily menu. There is little credible human data that lends support to the notion that eating fats makes us fat. Rather, only when fat is combined with refined carbohydrates in processed foods (pizza, potato chips, doughnuts, ice cream, cookies, french fries, bread, etc.) does it end up promoting excess weight problems and obesity. When your carbohydrates come almost exclusively from fresh fruits and veggies, they reduce the overall glycemic index of your diet. This effect, along with The Paleo Diet's® high protein content, normalizes blood sugar and insulin levels while it simultaneously reduces hunger. Accordingly, the most recent human randomized controlled trials of The Paleo Diet® show that it is one of the most effective nutritional plans to get weight off and keep it off while simultaneously reducing your risk of heart disease.

As more and more people from diverse walks of life are attracted to this lifetime program of eating, it is not surprising that the original Paleo Diet message has become diluted and somewhat splintered. For instance, as I mentioned in "Paleo Principles," some "Paleo" dieters believe that milk and dairy products are OK. Others think legumes shouldn't be excluded, and a certain segment of the "Paleosphere" believes that salt is not a problem, particularly if it is replaced with sea salt.

Bacon appears to have widespread acceptance in the Paleo community, judging from its popularity in a number of Paleo blogs and recipe books. There is no doubt that bacon is a savory, modern food that few people can resist, but is it Paleo? Absolutely not! Bacon is cured pork, whose high salt content should immediately disqualify it as a component of contemporary Paleo diets. A single, medium slice of bacon contains 192 mg of sodium; a thick slice totals 277 mg. But who eats a single slice of bacon? How about four slices? The sodium total for four slices of medium-to-thick bacon ranges from 768 mg to 1,108 mg. The USDA recommends that we limit our sodium intake to 2,300 mg/day, whereas calculations I have published in the scientific literature show that contemporary Paleo diets only total 726 mg/sodium per day. You can do the math comparisons yourself. It becomes obvious that bacon added to The Paleo Diet® blows healthful sodium intakes right out the window.

Rest assured that each and every recipe in *The Real Paleo Diet® Cookbook* is a low-sodium recipe. Moreover, following the guidelines in this book will help you to overcome lifelong addictions most people have to this toxic substance. After a few weeks of getting salt out of your diet, foods that you may have formerly shunned will become new favorites, with their recently discovered subtle flavors and aromas. The foods and recipes in *The Real Paleo Diet® Cookbook* will awaken your taste buds to an entirely new world. Enjoy!

TUNISIAN SPICE-RUBBED PORK SHOULDER WITH SPICY SWEET POTATO FRIES

PREP: 25 minutes   ROAST: 4 hours   BAKE: 30 minutes   MAKES: 4 servings

THIS IS A GREAT DISH TO MAKE ON A COOL FALL DAY. THE MEAT ROASTS FOR HOURS IN THE OVEN, MAKING YOUR HOUSE SMELL WONDERFUL AND GIVING YOU TIME TO DO OTHER THINGS. OVEN-BAKED SWEET POTATO FRIES DON'T GET CRISP IN THE SAME WAY THAT WHITE POTATOES DO, BUT THEY ARE DELICIOUS IN THEIR OWN WAY, ESPECIALLY WHEN DIPPED IN GARLICKY MAYONNAISE.

PORK

- 1   2½- to 3-pound bone-in pork shoulder roast
- 2   teaspoons ground ancho chile pepper
- 2   teaspoons ground cumin
- 1   teaspoon caraway seeds, lightly crushed
- 1   teaspoon ground coriander
- ½   teaspoon ground turmeric
- ¼   teaspoon ground cinnamon
- 3   tablespoons olive oil

FRIES

- 4   medium sweet potatoes (about 2 pounds), peeled and cut into ½-inch-thick wedges
- ½   teaspoon crushed red pepper
- ½   teaspoon onion powder
- ½   teaspoon garlic powder
    Olive oil

- 1   onion, thinly sliced
    Paleo Aïoli (Garlic Mayo) (see recipe, page 323)

1. Preheat oven to 300°F. Trim fat from meat. In a small bowl combine ground ancho chile pepper, ground cumin, caraway seeds, coriander, turmeric, and cinnamon. Sprinkle meat with spice mixture; using your fingers, rub evenly into meat.

2. In an ovenproof 5- to 6-quart Dutch oven heat 1 tablespoon of the olive oil over medium-high heat. Brown pork on all sides in hot oil. Cover and roast about 4 hours or until very tender and meat thermometer registers 190°F. Remove Dutch oven from oven. Let stand, covered, while you prepare the sweet potato fries and the onions, reserving 1 tablespoon of the fat in the Dutch oven.

3. Increase oven temperature to 400°F. For the sweet potato fries, in a large bowl combine sweet potatoes, the remaining 2 tablespoons olive oil, crushed red pepper, onion powder, and garlic powder; toss to coat. Line one large or two small baking sheets with foil; brush with additional olive oil. Arrange sweet potatoes in a single layer on the prepared baking sheet(s). Bake about 30 minutes or until tender, turning the sweet potatoes once halfway through baking.

4. Meanwhile, remove meat from Dutch oven; cover with foil to keep warm. Drain drippings, reserving 1 tablespoon fat. Return the reserved fat to Dutch oven. Add onion; cook over medium heat about 5 minutes or until just softened, stirring occasionally.

5. Transfer the pork and onion to a serving platter. Using two forks, pull the pork into large shreds. Serve pork and fries with Paleo Aïoli.

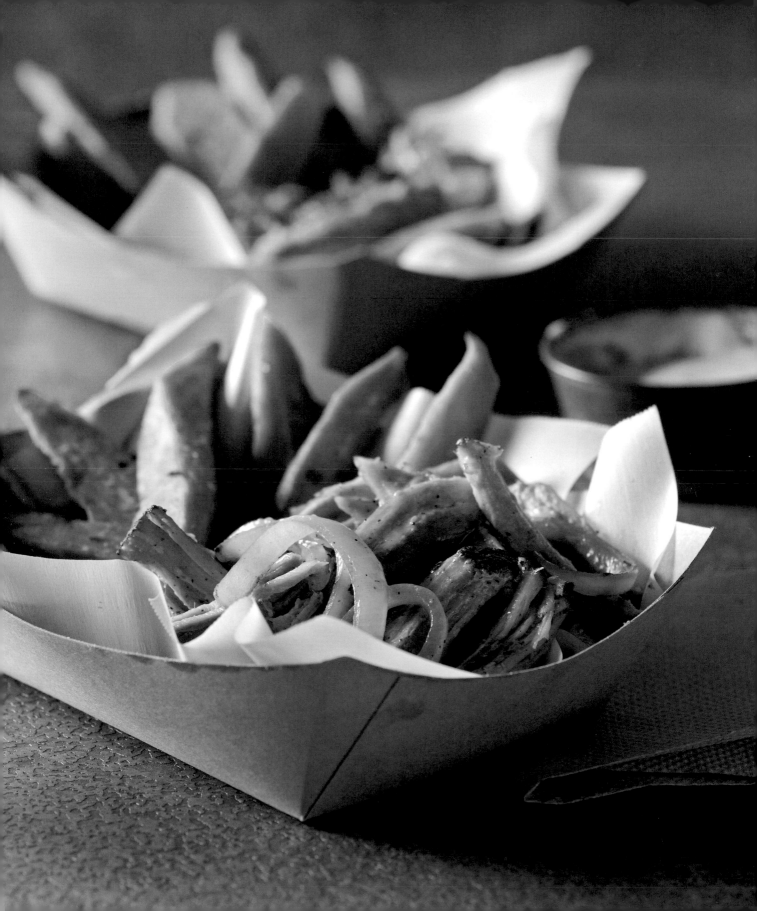

CUBAN GRILLED PORK SHOULDER

PREP: 15 minutes   MARINATE: 24 hours   GRILL: 2 hours 30 minutes   STAND: 10 minutes
MAKES 6 to 8 servings

KNOWN AS "LECHON ASADO" IN ITS COUNTRY OF ORIGIN, THIS PORK ROAST IS MARINATED IN A COMBINATION OF FRESH CITRUS JUICES, SPICES, CRUSHED RED PEPPER, AND AN ENTIRE BULB OF MINCED GARLIC. COOKING IT OVER HOT COALS AFTER AN OVERNIGHT SOAK IN THE MARINADE INFUSES IT WITH AMAZING FLAVOR.

 1 bulb garlic, cloves separated, peeled, and minced
 1 cup coarsely chopped onions
 1 cup olive oil
1⅓ cups fresh lime juice
 ⅔ cup fresh orange juice
 1 tablespoon ground cumin
 1 tablespoon dried oregano, crushed
 2 teaspoons freshly ground black pepper
 1 teaspoon crushed red pepper
 1 4- to 5-pound boneless pork shoulder roast

1. For marinade, separate garlic head into cloves. Peel and mince cloves; place in a large bowl. Add onions, olive oil, lime juice, orange juice, cumin, oregano, black pepper, and crushed red pepper. Stir well and set aside.

2. Using a boning knife, deeply puncture pork roast all over. Carefully lower roast into the marinade, submerging it as much as possible in the liquid. Cover bowl tightly with plastic wrap. Marinate in the refrigerator for 24 hours, turning once.

3. Remove pork from marinade. Pour marinade into a medium saucepan. Bring to boiling; boil for 5 minutes. Remove from heat and let cool. Set aside.

4. For a charcoal grill, arrange medium-hot coals around a drip pan. Test for medium heat above the pan. Place meat on grill rack over drip pan. Cover and grill for 2½ to 3 hours or until an instant-read thermometer inserted into center of roast registers 140°F. (For a gas grill, preheat grill. Reduce heat to medium. Adjust for indirect cooking. Place meat on grill rack over burner that is turned off. Cover and grill as directed.) Remove meat from grill. Cover loosely with foil and let stand for 10 minutes before carving or pulling.

ITALIAN SPICE-RUBBED PORK ROAST WITH VEGETABLES

PREP: 20 minutes   ROAST: 2 hours 25 minutes   STAND: 10 minutes   MAKES: 8 servings

"FRESH IS BEST" IS A GOOD MANTRA TO FOLLOW WHEN IT COMES TO COOKING MOST OF THE TIME. HOWEVER, DRIED HERBS WORK VERY WELL IN RUBS FOR MEATS. WHEN HERBS ARE DRIED, THEIR FLAVORS ARE CONCENTRATED. WHEN THEY COME INTO CONTACT WITH MOISTURE FROM THE MEAT, THEY RELEASE THEIR FLAVORS INTO IT, AS IN THIS ITALIAN-STYLE ROAST FLAVORED WITH PARSLEY, FENNEL, OREGANO, GARLIC, AND SPICY CRUSHED RED PEPPER.

2   tablespoons dried parsley, crushed
2   tablespoons fennel seeds, crushed
4   teaspoons dried oregano, crushed
1   teaspoon freshly ground black pepper
½   teaspoon crushed red pepper
4   cloves garlic, minced
1   4-pound bone-in pork shoulder roast
1   to 2 tablespoons olive oil
1¼ cups water
2   medium onions, peeled and cut into wedges
1   large fennel bulb, trimmed, cored, and cut into wedges
2   pounds Brussels sprouts

1. Preheat oven to 325°F. In a small bowl combine parsley, fennel seeds, oregano, black pepper, crushed red pepper, and garlic; set aside. Untie pork roast if necessary. Trim fat from meat. Rub the meat on all sides with the seasoning mixture. If desired, retie roast to hold it together.

2. In a Dutch oven heat oil over medium-high heat. Brown meat on all sides in the hot oil. Drain off fat. Pour the water into Dutch oven around roast. Roast, uncovered, for 1½ hours. Arrange onions and fennel around pork roast. Cover and roast for 30 minutes more.

3. Meanwhile, trim Brussels sprouts stems and remove any wilted outer leaves. Cut Brussels sprouts in half. Add Brussels sprouts to Dutch oven, arranging them over other vegetables. Cover and roast for 30 to 35 minutes more or until vegetables and meat are tender. Transfer meat to a serving platter and cover with foil. Let stand for 15 minutes before slicing. Toss vegetables with pan juices to coat. Using a slotted spoon, remove vegetables to the serving platter or a bowl; cover to keep warm.

4. Using a large spoon, skim fat from pan juices. Pour remaining pan juices through a sieve. Slice pork, removing the bone. Serve meat with vegetables and pan juices.

SLOW COOKER PORK MOLE

PREP: 20 minutes   SLOW COOK: 8 to 10 hours (low) or 4 to 5 hours (high)   MAKES: 8 servings

WITH CUMIN, CORIANDER, OREGANO, TOMATOES, ALMONDS, RAISINS, CHILE, AND CHOCOLATE, THIS RICH AND SPICY SAUCE HAS A LOT GOING ON—IN A VERY GOOD WAY. IT'S AN IDEAL MEAL TO START IN THE MORNING BEFORE YOU HEAD OUT FOR THE DAY. WHEN YOU COME HOME, DINNER IS NEARLY DONE—AND YOUR HOUSE SMELLS AMAZING.

1 3-pound boneless pork shoulder roast
1 cup coarsely chopped onion
3 cloves garlic, sliced
1½ cups Beef Bone Broth (see recipe, page 131), Chicken Bone Broth (see recipe, page 235), or no-salt-added beef or chicken broth
1 tablespoon ground cumin
1 tablespoon ground coriander
2 teaspoons dried oregano, crushed
1 15-ounce can diced no-salt-added tomatoes, drained
1 6-ounce can no-salt-added tomato paste
½ cup slivered almonds, toasted (see tip, page 57)
¼ cup unsulfured golden raisins or currants
2 ounces unsweetened chocolate (such as Scharffen Berger 99% cacao bar), coarsely chopped
1 dried whole ancho or chipotle chile pepper
2 4-inch cinnamon sticks
¼ cup snipped fresh cilantro
1 avocado, peeled, seeded, and thinly sliced
1 lime, cut into wedges
⅓ cup toasted unsalted green pumpkin seeds (optional) (see tip, page 57)

1. Trim fat from pork roast. If necessary, cut meat to fit a 5- to 6-quart slow cooker; set aside.

2. In the slow cooker combine onion and garlic. In a 2-cup glass measuring cup stir together Beef Bone Broth, cumin, coriander, and oregano; pour into cooker. Stir in diced tomatoes, tomato paste, almonds, raisins, chocolate, dried chile pepper, and cinnamon sticks. Place meat in cooker. Spoon some of the tomato mixture over the top. Cover and cook on low-heat setting for 8 to 10 hours or on high-heat setting for 4 to 5 hours or until pork is tender.

3. Transfer pork to a cutting board; cool slightly. Using two forks, pull meat apart into shreds. Cover meat with foil and set aside.

4. Remove and discard dried chile pepper and cinnamon sticks. Using a large spoon, skim fat from tomato mixture. Transfer the tomato mixture to a blender or food processor. Cover and blend or process until almost smooth. Return pulled pork and sauce into slow cooker. Keep warm on low-heat setting until serving time, up to 2 hours.

5. Just before serving, stir in cilantro. Serve mole in bowls and garnish with avocado slices, lime wedges, and, if desired, pumpkin seeds.

CARAWAY-SPICED PORK AND SQUASH STEW

PREP: 30 minutes   COOK: 1 hour   MAKES: 4 servings

PEPPERY MUSTARD GREENS AND BUTTERNUT SQUASH ADD VIBRANT COLOR AND A WHOLE HOST OF VITAMINS—
AS WELL AS FIBER AND FOLIC ACID—TO THIS STEW SPICED WITH EASTERN EUROPEAN FLAVORS.

1   1¼- to 1½-pound pork shoulder
    roast
1   tablespoon paprika
1   tablespoon caraway seeds,
    finely crushed
2   teaspoons dry mustard
¼   teaspoon cayenne pepper
2   tablespoon refined coconut oil
8   ounces fresh button
    mushrooms, thinly sliced
2   stalks celery, cut crosswise into
    1-inch slices
1   small red onion, cut into thin
    wedges
6   cloves garlic, minced
5   cups Chicken Bone Broth (see
    page 235) or no-salt-added
    chicken broth
2   cups cubed, peeled butternut
    squash
3   cups coarsely chopped,
    trimmed mustard greens or
    green cabbage
2   tablespoons snipped fresh sage
¼   cup fresh lemon juice

1. Trim fat from pork. Cut pork into 1½-inch cubes; place in a large bowl. In a small bowl combine paprika, caraway seeds, dry mustard, and cayenne pepper. Sprinkle over pork, tossing to coat evenly.

2. In a 4- to 5-quart Dutch oven heat coconut oil over medium heat. Add half of the meat; cook until browned, stirring occasionally. Remove meat from the pan. Repeat with the remaining meat. Set meat aside.

3. Add mushrooms, celery, red onion, and garlic to Dutch oven. Cook for 5 minutes, stirring occasionally. Return meat to the Dutch oven. Carefully add Chicken Bone Broth. Bring to boiling; reduce heat. Cover and simmer for 45 minutes. Stir in squash. Cover and simmer for 10 to 15 minutes more or until pork and squash are tender. Stir in mustard greens and sage. Cook for 2 to 3 minutes or until greens are just tender. Stir in lemon juice.

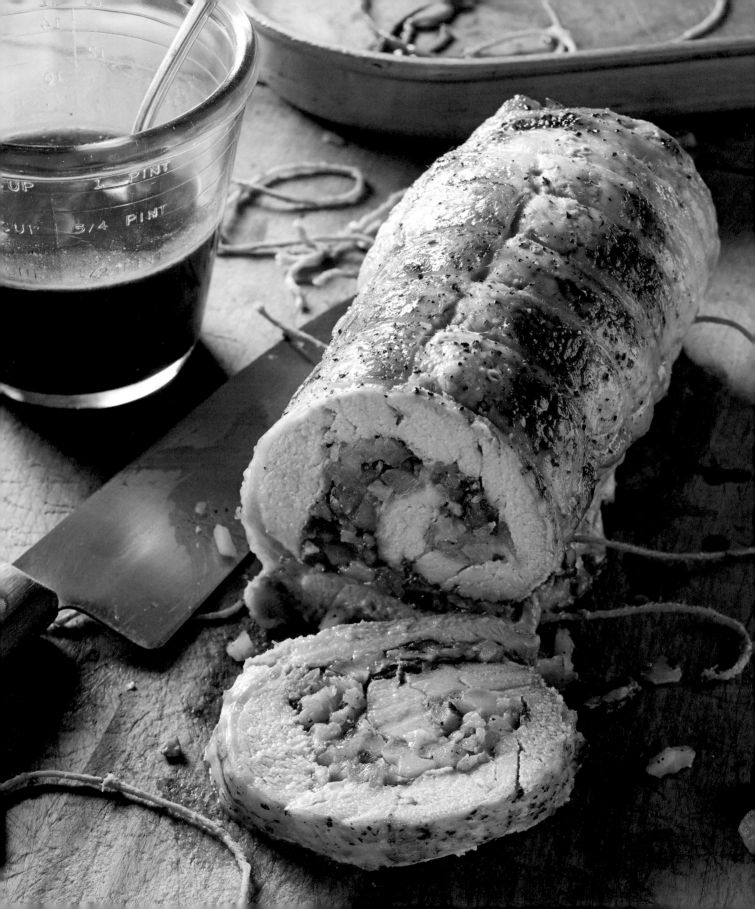

FRUIT-STUFFED TOP LOIN ROAST WITH BRANDY SAUCE

PREP: 30 minutes   COOK: 10 minutes   ROAST: 1 hour 15 minutes
STAND: 15 minutes   MAKES: 8 to 10 servings

THIS ELEGANT ROAST IS PERFECT FOR A SPECIAL OCCASION OR FAMILY GATHERING—PARTICULARLY IN THE FALL. ITS FLAVORS—APPLES, NUTMEG, DRIED FRUIT, AND PECANS—CAPTURE THE ESSENCE OF THAT SEASON. SERVE IT WITH MASHED SWEET POTATOES AND BLUEBERRY AND ROASTED BEET KALE SALAD (PAGE 296).

ROAST
- 1 tablespoon olive oil
- 2 cups chopped, peeled Granny Smith apples (about 2 medium)
- 1 shallot, finely chopped
- 1 tablespoon snipped fresh thyme
- ¾ teaspoon freshly ground black pepper
- ⅛ teaspoon ground nutmeg
- ½ cup snipped unsulfured dried apricots
- ¼ cup chopped pecans, toasted (see tip, page 57)
- 1 cup Chicken Bone Broth (see recipe, page 235) or no-salt-added chicken broth
- 1 3-pound boneless pork top loin roast (single loin)

BRANDY SAUCE
- 2 tablespoons apple cider
- 2 tablespoons brandy
- 1 teaspoon Dijoin-Style Mustard (see recipe, page 322)
  Freshly ground black pepper

1. For the stuffing, in a large skillet heat olive oil over medium heat. Add apples, shallot, thyme, ¼ teaspoon of the pepper, and nutmeg; cook for 2 to 4 minutes or until apples and shallot are tender and light golden, stirring occasionally. Stir in apricots, pecans, and 1 tablespoon of the broth. Cook, uncovered, for 1 minute to soften apricots. Remove from heat and set aside.

2. Preheat oven to 325°F. Butterfly the pork roast by making a lengthwise cut down the center of the roast, cutting to within ½ inch of the other side. Spread the roast open. Place the knife in the V cut, facing it horizontally toward one side of the V, and cut to within ½ inch of the side. Repeat on the other side of the V. Spread the roast open and cover with plastic wrap. Working from the center to the edges, pound the roast with a meat mallet until it is about ¾ inch thick. Remove and discard plastic wrap. Spread the stuffing over the top of the roast. Starting from a short side, roll the roast into a spiral. Tie with 100%-cotton kitchen string in several places to hold the roast together. Sprinkle roast with the remaining ½ teaspoon pepper.

3. Place roast on a rack in a shallow roasting pan. Insert an oven-going thermometer into the center of the roast (not in the stuffing). Roast, uncovered, for 1 hour 15 minutes to 1 hour 30 minutes or until thermometer registers 145°F. Remove roast and cover loosely with foil; let stand for 15 minutes before slicing.

4. Meanwhile, for Brandy Sauce, stir the remaining broth and apple cider into drippings in pan, whisking to scrape up browned bits. Strain drippings into a medium saucepan. Bring to boiling; cook about 4 minutes or until sauce is reduced by one-third. Stir in brandy and Dijon-Style Mustard. Season to taste with additional pepper. Serve sauce with the pork roast.

PORCHETTA-STYLE PORK ROAST

PREP: 15 minutes   MARINATE: overnight   STAND: 40 minutes   ROAST: 1 hour   MAKES: 6 servings

TRADITIONAL ITALIAN PORCHETTA (SOMETIMES SPELLED PORKETTA IN AMERICAN ENGLISH) IS A BONELESS SUCKLING PIG STUFFED WITH GARLIC, FENNEL, PEPPER, AND HERBS SUCH AS SAGE OR ROSEMARY, THEN PUT ON A SPIT AND ROASTED OVER WOOD. IT'S ALSO USUALLY HEAVILY SALTED. THIS PALEO VERSION IS SIMPLIFIED AND VERY TASTY. SUBSTITUTE FRESH ROSEMARY FOR THE SAGE, IF YOU LIKE, OR USE A BLEND OF THE TWO HERBS.

1 2- to 3-pound boneless pork loin roast
2 tablespoons fennel seeds
1 teaspoon black peppercorns
½ teaspoon crushed red pepper
6 cloves garlic, minced
1 tablespoon finely shredded orange peel
1 tablespoon snipped fresh sage
3 tablespoon olive oil
½ cup dry white wine
½ cup Chicken Bone Broth (see recipe, page 235) or no-salt-added chicken broth

1. Remove pork roast from refrigerator; let stand at room temperature for 30 minutes. Meanwhile, in a small skillet toast fennel seeds over medium heat, stirring frequently, about 3 minutes or until dark in color and fragrant; cool. Transfer to a spice mill or clean coffee grinder. Add peppercorns and crushed red pepper. Grind to medium-fine consistency. (Do not grind to a powder.)

2. Preheat oven to 325°F. In a small bowl combine ground spices, garlic, orange peel, sage, and olive oil to make a paste. Place pork roast on a rack in a small roasting pan. Rub mixture all over pork. (If desired, place seasoned pork in a 9×13×2-inch glass baking dish. Cover with with plastic wrap and refrigerate overnight to marinate. Transfer meat to a roasting pan before cooking and let stand at room temperature for 30 minutes before cooking.)

3. Roast pork for 1 to 1½ hours or until an instant-read thermometer inserted into center of roast registers 145°F. Transfer roast to a cutting board and cover loosely with foil. Let stand for 10 to 15 minutes before slicing.

4. Meanwhile, pour pan juices into a glass measuring cup. Skim fat from top; set aside. Place roasting pan on stovetop burner. Pour wine and Chicken Bone Broth into pan. Bring to boiling over medium-high heat, stirring to scrape up any browned bits. Boil about 4 minutes or until mixture is slightly reduced. Whisk in reserved pan juices; strain. Slice pork and serve with sauce.

TOMATILLO-BRAISED PORK LOIN

PREP: 40 minutes   BROIL: 10 minutes   COOK: 20 minutes
ROAST: 40 minutes   STAND: 10 minutes   MAKES: 6 to 8 servings

TOMATILLOS HAVE A STICKY, SAPPY COATING UNDER THEIR PAPER SKINS. AFTER YOU REMOVE THE SKINS, GIVE THEM A QUICK RINSE UNDER RUNNING WATER AND THEY ARE READY TO USE.

1   pound tomatillos, husked, stemmed, and rinsed
4   serrano chiles, stemmed, seeded, and halved (see tip, page 56)
2   jalapeños, stemmed, seeded, and halved (see tip, page 56)
1   large yellow sweet pepper, stemmed, seeded, and halved
1   large orange sweet pepper, stemmed, seeded, and halved
2   tablespoons olive oil
1   2- to 2½-pound boneless pork loin roast
1   large yellow onion, peeled, halved, and thinly sliced
4   cloves garlic, minced
¾   cup water
¼   cup fresh lime juice
¼   cup snipped fresh cilantro

1. Preheat broiler to high. Line a baking sheet with foil. Arrange tomatillos, serrano chiles, jalapeños, and sweet peppers on prepared baking sheet. Broil vegetables 4 inches from heat until well charred, turning tomatillos occasionally and removing vegetables as they become charred, about 10 to 15 minutes. Place serranos, jalapeños, and tomatillos in a bowl. Place sweet peppers on a plate. Set vegetables aside to cool.

2. In a large skillet heat oil over medium-high heat until it shimmers. Pat pork roast dry with clean paper towels and add to skillet. Cook until well browned on all sides, turning roast to brown evenly. Transfer roast to a platter. Reduce heat to medium. Add onion to skillet; cook and stir for 5 to 6 minutes or until golden. Add garlic; cook for 1 minute more. Remove skillet from heat.

3. Preheat oven to 350°F. For tomatillo sauce, in a food processor or blender combine tomatillos, serranos, and jalapeños. Cover and blend or process until smooth; add to onion in skillet. Return skillet to heat. Bring to boiling; cook for 4 to 5 minutes or until mixture is dark and thick. Stir in the water, lime juice, and cilantro.

4. Spread tomatillo sauce in a shallow roasting pan or 3-quart rectangular baking dish. Place pork roast in the sauce. Cover tightly with foil. Roast for 40 to 45 minutes or until an instant-read thermometer inserted into the center of the roast reads 140°F.

5. Cut sweet peppers into strips. Stir into the tomatillo sauce in pan. Tent loosely with foil; let stand for 10 minutes. Slice meat; stir sauce. Serve sliced pork topped generously with tomatillo sauce.

5 WAYS WITH PORK TENDERLOIN

PORK TENDERLOIN LIVES UP TO ITS NAME. IT IS THE TENDEREST CUT TAKEN FROM THE PIG. IT IS ALSO LEAN AND JUICY IF NOT OVERCOOKED. PORK TENDERLOIN COOKS QUICKLY—EVEN WHEN IT'S ROASTED—WHICH IS PERHAPS THE MOST COMMON COOKING METHOD. IT TAKES BEAUTIFULLY TO OTHER METHODS AS WELL. SLICE IT INTO MEDALLIONS AND PAN-SEAR, GRILL IT—EVEN CUT IT INTO THIN STRIPS AND STIR-FRY IT.

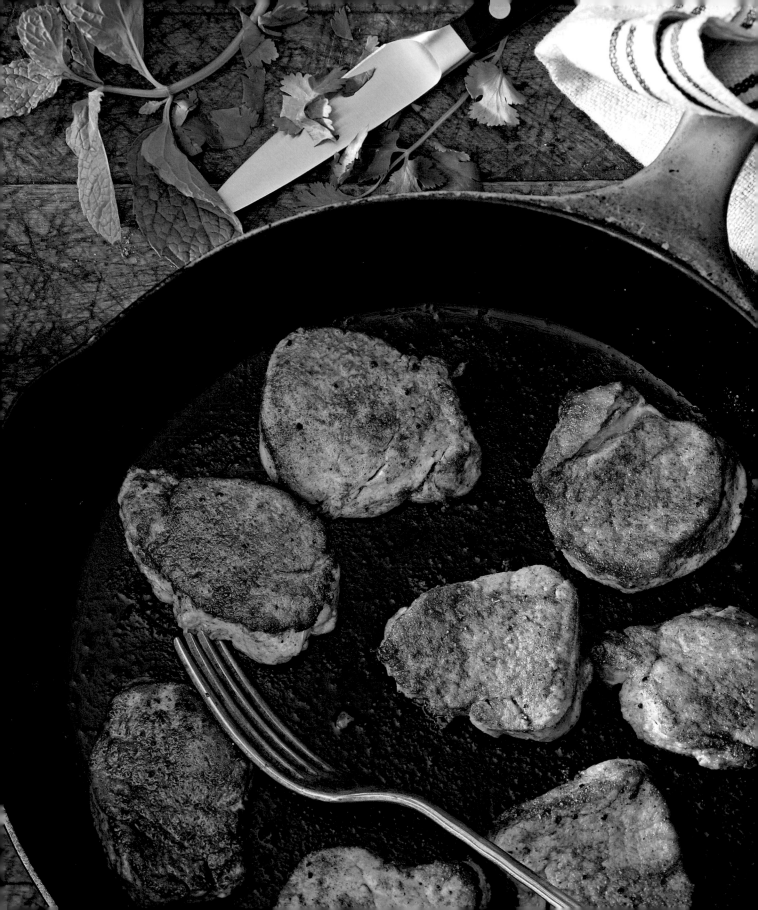

5 WAYS WITH PORK TENDERLOIN

BECAUSE PORK TENDERLOIN IS SO LEAN, THE MAIN CAUTION IN COOKING IT IS NOT TO OVERDO IT. IT HAS A MILD FLAVOR THAT PAIRS WELL WITH ALL KINDS OF SEASONINGS AND IT GOES PARTICULARLY WELL WITH FRUITS SUCH AS APPLES, APRICOTS, PEACHES, AND PLUMS. PORK TENDERLOIN CAN COME WITH CONNECTIVE TISSUE CALLED SILVERSKIN STILL ATTACHED. ASK THE BUTCHER TO REMOVE IT OR DO IT YOURSELF: SLIP A KNIFE UNDER ONE END AND CONTINUE SLICING DOWN THE LENGTH OF IT, HOLDING IT TAUT WITH ONE HAND AS YOU CUT WITH THE OTHER.

1. APRICOT-STUFFED PORK TENDERLOIN

PREP: 20 minutes
ROAST: 45 minutes
STAND: 5 minutes
MAKES: 2 to 3 servings

- 2 medium fresh apricots, coarsely chopped
- 2 tablespoons unsulfured raisins
- 2 tablespoons chopped walnuts
- 2 teaspoons grated fresh ginger
- ¼ teaspoon ground cardamom
- 1 12-ounce pork tenderloin
- 1 tablespoon olive oil
- 1 tablespoon Dijon-Style Mustard (see recipe, page 322)
- ¼ teaspoon black pepper

1. Preheat oven to 375°F. Line a baking sheet with foil; place a roasting rack on the baking sheet.

2. In a small bowl stir together the apricots, raisins, walnuts, ginger, and cardamom.

3. Make a lengthwise cut down the center of the pork, cutting to within ½ inch of the other side. Butterfly it open. Place the pork between two layers of plastic wrap. Using the flat side of a meat mallet, lightly pound meat until about ⅓ inch thick. Fold in the tail end to make an even rectangle. Lightly pound meat to make even thickness.

4. Spread the apricot mixture over the pork. Beginning at the narrow end, roll up the pork. Tie with 100%-cotton kitchen string, first in the center, then at 1-inch intervals. Place roast on the rack.

5. Stir together the olive oil and Dijon-Style Mustard; brush over the roast. Sprinkle roast with pepper. Roast for 45 to 55 minutes or until an instant-read thermometer inserted into center of roast registers 140°F. Let stand for 5 to 10 minutes before slicing.

2. HERB-CRUSTED PORK TENDERLOIN WITH CRISPY GARLIC OIL

PREP: 15 minutes
ROAST: 30 minutes
COOK: 8 minutes
STAND: 5 minutes
makes: 6 servings

- ⅓ cup Dijon-Style Mustard (see recipe, page 322)
- ¼ cup snipped fresh parsley
- 2 tablespoons snipped fresh thyme
- 1 tablespoon snipped fresh rosemary
- ½ teaspoon black pepper
- 2 12-ounce pork tenderloins
- ½ cup olive oil
- ¼ cup minced fresh garlic
- ¼ to 1 teaspoon crushed red pepper

1. Preheat oven to 450°F. Line a baking sheet with foil; place a roasting rack on the baking sheet.

2. In a small bowl stir together the mustard, parsley, thyme, rosemary, and black pepper to make a paste. Spread the mustard-herb mixture over the top and sides of the pork. Transfer pork to the roasting rack. Place roast in the oven; decrease temperature to 375°F. Roast for 30 to 35 minutes or until an instant-read thermometer inserted into center of roast registers 140°F. Let stand for 5 to 10 minutes before slicing.

3. Meanwhile, for garlic oil, in a small saucepan combine the olive oil and garlic. Cook over medium-low heat for 8 to 10 minutes or until garlic is golden and begins to crisp (do not let garlic burn). Remove from heat; stir in crushed red pepper. Slice pork; spoon garlic oil over the slices before serving.

3. INDIAN-SPICED PORK WITH COCONUT PAN SAUCE

START TO FINISH: 20 minutes
MAKES: 2 servings

- 3 teaspoons curry powder
- 2 teaspoons salt-free garam masala
- 1 teaspoon ground cumin
- 1 teaspoon ground coriander
- 1 12-ounce pork tenderloin
- 1 tablespoon olive oil
- ½ cup natural coconut milk (such as Nature's Way brand)
- ¼ cup snipped fresh cilantro
- 2 tablespoons snipped fresh mint

1. In a small bowl stir together 2 teaspoons of the curry powder, garam masala, cumin, and coriander. Slice pork into ½-inch-thick slices; sprinkle with spices. .

2. In a large skillet heat olive oil over medium heat. Add pork slices to skillet; cook for 7 minutes, turning once. Remove pork from skillet; cover to keep warm. For sauce, add coconut milk and the remaining 1 teaspoon curry powder to the skillet, stirring to scrape up any bits. Simmer for 2 to 3 minutes. Stir in cilantro and mint. Add pork; cook until heated through, spooning sauce over the pork.

4. PORK SCALOPPINI WITH SPICED APPLES AND CHESTNUTS

PREP: 20 minutes
COOK: 15 minutes
MAKES: 4 servings

- 2 12-ounce pork tenderloins
- 1 tablespoon onion powder
- 1 tablespoon garlic powder
- ½ teaspoon black pepper
- 2 to 4 tablespoons olive oil
- 2 Fuji or Pink Lady apples, peeled, cored, and coarsely chopped
- ¼ cup finely chopped shallots
- ¾ teaspoon ground cinnamon
- ⅛ teaspoon ground cloves
- ⅛ teaspoon ground nutmeg
- ½ cup Chicken Bone Broth (see page 235) or no-salt added chicken broth
- 2 tablespoons fresh lemon juice
- ½ cup peeled roasted chestnuts, chopped,* or chopped pecans
- 1 tablespoon snipped fresh sage

1. Cut the tenderloins into ½-inch- thick slices on a bias. Place pork slices between two sheets of plastic wrap. Using the flat side of a meat mallet, pound until thin. Sprinkle slices with onion powder, garlic powder, and black pepper.

2. In a large skillet heat 2 tablespoons olive oil over medium heat. Cook pork, in batches, for 3 to 4 minutes, turning once and adding oil if necessary. Transfer pork to a plate; cover and keep warm.

3. Increase heat to medium-high. Add the apples, shallots, cinnamon, cloves, and nutmeg. Cook and stir for 3 minutes. Stir in Chicken Bone Broth and lemon juice. Cover and cook for 5 minutes. Remove from heat; stir in the chestnuts and sage. Serve apple mixture over pork.

*Note: To roast chestnuts, preheat oven to 400°F. Cut an X in one side of the chestnut shell. This will let the shell loosen as it cooks. Place chestnuts on a baking pan and roast for 30 minutes or until the shell pulls apart from the nut and the nuts are tender. Wrap the roasted chestnuts in a clean kitchen towel. Peel shells and skin from the yellow-white nut.

5. PORK FAJITA STIR-FRY

PREP: 20 minutes
COOK: 22 minutes
MAKES: 4 servings

- 1 pound pork tenderloin, cut into 2-inch strips
- 3 tablespoons salt-free fajita seasoning or Mexican Seasoning (page 324)
- 2 tablespoons olive oil
- 1 small onion, thinly sliced
- ½ of a red sweet pepper, seeded and thinly sliced
- ½ of an orange sweet pepper, seeded and thinly sliced
- 1 jalapeño, stemmed and thinly sliced (see tip, page 56) (optional)
- ½ teaspoon cumin seeds
- 1 cup thinly sliced fresh mushrooms
- 3 tablespoons fresh lime juice
- ½ cup snipped fresh cilantro
- 1 avocado, seeded, peeled, and diced
   Desired salsa (see recipes, pages 326–327)

1. Sprinkle the pork with 2 tablespoons fajita seasoning. In an extra-large skillet heat 1 tablespoon of the oil over medium-high heat. Add half the pork; cook and stir about 5 minutes or until no longer pink. Transfer meat to a bowl and cover to keep warm. Repeat with remaining oil and pork.

2. Turn heat to medium. Add the remaining 1 tablespoon fajita seasoning, onion, sweet peppers, jalapeño, and cumin. Cook and stir about 10 minutes or until vegetables are tender. Return all the meat and accumulated juices to skillet. Stir in mushrooms and lime juice. Cook until heated through. Remove skillet from heat; stir in the cilantro. Serve with avocado and desired salsa.

PORK TENDERLOIN WITH PORT AND PRUNES

PREP: 10 minutes   ROAST: 12 minutes   STAND: 5 minutes   MAKES: 4 servings

PORT IS A FORTIFIED WINE, WHICH MEANS IT HAS A SPIRIT SIMILAR TO BRANDY ADDED TO IT TO STOP THE FERMENTATION PROCESS. THIS MEANS THERE IS MORE RESIDUAL SUGAR IN IT THAN RED TABLE WINE AND CONSEQUENTLY IT HAS A SWEETER TASTE. IT ISN'T SOMETHING YOU WANT TO DRINK EVERY DAY, BUT A LITTLE BIT USED IN COOKING ONCE IN A WHILE IS FINE.

2	12-ounce pork tenderloins
2½	teaspoons ground coriander
¼	teaspoon black pepper
2	tablespoons olive oil
1	shallot, sliced
½	cup port wine
½	cup Chicken Bone Broth (see recipe, page 235) or no-salt-added chicken broth
20	pitted unsulfured dried plums (prunes)
½	teaspoon crushed red pepper
2	teaspoons snipped fresh tarragon

1. Preheat oven to 400°F. Sprinkle pork with 2 teaspoons of the coriander and the black pepper.

2. In a large ovenproof skillet heat olive oil over medium-high heat. Add tenderloins to skillet. Cook until browned on all sides, turning to brown evenly, about 8 minutes. Place skillet in oven. Roast, uncovered, about 12 minutes or until an instant-read thermometer inserted into center of roasts registers 140°F. Transfer tenderloins to a cutting board. Cover loosely with aluminum foil and let stand for 5 minutes.

3. Meanwhile, for sauce, drain fat from skillet, reserving 1 tablespoon. Cook shallot in the reserved drippings in skillet over medium heat about 3 minutes or until browned and tender. Add port to skillet. Bring to boiling, stirring to scrape up any browned bits. Add Chicken Bone Broth, dried plums, crushed red pepper, and the remaining ½ teaspoon coriander. Cook over medium-high heat to reduce slightly, about 1 to 2 minutes. Stir in tarragon.

4. Slice pork and serve with prunes and sauce.

MOO SHU-STYLE PORK IN LETTUCE CUPS WITH QUICK PICKLED VEGETABLES

START TO FINISH: **45 minutes**   MAKES: **4 servings**

IF YOU'VE HAD A TRADITIONAL MOO SHU DISH IN A CHINESE RESTAURANT, YOU KNOW IT IS A SAVORY MEAT AND VEGETABLE FILLING EATEN IN THIN PANCAKES WITH A SWEET PLUM OR HOISIN SAUCE. THIS LIGHTER AND FRESHER PALEO VERSION FEATURES PORK, CHINESE CABBAGE, AND SHIITAKE MUSHROOMS STIR-FRIED IN GINGER AND GARLIC AND ENJOYED IN LETTUCE WRAPS WITH CRUNCHY PICKLED VEGETABLES.

PICKLED VEGETABLES

- 1 cup julienne-cut carrots
- 1 cup julienne-cut daikon radish
- ¼ cup slivered red onion
- 1 cup unsweetened apple juice
- ½ cup cider vinegar

PORK

- 2 tablespoons olive oil or refined coconut oil
- 3 eggs, lightly beaten
- 8 ounces pork loin, cut into 2×½-inch strips
- 2 teaspoons minced fresh ginger
- 4 cloves garlic, minced
- 2 cups thinly sliced napa cabbage
- 1 cup thinly sliced shiitake mushrooms
- ¼ cup thinly sliced scallions
- 8 Boston lettuce leaves

1. For quick pickled vegetables, in a large bowl toss together the carrots, daikon, and onion. For brine, in a saucepan heat the apple juice and vinegar just until steam rises. Pour the brine over the vegetables in bowl; cover and chill until ready to serve.

2. In a large skillet heat 1 tablespoon of the oil over medium-high heat. Using a whisk, lightly beat eggs. Add eggs to skillet; cook, without stirring, until set on the bottom, about 3 minutes. Using a flexible spatula, carefully turn the egg over and cook on the other side. Slide the egg out of the pan onto a platter.

3. Return the skillet to heat; add the remaining 1 tablespoon oil. Add the pork strips, ginger, and garlic. Cook and stir over medium-high heat about 4 minutes or until pork is no longer pink. Add the cabbage and mushrooms; cook and stir about 4 minutes or until cabbage wilts, mushrooms soften, and pork is cooked through. Remove skillet from heat. Cut the cooked egg into strips. Gently stir egg strips and scallions into pork mixture. Serve in lettuce leaves and top with pickled vegetables.

PORK CHOPS WITH MACADAMIAS, SAGE, FIGS, AND MASHED SWEET POTATOES

PREP: 15 minutes   COOK: 25 minutes   MAKES: 4 servings

PAIRED WITH MASHED SWEET POTATOES, THESE JUICY SAGE-TOPPED CHOPS MAKE A PERFECT FALL MEAL—AND ONE THAT'S QUICK TO FIX, MAKING IT A PERFECT FOR A BUSY WEEKNIGHT.

4 boneless pork loin chops, cut 1¼ inches thick
3 tablespoons snipped fresh sage
¼ teaspoon black pepper
3 tablespoons macadamia nut oil
2 pounds sweet potatoes, peeled and cut into 1-inch pieces
¾ cup chopped macadamia nuts
½ cup chopped dried figs
⅓ cup Beef Bone Broth (see recipe page 131) or no-salt-added beef broth
1 tablespoon fresh lemon juice

1. Sprinkle both sides of pork chops with 2 tablespoons of the sage and the pepper; rub in with your fingers. In a large skillet heat 2 tablespoons of the oil over medium heat. Add chops to skillet; cook for 15 to 20 minutes or until done (145°F), turning once halfway through cooking. Transfer chops to a plate; cover to keep warm.

2. Meanwhile, in a large saucepan combine sweet potatoes and enough water to cover. Bring to boiling; reduce heat. Cover and simmer for 10 to 15 minutes or until potatoes are tender. Drain potatoes. Add the remaining tablespoon macadamia oil to potatoes and mash until creamy; keep warm.

3. For sauce, add macadamia nuts to skillet; cook over medium heat just until toasted. Add dried figs and the remaining 1 tablespoon sage; cook for 30 seconds. Add Beef Bone Broth and lemon juice to skillet, stirring to scrape up any browned bits. Spoon sauce over pork chops and serve with mashed sweet potatoes.

SKILLET-ROASTED ROSEMARY-LAVENDER PORK CHOPS WITH GRAPES AND TOASTED WALNUTS

PREP: 10 minutes   COOK: 6 minutes   ROAST: 25 minutes   MAKES: 4 servings

ROASTING THE GRAPES ALONG WITH THE PORK CHOPS INTENSIFIES THEIR FLAVOR AND SWEETNESS. ALONG WITH THE CRUNCHY TOASTED WALNUTS AND A SPRINKLING OF FRESH ROSEMARY, THEY MAKE A WONDERFUL TOPPING FOR THESE HEARTY CHOPS.

2   tablespoons snipped fresh rosemary
1   tablespoon snipped fresh lavender
½   teaspoon garlic powder
½   teaspoon black pepper
4   pork loin chops, cut 1¼ inches thick (about 3 pounds)
1   tablespoon olive oil
1   large shallot, thinly sliced
1½ cups red and/or green seedless grapes
½   cup dry white wine
¾   cup coarsely chopped walnuts
    Snipped fresh rosemary

1. Preheat oven to 375°F. In a small bowl combine 2 tablespoons rosemary, lavender, garlic powder, and pepper. Rub herb mixture evenly into pork chops. In an extra-large ovenproof skillet heat olive oil over medium heat. Add chops to skillet; cook for 6 to 8 minutes or until browned on both sides. Transfer chops to a plate; cover with foil.

2. Add the shallot to the skillet. Cook and stir over medium heat for 1 minute. Add grapes and wine. Cook about 2 minutes more, stirring to scrape up any browned bits. Return pork chops to skillet. Place the skillet in the oven; roast for 25 to 30 minutes or until chops are done (145°F).

3. Meanwhile, spread the walnuts in a shallow baking pan. Add to oven with chops. Roast about 8 minutes or until toasted, stirring once to toast evenly.

4. To serve, top pork chops with grapes and toasted walnuts. Sprinkle with additional fresh rosemary.

PORK CHOPS ALLA FIORENTINA WITH GRILLED BROCCOLI RABE

PREP: 20 minutes   GRILL: 20 minutes   MARINATE: 3 minutes   MAKES: 4 servings

"ALLA FIORENTINA" ESSENTIALLY MEANS "IN THE STYLE OF FLORENCE." THIS RECIPE IS STYLED AFTER *BISTECCA ALLA FIORENTINA*, A TUSCAN T-BONE GRILLED OVER A WOOD FIRE WITH THE SIMPLEST FLAVORINGS—USUALLY JUST OLIVE OIL, SALT, BLACK PEPPER, AND A SQUEEZE OF FRESH LEMON TO FINISH.

1   pound broccoli rabe
1   tablespoon olive oil
4   6- to 8-ounce bone-in pork loin
    chops, cut 1½ to 2 inches thick
    Coarsely ground black pepper
1   lemon
4   cloves garlic, thinly sliced
2   tablespoons snipped fresh
    rosemary
6   fresh sage leaves, chopped
1   teaspoon crushed red pepper
    flakes (or to taste)
½   cup olive oil

1. In a large saucepan blanch the broccoli rabe in boiling water for 1 minute. Immediately transfer to a bowl of ice water. When cool, drain the broccoli rabe on a paper towel-lined baking sheet, blotting as dry as possible with additional paper towels. Remove paper towels from baking sheet. Drizzle the broccoli rabe with 1 tablespoon olive oil, tossing to coat; set aside until ready to grill.

2. Sprinkle both sides of the pork chops with coarsely ground pepper; set aside. Using a vegetable peeler, remove strips of peel from lemon (save lemon for another use). Scatter lemon peel strips, sliced garlic, rosemary, sage, and crushed red pepper on a large serving platter; set aside.

3. For a charcoal grill, move most hot coals to one side of the grill, leaving some coals under the other side of the grill. Sear the chops directly over the hot coals for 2 to 3 minutes or until a brown crust forms. Turn the chops over and sear on the second side for 2 minutes more. Move the chops to the other side of the grill. Cover and grill for 10 to 15 minutes or until done (145°F). (For a gas grill, preheat grill; reduce heat on one side of grill to medium. Sear chops as directed above over high heat. Move to medium heat side of grill; continue as directed above.)

4. Transfer the chops to the platter. Drizzle chops with the ½ cup olive oil, turning to coat both sides. Let the chops marinate for 3 to 5 minutes before serving, turning once or twice to infuse the meat with the flavors of the lemon peel, garlic, and herbs.

5. While the chops rest, grill the broccoli rabe to char lightly and warm through. Arrange broccoli rabe on the platter with the pork chops; spoon some of the marinade over each chop and broccoli rabe before serving.

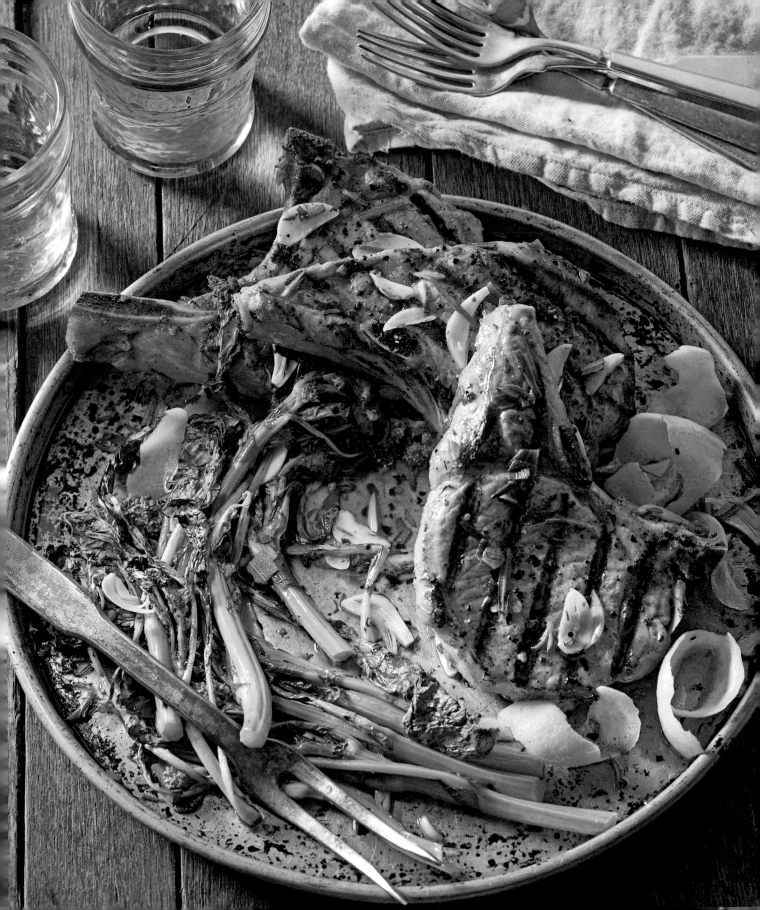

ESCAROLE-STUFFED PORK CHOPS

PREP: 20 minutes   COOK: 9 minutes   MAKES: 4 servings

ESCAROLE CAN BE EATEN AS A SALAD GREEN OR LIGHTLY SAUTÉED WITH GARLIC IN OLIVE OIL FOR A QUICK SIDE DISH. HERE, COMBINED WITH OLIVE OIL, GARLIC, BLACK PEPPER, CRUSHED RED PEPPER, AND LEMON, IT MAKES A BEAUTIFUL BRIGHT-GREEN FILLING FOR JUICY PAN-SEARED PORK CHOPS.

4 6- to 8-ounce bone-in pork chops, cut ¾ inch thick
½ of a medium head escarole, finely chopped
4 tablespoons olive oil
1 tablespoon fresh lemon juice
¼ teaspoon black pepper
¼ teaspoon crushed red pepper
2 large cloves garlic, minced
   Olive oil
1 tablespoon snipped fresh sage
¼ teaspoon black pepper
⅓ cup dry white wine

1. Using a paring knife, cut a deep pocket, about 2 inches wide, into the curved side of each pork chop; set aside.

2. In a large bowl combine escarole, 2 tablespoons of the olive oil, lemon juice, ¼ teaspoon black pepper, crushed red pepper, and garlic. Stuff each chop with one-fourth of the mixture. Brush chops with olive oil. Sprinkle with sage and ¼ teaspoon ground black pepper.

3. In an extra-large skillet heat remaining 2 tablespoons olive oil over medium-high heat. Sear pork for 4 minutes on each side until golden brown. Transfer chops to a plate. Add wine to skillet, scraping up any browned bits. Reduce pan juices for 1 minute.

4. Drizzle chops with pan juices before serving.

PORK CHOPS WITH A DIJON-PECAN CRUST

pictured on page 309

PREP: 15 minutes   COOK: 6 minutes   BAKE: 3 minutes   MAKES: 4 servings

THESE MUSTARD-AND-NUT-CRUSTED CHOPS COULDN'T BE **SIMPLER** TO MAKE—AND THE TASTE PAY-OFF FAR EXCEEDS THE EFFORT. TRY THEM WITH CINNAMON-ROASTED BUTTERNUT SQUASH (PAGE 288), NEO-CLASSIC WALDORF SALAD (PAGE 303), OR BRUSSELS SPROUTS AND APPLE SALAD (PAGE 310).

⅓ cup finely chopped pecans, toasted (see tip, page 57)
1 tablespoon snipped fresh sage
3 tablespoons olive oil
4 bone-in center-cut pork chops, about 1 inch thick (about 2 pounds total)
½ teaspoon black pepper
2 tablespoons olive oil
3 tablespoons Dijon-Style Mustard (see recipe, page 322)

1. Preheat oven to 400°F. In a small bowl combine pecans, sage, and 1 tablespoon of the olive oil.

2. Sprinkle pork chops with pepper. In a large ovenproof skillet heat the remaining 2 tablespoons olive oil over high heat. Add chops; cook about 6 minutes or until browned on both sides, turning once. Remove skillet from heat. Spread Dijon-Style Mustard on tops of chops; sprinkle with pecan mixture, lightly pressing into mustard.

3. Place skillet in oven. Bake for 3 to 4 minutes or until chops are done (145°F).

WALNUT-CRUSTED PORK WITH BLACKBERRY SPINACH SALAD

PREP: 30 minutes   COOK: 4 minutes   MAKES: 4 servings

PORK HAS A NATURALLY SWEET TASTE THAT PAIRS WELL WITH FRUIT. ALTHOUGH THE USUAL SUSPECTS ARE FALL FRUITS SUCH AS APPLES AND PEARS—OR STONE FRUITS SUCH AS PEACHES, PLUMS, AND APRICOTS—PORK IS ALSO DELICIOUS WITH BLACKBERRIES, WHICH HAVE A SWEET-TART, WINELIKE FLAVOR.

1⅔ cups blackberries

1 tablespoon plus 1½ teaspoons water

3 tablespoons walnut oil

1 tablespoon plus 1½ teaspoons white wine vinegar

2 eggs

¾ cup almond meal

⅓ cup finely chopped walnuts

1 tablespoon plus 1½ teaspoons Mediterranean Seasoning (see recipe, page 324)

4 pork cutlets or boneless pork loin chops (1 to 1½ pounds total)

6 cups fresh baby spinach leaves

½ cup torn fresh basil leaves

½ cup slivered red onion

½ cup chopped walnuts, toasted (see tip, page 57)

¼ cup refined coconut oil

1. For blackberry vinaigrette, in a small saucepan combine 1 cup of the blackberries and the water. Bring to boiling; reduce heat. Simmer, covered, for 4 to 5 minutes or just until berries are softened and color turns to a bright maroon, stirring occasionally. Remove from the heat; cool slightly. Pour undrained blackberries into a blender or food processor; cover and blend or process until smooth. Using the back of a spoon, press pureed berries through a fine-mesh sieve; discard seeds and solids. In a medium bowl whisk together strained berries, walnut oil, and vinegar; set aside.

2. Line a large baking sheet with parchment paper; set aside. In a shallow dish lightly beat eggs well with a fork. In another shallow dish combine almond meal, the ⅓ cup finely chopped walnuts, and Mediterranean Seasoning. Dip pork cutlets, one at a time, in eggs and then in walnut mixture, turning to coat evenly. Place coated pork cutlets on a prepared baking sheet; set aside.

3. In a large bowl combine spinach and basil. Divide greens among four serving plates, arranging them along one side of the plates. Top with remaining ⅔ cup berries, the red onion, and the ½ cup toasted walnuts. Drizzle with blackberry vinaigrette.

4. In an extra-large skillet heat coconut oil over medium-high heat. Add pork cutlets to skillet; cook about 4 minutes or until done (145°F), turning once. Add pork cutlets to plates with salad.

PORK SCHNITZEL WITH SWEET-AND-SOUR RED CABBAGE

PREP: 20 minutes   COOK: 45 minutes   MAKES: 4 servings

IN THE "PALEO PRINCIPLES" SECTION OF THIS BOOK, ALMOND FLOUR (ALSO CALLED ALMOND MEAL) IS LISTED AS A NON-PALEO INGREDIENT (PAGE 19)—NOT BECAUSE ALMOND FLOUR IS INHERENTLY BAD, BUT BECAUSE IT IS FREQUENTLY USED TO CREATE ANALOGS OF WHEAT-FLOUR BROWNIES, CAKES, COOKIES, ETC., THAT SHOULD NOT BE A REGULAR PART OF A REAL PALEO DIET®. USED IN MODERATION AS COATING FOR A THIN SCALLOP OF PAN-FRIED PORK OR POULTRY, AS IT IS HERE, IS NOT A PROBLEM.

CABBAGE

- 2 tablespoons olive oil
- 1 cup chopped red onion
- 6 cups thinly sliced red cabbage (about ½ of a head)
- 2 Granny Smith apples, peeled, cored, and diced
- ¾ cup fresh orange juice
- 3 tablespoons cider vinegar
- ½ teaspoon caraway seeds
- ½ teaspoon celery seeds
- ½ teaspoon black pepper

PORK

- 4 boneless pork loin chops, cut ½ inch thick
- 2 cups almond flour
- 1 tablespoon dried lemon peel
- 2 teaspoons black pepper
- ¾ teaspoon ground allspice
- 1 large egg
- ¼ cup almond milk
- 3 tablespoons olive oil
  Lemon wedges

1. For sweet-and-sour cabbage, in a 6-quart Dutch oven heat olive oil over medium-low heat. Add onion; cook for 6 to 8 minutes or until tender and lightly browned. Add cabbage; cook and stir for 6 to 8 minutes or until cabbage is crisp-tender. Add apples, orange juice, vinegar, caraway seeds, celery seeds, and ½ teaspoon pepper. Bring to boiling; reduce heat to low. Cover and cook for 30 minutes, stirring occasionally. Uncover and cook until liquid is reduced slightly.

2. Meanwhile, for pork, place chops between two sheets of plastic wrap or waxed paper. Using the flat side of a meat mallet or rolling pin, pound to about ¼ inch thickness; set aside.

3. In a shallow dish combine almond flour, dried lemon peel, 2 teaspoons pepper, and allspice. In another shallow dish whisk together the egg and almond milk. Lightly coat the pork cutlets in the seasoned flour, shaking off excess. Dip in the egg mixture, then again into the seasoned flour, shaking off excess. Repeat with remaining cutlets.

4. In a large skillet heat olive oil over medium-high heat. Add 2 cutlets to the pan. Cook for 6 to 8 minutes or until cutlets are golden brown and cooked through, turning once. Transfer cutlets to a warm platter. Repeat with remaining 2 cutlets.

5. Serve cutlets with cabbage and lemon wedges.

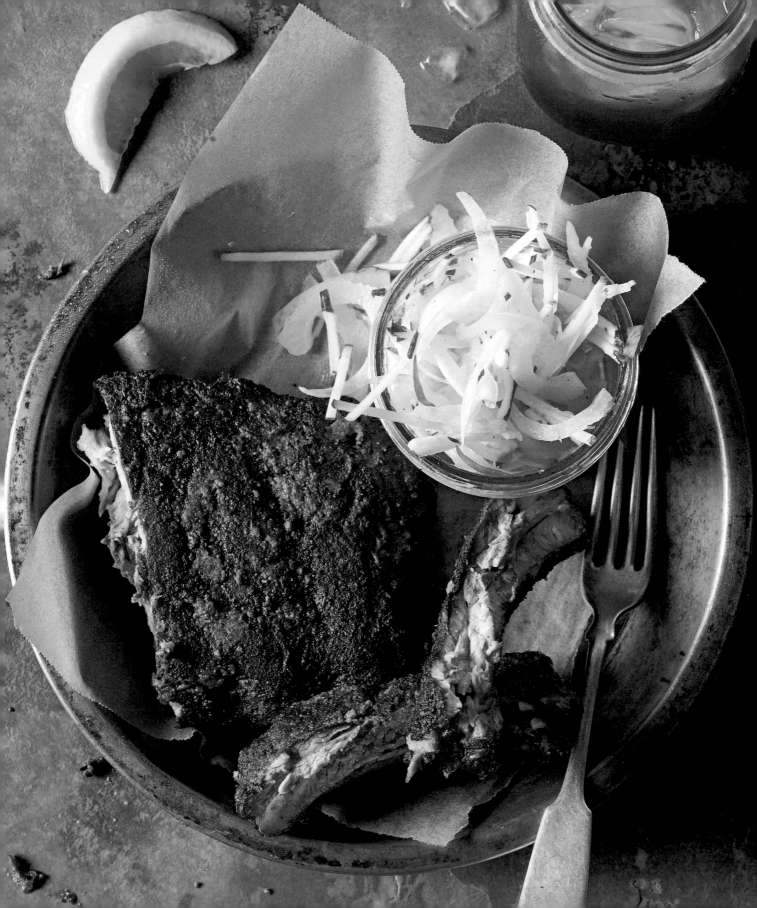

SMOKED BABY BACK RIBS WITH APPLE-MUSTARD MOP SAUCE

SOAK: 1 hour   STAND: 15 minutes   SMOKE: 4 hours   COOK: 20 minutes   MAKES: 4 servings

THE RICH FLAVOR AND MEATY TEXTURE OF SMOKED RIBS CALLS FOR SOMETHING COOL AND CRISP TO GO ALONG WITH IT. ALMOST ANY SLAW WILL DO, BUT THE FENNEL SLAW (PAGE 313 AND PICTURED HERE), IS ESPECIALLY GOOD.

RIBS

- 8 to 10 apple or hickory wood chunks
- 3 to 3½ pounds pork loin baby back ribs
- ¼ cup Smoky Seasoning (see recipe, page 324)

SAUCE

- 1 medium cooking apple, peeled, cored, and thinly sliced
- ¼ cup chopped onion
- ¼ cup water
- ¼ cup cider vinegar
- 2 tablespoons Dijon-Style Mustard (see recipe, page 322)
- 2 to 3 tablespoons water

1. At least 1 hour before smoke-cooking, soak wood chunks in enough water to cover. Drain before using. Trim visible fat from ribs. If necessary, peel off the thin membrane from the back of the ribs. Place ribs in a large shallow pan. Sprinkle evenly with Smoky Seasoning; rub in with your fingers. Let stand at room temperature for 15 minutes.

2. In a smoker arrange preheated coals, drained wood chunks, and water pan according to the manufacturer's directions. Pour water into pan. Place ribs, bone sides down, on grill rack over water pan. (Or place ribs in a rib rack; place rib rack on grill rack.) Cover and smoke for 2 hours. Maintain a temperature of about 225°F in the smoker for the duration of smoking. Add additional coals and water as needed to maintain temperature and moisture.

3. Meanwhile, for mop sauce, in a small saucepan combine apple slices, onion, and the ¼ cup water. Bring to boiling; reduce heat. Simmer, covered, for 10 to 12 minutes or until apple slices are very tender, stirring occasionally. Cool slightly; transfer undrained apple and onion to a food processor or blender. Cover and process or blend until smooth. Return puree to saucepan. Stir in vinegar and Dijon-Style Mustard. Cook over medium-low heat for 5 minutes, stirring occasionally. Add 2 to 3 tablespoons of water (or more, as needed) to make the sauce the consistency of a vinaigrette. Divide the sauce into thirds.

4. After 2 hours, brush ribs generously with one-third of the mop sauce. Cover and smoke 1 hour more. Brush again with another one-third of the mop sauce. Wrap each slab of ribs in heavy foil and place the ribs back on the smoker, layering them on top of each other if needed. Cover and smoke for 1 to 1½ hours more or until ribs are tender.*

5. Unwrap ribs and brush with the remaining one-third of the mop sauce. Cut ribs between bones to serve.

*Tip: To test tenderness of the ribs, carefully remove the foil from one of the slabs of ribs. Pick up the rib slab with tongs, holding the slab by the top one-fourth of the slab. Turn the rib slab over so the meaty side is facing down. If the ribs are tender, the slab should begin to fall apart as you pick it up. If it is not tender, wrap again in foil and continue to smoke ribs until tender.

OVEN BBQ COUNTRY-STYLE PORK RIBS WITH FRESH PINEAPPLE SLAW

PREP: 20 minutes   COOK: 8 minutes   BAKE: 1 hour 15 minutes   MAKES: 4 servings

COUNTRY-STYLE PORK RIBS ARE MEATY, INEXPENSIVE, AND, IF TREATED THE RIGHT WAY—SUCH AS COOKED LOW AND SLOW IN A MESS OF BARBECUE SAUCE—GET MELTINGLY TENDER.

2 pounds boneless country-style pork ribs
¼ teaspoon black pepper
1 tablespoon refined coconut oil
½ cup fresh orange juice
1½ cups BBQ Sauce (see recipe, page 323)
3 cups shredded green and/or red cabbage
1 cup shredded carrots
2 cups finely chopped pineapple
⅓ cup Bright Citrus Vinaigrette (see recipe, page 320)
BBQ Sauce (see recipe, page 323) (optional)

1. Preheat oven to 350°F. Sprinkle pork with pepper. In an extra-large skillet heat coconut oil over medium-high heat. Add pork ribs; cook for 8 to 10 minutes or until browned, turning to brown evenly. Place ribs in a 3-quart rectangular baking dish.

2. For sauce, add orange juice to skillet, stirring to scrape up any browned bits. Stir in the 1½ cups BBQ Sauce. Pour sauce over ribs. Turn ribs to coat with sauce (if necessary, use a pastry brush to brush sauce over ribs). Cover baking dish tightly with aluminum foil.

3. Bake ribs for 1 hour. Remove foil and brush ribs with sauce from baking dish. Bake about 15 minutes more or until ribs are tender and browned and sauce has thickened slightly.

4. Meanwhile, for pineapple slaw, combine cabbage, carrots, pineapple, and Bright Citrus Vinaigrette. Cover and refrigerate until serving time.

5. Serve ribs with slaw and, if desired, additional BBQ Sauce.

SPICY PORK GOULASH

PREP: 20 minutes   COOK: 40 minutes   MAKES: 6 servings

THIS HUNGARIAN-STYLE STEW IS SERVED ON A BED OF CRUNCHY, BARELY WILTED CABBAGE FOR A ONE-DISH MEAL. CRUSH THE CARAWAY SEEDS IN A MORTAR AND PESTLE IF YOU HAVE ONE. IF NOT, CRUSH THEM UNDER THE BROAD SIDE OF A CHEF'S KNIFE BY PRESSING DOWN ON KNIFE GENTLY WITH YOUR FIST.

GOULASH

1½ pounds ground pork
2 cups chopped red, orange, and/ or yellow sweet peppers
¾ cup finely chopped red onion
1 small fresh red chile, seeded and finely chopped (see tip, page 56)
4 teaspoons Smoky Seasoning (see recipe, page 324)
1 teaspoon caraway seeds, crushed
¼ teaspoon ground marjoram or oregano
1 14-ounce can no-salt-added diced tomatoes, undrained
2 tablespoons red wine vinegar
1 tablespoon finely shredded lemon peel
⅓ cup snipped fresh parsley

CABBAGE

2 tablespoons olive oil
1 medium onion, sliced
1 small head green or red cabbage, cored and thinly sliced

1. For the goulash, in a large Dutch oven cook ground pork, sweet peppers, and onion over medium-high heat for 8 to 10 minutes or until the pork is no longer pink and vegetables are crisp-tender, stirring with a wooden spoon to break up meat. Drain off fat. Reduce heat to low; add red chile, Smoky Seasoning, caraway seeds, and marjoram. Cover and cook for 10 minutes. Add undrained tomatoes and vinegar. Bring to boiling; reduce heat. Simmer, covered, for 20 minutes.

2. Meanwhile, for cabbage, in an extra-large skillet heat oil over medium heat. Add onion and cook until softened, about 2 minutes. Add cabbage; stir to combine. Reduce heat to low. Cook about 8 minutes or until cabbage is just tender, stirring occasionally.

3. To serve, place some of the cabbage mixture on a plate. Top with goulash and sprinkle with lemon zest and parsley.

ITALIAN SAUSAGE MEATBALLS MARINARA WITH SLICED FENNEL AND ONION SAUTÉ

PREP: 30 minutes   BAKE: 30 minutes   COOK: 40 minutes   MAKES: 4 to 6 servings

THIS RECIPE IS A RARE EXAMPLE OF A CANNED PRODUCT WORKING AS WELL AS—IF NOT BETTER THAN—THE FRESH VERSION. UNLESS YOU HAVE TOMATOES THAT ARE VERY, VERY RIPE, YOU WILL NOT GET AS GOOD A CONSISTENCY IN A SAUCE USING FRESH TOMATOES AS YOU CAN USING CANNED TOMATOES. JUST BE SURE YOU USE A NO-SALT-ADDED PRODUCT—AND, EVEN BETTER, ORGANIC.

MEATBALLS

- 2 large eggs
- ½ cup almond meal
- 8 cloves garlic, minced
- 6 tablespoons dry white wine
- 1 tablespoon paprika
- 2 teaspoons black pepper
- 1 teaspoon fennel seeds, lightly crushed
- 1 teaspoon dried oregano, crushed
- 1 teaspoon dried thyme, crushed
- ¼ to ½ teaspoon cayenne pepper
- 1½ pounds ground pork

MARINARA

- 2 tablespoons olive oil
- 2 15-ounce cans no-salt-added crushed tomatoes or one 28-ounce can no-salt-added crushed tomatoes
- ½ cup snipped fresh basil
- 3 medium fennel bulbs, halved, cored, and thinly sliced
- 1 large sweet onion, halved and thinly sliced

1. Preheat oven to 375°F. Line a large rimmed baking sheet with parchment paper; set aside. In a large bowl whisk together the eggs, almond meal, 6 cloves of the minced garlic, 3 tablespoons of the wine, the paprika, 1½ teaspoons of the black pepper, the fennel seeds, oregano, thyme, and cayenne pepper. Add the pork; mix well. Shape pork mixture into 1½-inch meatballs (should have about 24 meatballs); arrange in a single layer on the prepared baking sheet. Bake about 30 minutes or until lightly browned, turning once while baking.

2. Meanwhile, for marinara sauce, in a 4- to 6-quart Dutch oven heat 1 tablespoon of the olive oil. Add the 2 remaining cloves minced garlic; cook about 1 minute or until just starting to brown. Quickly add the remaining 3 tablespoons wine, the crushed tomatoes, and the basil. Bring to boiling; reduce heat. Simmer, uncovered, for 5 minutes. Carefully stir the cooked meatballs into the marinara sauce. Cover and simmer for 25 to 30 minutes.

3. Meanwhile, in a large skillet heat the remaining 1 tablespoon olive oil over medium heat. Stir in the sliced fennel and onion. Cook for 8 to 10 minutes or until just tender and lightly browned, stirring frequently. Season with the remaining ½ teaspoon black pepper. Serve the meatballs and marinara sauce over the fennel and onion sauté.

PORK-STUFFED ZUCCHINI BOATS WITH BASIL AND PINE NUTS

PREP: 20 minutes   COOK: 22 minutes   BAKE: 20 minutes   MAKES: 4 servings

KIDS WILL LOVE THIS FUN-TO-EAT DISH OF HOLLOWED-OUT ZUCCHINI STUFFED WITH GROUND PORK, TOMATOES, AND SWEET PEPPERS. IF YOU LIKE, STIR IN 3 TABLESPOONS OF BASIL PESTO (PAGE 320) IN PLACE OF THE FRESH BASIL, PARSLEY, AND PINE NUTS.

2 medium zucchini
1 tablespoon extra virgin olive oil
12 ounces ground pork
¾ cup chopped onion
2 cloves garlic, minced
1 cup chopped tomatoes
⅔ cup finely chopped yellow or orange sweet pepper
1 teaspoon fennel seeds, lightly crushed
½ teaspoon crushed red pepper flakes
¼ cup snipped fresh basil
3 tablespoons snipped fresh parsley
2 tablespoons pine nuts, toasted (see tip, page 57) and coarsely chopped
1 teaspoon finely shredded lemon peel

1. Preheat oven to 350°F. Halve zucchini lengthwise and carefully scrape out the center, leaving ¼-inch-thick shell. Coarsely chop the zucchini pulp and set aside. Arrange zucchini halves, cut sides up, on a foil-lined baking sheet.

2. For filling, in a large skillet heat the olive oil over medium-high heat. Add ground pork; cook until no longer pink, stirring with a wooden spoon to break up meat. Drain off fat. Reduce heat to medium. Add the reserved zucchini pulp, onion, and garlic; cook and stir about 8 minutes or until onion is soft. Stir in the tomatoes, sweet pepper, fennel seeds, and crushed red pepper. Cook about 10 minutes or until tomatoes are soft and beginning to break down. Remove pan from heat. Stir in the basil, parsley, pine nuts, and lemon peel. Divide filling among zucchini shells, mounding slightly. Bake for 20 to 25 minutes or until zucchini shells are crisp-tender.

CURRIED PORK AND PINEAPPLE "NOODLE" BOWLS WITH COCONUT MILK AND HERBS

PREP: 30 minutes   COOK: 15 minutes   BAKE: 40 minutes   MAKES: 4 servings

THIS DISH PACKS A POWERFUL PUNCH—DUE IN LARGE PART TO THE COMPLEX FLAVORS AND HEAT OF THAI-STYLE RED CURRY POWDER. LOOK FOR A SALT-FREE VERSION AT ASIAN MARKETS OR SPECIALTY SHOPS. IT'S ALSO AVAILABLE ONLINE AT WWW.MYSPICESAGE.COM.

1 large spaghetti squash
2 tablespoons refined coconut oil
1 pound ground pork
2 tablespoons finely chopped scallions
2 tablespoons fresh lime juice
1 tablespoon minced fresh ginger
6 cloves garlic, minced
1 tablespoon minced lemongrass
1 tablespoon no-salt-added Thai-style red curry powder
1 cup chopped red sweet pepper
1 cup chopped onion
½ cup julienne-cut carrot
1 baby bok choy, sliced (3 cups)
1 cup sliced fresh button mushrooms
1 or 2 Thai bird chiles, thinly sliced (see tip, page 56)
1 13.5-ounce can natural coconut milk (such as Nature's Way)
½ cup Chicken Bone Broth (see recipe, page 235) or no-salt-added chicken broth
¼ cup fresh pineapple juice
3 tablespoons unsalted no-oil-added cashew butter
1 cup cubed fresh pineapple, cubed
  Lime wedges
  Fresh cilantro, mint, and/or Thai basil
  Chopped roasted cashews

1. Preheat oven to 400°F. Microwave spaghetti squash on high for 3 minutes. Carefully cut the squash in half lengthwise and scrape out the seeds. Rub 1 tablespoon of the coconut oil over the cut sides of the squash. Place squash halves, cut sides down, on a baking sheet. Bake for 40 to 50 minutes or until squash can be pierced easily with a knife. Using the tines of a fork, scrape the flesh from the shells and keep warm until ready to serve.

2. Meanwhile, in a medium bowl combine the pork, scallions, lime juice, ginger, garlic, lemongrass, and curry powder; mix well. In an extra-large skillet heat the remaining 1 tablespoon of the coconut oil over medium-high heat. Add pork mixture; cook until no longer pink, stirring with a wooden spoon to break up meat. Add the sweet pepper, onion, and carrot; cook and stir about 3 minutes or until vegetables are crisp-tender. Stir in the bok choy, mushrooms, chiles, coconut milk, Chicken Bone Broth, pineapple juice, and cashew butter. Bring to boiling; reduce heat. Add pineapple; simmer, uncovered, until heated through.

3. To serve, divide the spaghetti squash among four serving bowls. Ladle the curried pork over the squash. Serve with lime wedges, herbs, and cashews.

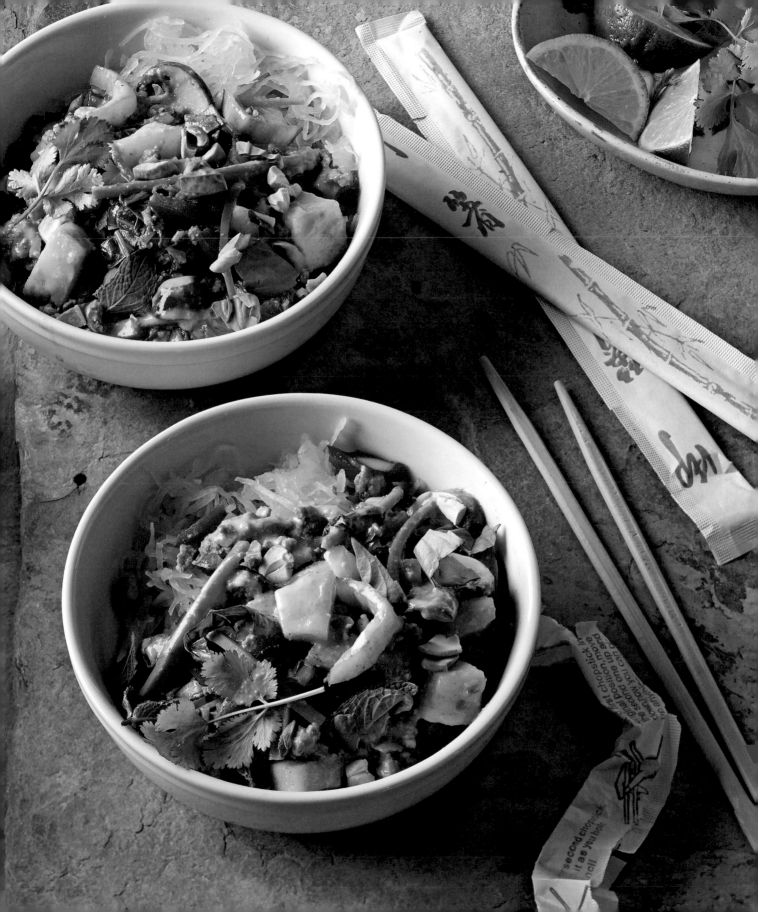

SPICY GRILLED PORK PATTIES WITH TANGY CUCUMBER SALAD

PREP: 30 minutes   GRILL: 10 minutes   STAND: 10 minutes   MAKES: 4 servings

THE CRUNCHY CUCUMBER SALAD FLAVORED WITH FRESH MINT IS A COOLING AND REFRESHING COMPLEMENT TO THE SPICY PORK BURGERS.

⅓ cup olive oil
¼ cup chopped fresh mint
3 tablespoons white wine vinegar
8 cloves garlic, minced
¼ teaspoon black pepper
2 medium cucumbers, very thinly sliced
1 small onion, cut into thin slivers (about ½ cup)
1¼ to 1½ pounds ground pork
¼ cup chopped fresh cilantro
1 to 2 medium fresh jalapeño or serrano chile peppers, seeded (if desired) and finely chopped (see tip, page 56)
2 medium red sweet peppers, seeded and quartered
2 teaspoons olive oil

1. In a large bowl whisk together ⅓ cup olive oil, mint, vinegar, 2 cloves minced garlic, and the black pepper. Add sliced cucumbers and onion. Toss until well coated. Cover and chill until ready to serve, stirring once or twice.

2. In a large bowl combine pork, cilantro, chile pepper, and the remaining 6 cloves minced garlic. Shape into four ¾-inch-thick patties. Brush pepper quarters lightly with the 2 teaspoons olive oil.

3. For a charcoal or gas grill, place patties and sweet pepper quarters directly over medium heat. Cover and grill until an instant-read thermometer inserted into sides of pork patties registers 160°F and pepper quarters are tender and lightly charred, turning patties and pepper quarters once halfway through grilling. Allow 10 to 12 minutes for patties and 8 to 10 minutes for the pepper quarters.

4. When pepper quarters are done, wrap them in a piece of foil to completely enclose. Let stand about 10 minutes or until cool enough to handle. Using a sharp knife, carefully peel off the pepper skins. Thinly slice pepper quarters lengthwise.

5. To serve, stir cucumber salad and spoon evenly onto four large serving plates. Add a pork patty to each plate. Pile the red pepper slices evenly on top of patties.

ZUCCHINI-CRUST PIZZA WITH SUN-DRIED TOMATO PESTO, SWEET PEPPERS, AND ITALIAN SAUSAGE

PREP: 30 minutes   COOK: 15 minutes   BAKE: 30 minutes   MAKES: 4 servings

THIS IS KNIFE-AND-FORK PIZZA. BE SURE TO PRESS THE SAUSAGE AND PEPPERS LIGHTLY INTO THE PESTO-COATED CRUST SO THAT THE TOPPINGS ADHERE ENOUGH FOR THE PIZZA TO CUT NEATLY.

2 tablespoons olive oil
1 tablespoon finely ground almonds
1 large egg, lightly beaten
½ cup almond flour
1 tablespoon snipped fresh oregano
¼ teaspoon black pepper
3 cloves garlic, minced
3½ cups shredded zucchini (2 medium)
Italian Sausage (see recipe, right)
1 tablespoon extra virgin olive oil
1 sweet pepper (yellow, red, or half of each), seeded and cut into very thin strips
1 small onion, thinly sliced
Sun-Dried Tomato Pesto (see recipe, right)

1. Preheat oven to 425°F. Brush a 12-inch pizza pan with the 2 tablespoons olive oil. Sprinkle with ground almonds; set aside.

2. For crust, in a large bowl combine egg, almond flour, oregano, black pepper, and garlic. Place shredded zucchini in a clean towel or piece of cheesecloth. Wrap tightly around zucchini and twist to wring out excess water. Repeat until no more water comes out of the zucchini. Add drained zucchini to bowl; mix well. Transfer zucchini mixture to the prepared pan and press to an even thickness to form a crust. Bake about 20 minutes or until golden. Using a thin spatula, loosen the crust from the pan (this keeps the crust from sticking to pan after adding toppings).

3. Meanwhile, in a large skillet cook Italian Sausage over medium-high heat about 5 minutes or until browned, stirring with a wooden spoon to break up meat as it cooks. Using a slotted spoon, transfer sausage to a plate lined with paper towels. Heat 1 tablespoon olive oil in the skillet. Add pepper strips and onion slices; cook over medium-low heat about 10 minutes or until onion slices are golden brown.

4. Spread Sun-Dried Tomato Pesto over crust. Top with sausage, pressing lightly into the pesto. Add pepper strips and onion, pressing lightly. Reduce oven temperature to 400°F. Bake about 10 minutes or until edges of crust are golden brown and pizza is heated through. Using a pizza wheel, cut into eight pieces.

Italian Sausage: In a large bowl combine 8 ounces ground pork; 2 teaspoons red wine vinegar; ¾ teaspoon dried parsley flakes; ¾ teaspoon garlic powder; ¾ teaspoon onion powder; ¾ teaspoon dried basil, crushed; ¾ teaspoon paprika; ½ teaspoon crushed red pepper; ½ teaspoon black pepper; ½ teaspoon fennel seeds; ⅛ teaspoon dried oregano, crushed; and ⅛ teaspoon dried thyme, crushed. Mix well.

Sun-Dried Tomato Pesto: In a small bowl cover ½ cup unsulfured, no-salt-added sun-dried tomatoes (not oil-packed) with boiling water. Cover and let stand about 10 minutes or until softened; drain. In a food processor combine the drained tomatoes, ½ cup fresh basil leaves, ¼ cup olive oil, and 1 clove garlic. Pulse until tomatoes are finely chopped. Season with ⅛ teaspoon black pepper.

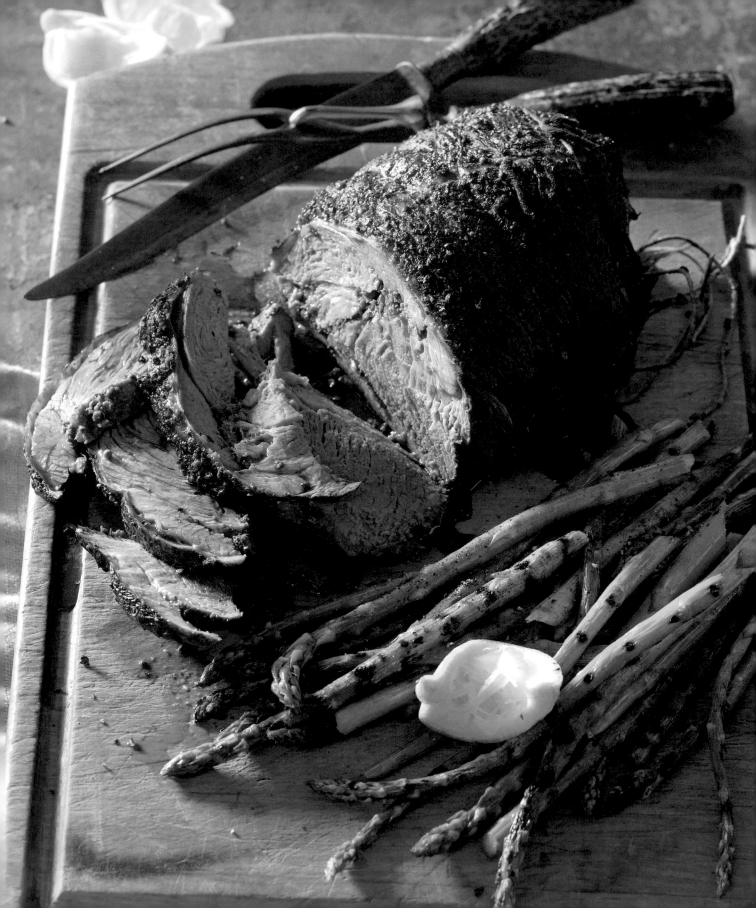

SMOKED LEMON-CORIANDER LAMB LEG WITH GRILLED ASPARAGUS

SOAK: 30 minutes   PREP: 20 minutes   GRILL: 45 minutes   STAND: 10 minutes   MAKES: 6 to 8 servings

SIMPLE BUT ELEGANT, THIS DISH FEATURES TWO INGREDIENTS THAT COME INTO THEIR OWN IN THE SPRING—LAMB AND ASPARAGUS. TOASTING THE CORIANDER SEEDS ENHANCES THE WARM, EARTHY, SLIGHTLY TANGY FLAVOR.

1 cup hickory wood chips
2 tablespoons coriander seeds
2 tablespoons finely shredded lemon peel
1½ teaspoons black pepper
2 tablespoons snipped fresh thyme
1 2- to 3-pound boneless leg of lamb
2 bunches fresh asparagus
1 tablespoon olive oil
¼ teaspoon black pepper
1 lemon, cut into quarters

1. At least 30 minutes before smoke-cooking, in a bowl soak hickory chips in enough water to cover; set aside. Meanwhile, in a small skillet toast coriander seeds over medium heat about 2 minutes or until fragrant and crackling, stirring frequently. Remove seeds from skillet; let cool. When seeds have cooled, coarsely crush in a mortar and pestle (or place seeds on a cutting board and crush them with the back of a wooden spoon). In a small bowl combine crushed coriander seeds, lemon peel, the 1½ teaspoons pepper, and thyme; set aside.

2. Remove netting from lamb roast if present. On a work surface open up the roast, fat side down. Sprinkle half of the spice mixture over meat; rub in with your fingers. Roll the roast up and tie with four to six pieces of 100%-cotton kitchen string. Sprinkle the remaining spice mixture over outside of roast, pressing lightly to adhere.

3. For a charcoal grill, arrange medium-hot coals around a drip pan. Test for medium heat above the pan. Sprinkle the drained wood chips over the coals. Place lamb roast on the grill rack over the drip pan. Cover and smoke for 40 to 50 minutes for medium (145°F). (For a gas grill, preheat grill. Reduce heat to medium. Adjust for indirect cooking. Smoke as above, except add drained wood chips according to manufacturer's directions.) Cover roast loosely with foil. Let stand for 10 minutes before slicing.

4. Meanwhile, trim woody ends from asparagus. In a large bowl toss asparagus with olive oil and the ¼ teaspoon pepper. Place asparagus around outer edges of grill, directly over the coals and perpendicular to the grill grate. Cover and grill for 5 to 6 minutes until crisp-tender. Squeeze lemon wedges over asparagus.

5. Remove string from lamb roast and thinly slice meat. Serve meat with grilled asparagus.

LAMB HOT POT

PREP: 30 minutes   COOK: 2 hours 40 minutes   MAKES: 4 servings

WARM UP WITH THIS SAVORY STEW ON A FALL OR WINTER NIGHT. THE STEW IS SERVED OVER A VELVETY CELERY ROOT-PARSNIP MASH FLAVORED WITH DIJON-STYLE MUSTARD, CASHEW CREAM, AND CHIVES. NOTE: CELERY ROOT IS SOMETIMES CALLED CELERIAC.

10 black peppercorns

6 sage leaves

3 whole allspice

2 2-inch strips orange peel

2 pounds boneless lamb shoulder

3 tablespoons olive oil

2 medium onions, coarsely chopped

1 14.5-ounce can no-salt-added diced tomatoes, undrained

1½ cups Beef Bone Broth (see recipe, page 131) or no-salt-added beef broth

¾ cup dry white wine

3 large cloves garlic, crushed and peeled

2 pounds celery root, peeled and cut into 1-inch cubes

6 medium parsnips, peeled and cut into 1-inch slices (about 2 pounds)

2 tablespoons olive oil

2 tablespoons Cashew Cream (see recipe, page 327)

1 tablespoon Dijon-Style Mustard (see recipe, page 322)

¼ cup snipped chives

1. For the bouquet garni, cut a 7-inch square of cheesecloth. Place peppercorns, sage, allspice, and orange peel in center of cheesecloth. Bring up the corners of the cheesecloth and tie securely with clean 100%-cotton kitchen string. Set aside.

2. Trim fat from lamb shoulder; cut lamb into 1-inch pieces. In a Dutch oven heat the 3 tablespoons olive oil over medium heat. Cook lamb, in batches if necessary, in hot oil until browned; remove from pan and keep warm. Add onions to pan; cook for 5 to 8 minutes or until softened and lightly browned. Add bouquet garni, undrained tomatoes, 1¼ cups of the Beef Bone Broth, wine, and garlic. Bring to boiling; reduce heat. Simmer, covered, for 2 hours, stirring occasionally. Remove and discard bouquet garni.

3. Meanwhile, for mash, place celery root and parsnips in a large stockpot; cover with water. Bring to boiling over medium-high heat; reduce heat to low. Cover and simmer gently for 30 to 40 minutes or until the vegetables are very tender when pierced with a fork. Drain; place vegetables in a food processor. Add the remaining ¼ cup Beef Bone Broth and the 2 tablespoons oil; pulse until mash is almost smooth but still has some texture, stopping once or twice to scrape down the sides. Transfer mash to a bowl. Stir in Cashew Cream, mustard, and chives.

4. To serve, divide mash among four bowls; top with Lamb Hot Pot.

LAMB STEW WITH CELERY-ROOT NOODLES

PREP: 30 minutes   BAKE: 1 hour 30 minutes   MAKES: 6 servings

CELERY ROOT TAKES AN ENTIRELY DIFFERENT FORM IN THIS STEW THAN IT DOES IN THE LAMB HOT POT, OPPOSITE. A MANDOLINE SLICER IS USED TO CREATE VERY THIN STRIPS OF THE SWEET AND NUTTY-TASTING ROOT. THE "NOODLES" SIMMER IN THE STEW UNTIL THEY ARE TENDER.

2 teaspoons Lemon-Herb Seasoning (see recipe, page 324)

1½ pounds lamb stew meat, cut into 1-inch cubes

2 tablespoons olive oil

2 cups chopped onions

1 cup chopped carrots

1 cup diced turnips

1 tablespoon minced garlic (6 cloves)

2 tablespoons no-salt-added tomato paste

½ cup dry red wine

4 cups Beef Bone Broth (see recipe, page 131) or no-salt-added beef broth

1 bay leaf

2 cups 1-inch cubes butternut squash

1 cup diced eggplant

1 pound celery root, peeled
Chopped fresh parsley

1. Preheat oven to 250°F. Sprinkle Lemon-Herb Seasoning evenly over lamb. Toss gently to coat. Heat a 6- to 8-quart Dutch oven over medium-high heat. Add 1 tablespoon of the olive oil and half of the seasoned lamb to the Dutch oven. Brown meat in hot oil on all sides; transfer browned meat to a plate and repeat with remaining lamb and olive oil. Reduce heat to medium.

2. Add onions, carrots, and turnips to pot. Cook and stir vegetables for 4 minutes; add garlic and tomato paste and cook 1 minute more. Add red wine, Beef Bone Broth, bay leaf, and reserved meat and any accumulated juices to pot. Bring mixture to a simmer. Cover and place Dutch oven in preheated oven. Bake for 1 hour. Stir in butternut squash and eggplant. Return to oven and bake for an additional 30 minutes.

3. While stew is in oven, use a mandoline to very thinly slice celery root. Cut celery root slices into ½-inch-wide strips. (You should have about 4 cups.) Stir celery root strips into stew. Simmer about 10 minutes or until tender. Remove and discard bay leaf before serving stew. Sprinkle each serving with chopped parsley.

Frenched Lamb Chops with
Pomegranate-Date Chutney,
recipe page 176

Spiced Carrot Slaw,
recipe page 315

FRENCHED LAMB CHOPS WITH POMEGRANATE-DATE CHUTNEY

pictured on page 174

PREP: 10 minutes   COOK: 18 minutes   COOL: 10 minutes   MAKES: 4 servings

THE TERM "FRENCHED" REFERS TO A RIB BONE FROM WHICH FAT, MEAT, AND CONNECTIVE TISSUE HAVE BEEN REMOVED WITH A SHARP PARING KNIFE. IT MAKES FOR AN ATTRACTIVE PRESENTATION. ASK YOUR BUTCHER TO DO IT OR YOU CAN DO IT YOURSELF.

CHUTNEY

- ½ cup unsweetened pomegranate juice
- 1 tablespoon fresh lemon juice
- 1 shallot, peeled and thinly sliced into rings
- 1 teaspoon finely shredded orange peel
- ⅓ cup chopped Medjool dates
- ¼ teaspoon crushed red pepper
- ¼ cup pomegranate arils*
- 1 tablespoon olive oil
- 1 tablespoon chopped fresh Italian (flat-leaf) parsley

LAMB CHOPS

- 2 tablespoons olive oil
- 8 frenched lamb rib chops

1. For the chutney, in a small skillet combine pomegranate juice, lemon juice, and shallot. Bring to boiling; reduce heat. Simmer, uncovered, for 2 minutes. Add orange peel, dates, and crushed red pepper. Let stand until cool, about 10 minutes. Stir in pomegranate arils, the 1 tablespoon olive oil, and the parsley. Set aside at room temperature until serving time.

2. For the chops, in a large skillet heat the 2 tablespoons olive oil over medium heat. Working in batches, add chops to skillet and cook for 6 to 8 minutes for medium rare (145°F), turning once. Top chops with chutney.

*Note: Fresh pomegranates and their arils, or seeds, are available from October through February. If you can't find them, use unsweetened dried seeds to add crunch to the chutney.

CHIMICHURRI LAMB LOIN CHOPS WITH SAUTÉED RADICCHIO SLAW

PREP: **30 minutes**   MARINATE: **20 minutes**   COOK: **20 minutes**   MAKES: **4 servings**

IN ARGENTINA, CHIMICHURRI IS THE MOST POPULAR CONDIMENT ACCOMPANYING THAT COUNTRY'S RENOWNED GAUCHO-STYLE GRILLED STEAK. THERE ARE LOTS OF VARIATIONS, BUT THE THICK HERB SAUCE IS USUALLY BUILT AROUND PARSLEY, CILANTRO OR OREGANO, SHALLOTS AND/OR GARLIC, CRUSHED RED PEPPER, OLIVE OIL, AND RED WINE VINEGAR. IT'S GREAT ON GRILLED STEAK BUT EQUALLY BRILLIANT ON ROASTED OR PAN-SEARED LAMB CHOPS, CHICKEN, AND PORK.

8 lamb loin chops, cut 1 inch thick
½ cup Chimichurri Sauce (see recipe, page 323)
2 tablespoons olive oil
1 sweet onion, halved and sliced
1 teaspoon cumin seeds, crushed*
1 clove garlic, minced
1 head radicchio, cored and sliced into thin ribbons
1 tablespoon balsamic vinegar

1. Place lamb chops in an extra-large bowl. Drizzle with 2 tablespoons of the Chimichurri Sauce. Using your fingers, rub the sauce over the entire surface of each chop. Let chops marinate at room temperature for 20 minutes.

2. Meanwhile, for sautéed radicchio slaw, in an extra-large skillet heat 1 tablespoon of the olive oil. Add onion, cumin seeds, and garlic; cook for 6 to 7 minutes or until onion softens, stirring frequently. Add radicchio; cook for 1 to 2 minutes or until radicchio just wilts slightly. Transfer slaw to a large bowl. Add balsamic vinegar and toss well to combine. Cover and keep warm.

3. Wipe out skillet. Add the remaining 1 tablespoon olive oil to the skillet and heat over medium-high heat. Add the lamb chops; reduce heat to medium. Cook for 9 to 11 minutes or until desired doneness, turning chops occasionally with tongs.

4. Serve chops with slaw and the remaining Chimichurri Sauce.

***Note:** To crush cumin seeds, use a mortar and pestle—or place seeds on a cutting board and crush with a chef's knife.

ANCHO-AND-SAGE-RUBBED LAMB CHOPS WITH CARROT-SWEET POTATO REMOULADE

PREP: 12 minutes   CHILL: 1 to 2 hours   GRILL: 6 minutes   MAKES: 4 servings

THERE ARE THREE TYPES OF LAMB CHOPS. THICK AND MEATY LOIN CHOPS LOOK LIKE SMALL T-BONE STEAKS. RIB CHOPS—CALLED FOR HERE—ARE CREATED BY CUTTING BETWEEN THE BONES OF A RACK OF LAMB. THEY ARE VERY TENDER AND HAVE A LONG, ATTRACTIVE BONE ON THE SIDE. THEY ARE OFTEN SERVED PAN-SEARED OR GRILLED. BUDGET-FRIENDLY SHOULDER CHOPS ARE A BIT FATTIER AND LESS TENDER THAN THE OTHER TWO TYPES. THEY ARE BEST BROWNED AND THEN BRAISED IN WINE, STOCK, AND TOMATOES—OR SOME COMBINATION OF THEM.

3 medium carrots, coarsely shredded

2 small sweet potatoes, julienne-cut* or coarsely shredded

½ cup Paleo Mayo (see recipe, page 323)

2 tablespoons fresh lemon juice

2 teaspoons Dijon-Style Mustard (see recipe, page 322)

2 tablespoons snipped fresh parsley

½ teaspoon black pepper

8 lamb rib chops, cut ½ to ¾ inch thick

2 tablespoon snipped fresh sage or 2 teaspoons dried sage, crushed

2 teaspoons ground ancho chile pepper

½ teaspoon garlic powder

1. For the remoulade, in a medium bowl combine carrots and sweet potatoes. In a small bowl stir together Paleo Mayo, lemon juice, Dijon-Style Mustard, parsley, and black pepper. Pour over carrots and sweet potatoes; toss to coat. Cover and chill for 1 to 2 hours.

2. Meanwhile, in a small bowl combine sage, ancho chile, and garlic powder. Rub spice mixture onto lamb chops.

3. For a charcoal or gas grill, place lamb chops on a grill rack directly over medium heat. Cover and grill for 6 to 8 minutes for medium rare (145°F) or 10 to 12 minutes for medium (150°F), turning once halfway through grilling.

4. Serve the lamb chops with the remoulade.

***Note:** Use a mandoline with a julienne attachment to cut the sweet potatoes.

LAMB CHOPS WITH SHALLOT, MINT, AND OREGANO RUB

PREP: 20 minutes   MARINATE: 1 to 24 hours   ROAST: 40 minutes   GRILL: 12 minutes   MAKES: 4 servings

AS WITH MOST MARINATED MEATS, THE LONGER YOU LEAVE THE HERB RUB ON THE LAMB CHOPS BEFORE COOKING, THE MORE FLAVORFUL THEY WILL BE. THERE IS AN EXCEPTION TO THIS RULE, AND THAT IS WHEN YOU ARE USING A MARINADE THAT CONTAINS HIGHLY ACIDIC INGREDIENTS SUCH AS CITRUS JUICE, VINEGAR, AND WINE. IF YOU LET THE MEAT SIT IN AN ACIDIC MARINADE TOO LONG, IT BEGINS TO BREAK DOWN AND GET MUSHY.

LAMB
- 2 tablespoons finely chopped shallot
- 2 tablespoons finely chopped fresh mint
- 2 tablespoons finely chopped fresh oregano
- 5 teaspoons Mediterranean Seasoning (see recipe, page 324)
- 4 teaspoons olive oil
- 2 cloves garlic, minced
- 8 lamb rib chops, cut about 1 inch thick

SALAD
- ¾ pound baby beets, trimmed
- 1 tablespoon olive oil
- ¼ cup fresh lemon juice
- ¼ cup olive oil
- 1 tablespoon finely chopped shallot
- 1 teaspoon Dijon-Style Mustard (see recipe, page 322)
- 6 cups mixed greens
- 4 teaspoons snipped chives

1. For the lamb, in a small bowl combine 2 tablespoons shallot, mint, oregano, 4 teaspoons of the Mediterranean seasoning, and 4 teaspoons olive oil. Sprinkle rub over all sides of the lamb chops; rub in with your fingers. Place chops on a plate; cover with plastic wrap and refrigerate for at least 1 hour or up to 24 hours to marinate.

2. For salad, preheat oven to 400°F. Scrub beets well; cut into wedges. Place in a 2-quart baking dish. Drizzle with the 1 tablespoon olive oil. Cover dish with foil. Roast about 40 minutes or until beets are tender. Cool completely. (Beets can be roasted up to 2 days ahead.)

3. In a screw-top jar combine lemon juice, ¼ cup olive oil, 1 tablespoon shallot, Dijon-Style Mustard, and the remaining 1 teaspoon Mediterranean Seasoning. Cover and shake well. In a salad bowl combine beets and greens; toss with some of the vinaigrette.

4. For a charcoal or gas grill, place chops on the greased grill rack directly over medium heat. Cover and grill to desired doneness, turning once halfway through grilling. Allow 12 to 14 minutes for medium rare (145°F) or 15 to 17 minutes for medium (160°F).

5. To serve, place 2 lamb chops and some of the salad on each of four serving plates. Sprinkle with chives. Pass remaining vinaigrette.

GARDEN-STUFFED LAMB BURGERS WITH RED PEPPER COULIS

PREP: 20 minutes   STAND: 15 minutes   GRILL: 27 minutes   MAKES: 4 servings

A COULIS IS NOTHING MORE THAN A SIMPLE, SMOOTH SAUCE MADE FROM PUREED FRUITS OR VEGETABLES. THE BRIGHT AND BEAUTIFUL RED PEPPER SAUCE FOR THESE LAMB BURGERS GETS A DOUBLE DOSE OF SMOKE—FROM GRILLING AND FROM A SHOT OF SMOKED PAPRIKA.

RED PEPPER COULIS

- 1 large red sweet pepper
- 1 tablespoon dry white wine or white wine vinegar
- 1 teaspoon olive oil
- ½ teaspoon smoked paprika

BURGERS

- ¼ cup snipped unsulfured dried tomatoes
- ¼ cup shredded zucchini
- 1 tablespoon snipped fresh basil
- 2 teaspoons olive oil
- ½ teaspoon black pepper
- 1½ pounds ground lamb
- 1 egg white, lightly beaten
- 1 tablespoon Mediterranean Seasoning (see recipe, page 324)

1. For the red pepper coulis, place the red pepper on the grill rack directly over medium heat. Cover and grill for 15 to 20 minutes or until charred and very tender, turning the pepper about every 5 minutes to char each side. Remove from the grill and immediately place in a paper bag or foil to completely enclose the pepper. Let stand for 15 minutes or until cool enough to handle. Using a sharp knife, gently pull off skins and discard. Quarter pepper lengthwise and remove stems, seeds, and membranes. In a food processor combine the roasted pepper, wine, olive oil, and smoked paprika. Cover and process or blend until smooth.

2. Meanwhile, for the filling, place dried tomatoes in a small bowl and cover with boiling water. Let stand for 5 minutes; drain. Pat tomatoes and shredded zucchini dry with paper towels. In the small bowl stir together tomatoes, zucchini, basil, olive oil, and ¼ teaspoon of the black pepper; set aside.

3. In a large bowl combine ground lamb, egg white, remaining ¼ teaspoon black pepper, and Mediterranean Seasoning; mix well. Divide meat mixture into eight equal portions and shape each into a ¼-inch-thick patty. Spoon filling onto four of the patties; top with remaining patties and pinch edges to seal in the filling.

4. Place patties on the grill rack directly over medium heat. Cover and grill for 12 to 14 minutes or until done (160°F), turning once halfway through grilling.

5. To serve, top burgers with red pepper coulis.

DOUBLE-OREGANO LAMB KABOBS WITH TZATZIKI SAUCE

SOAK: 30 minutes   PREP: 20 minutes   CHILL: 30 minutes   GRILL: 8 minutes   MAKES: 4 servings

THESE LAMB KABOBS ARE ESSENTIALLY WHAT IS KNOWN AS KOFTA IN THE MEDITERRANEAN AND MIDDLE EAST—SEASONED GROUND MEAT (USUALLY LAMB OR BEEF) IS SHAPED INTO BALLS OR AROUND A SKEWER AND THEN GRILLED. FRESH AND DRIED OREGANO GIVE THEM GREAT GREEK FLAVOR.

8 10-inch wooden skewers

LAMB KABOBS
1½ pounds lean ground lamb
1 small onion, shredded and squeezed dry
1 tablespoon snipped fresh oregano
2 teaspoon dried oregano, crushed
1 teaspoon black pepper

TZATZIKI SAUCE
1 cup Paleo Mayo (see recipe, page 323)
½ of a large cucumber, seeded and shredded and squeezed dry
2 tablespoons fresh lemon juice
1 clove garlic, minced

1. Soak skewers in enough water to cover for 30 minutes.

2. For lamb kabobs, in a large bowl combine ground lamb, onion, fresh and dried oregano, and pepper; mix well. Divide the lamb mixture into eight equal portions. Shape each portion around half of a skewer, creating a 5×1-inch log. Cover and chill for at least 30 minutes.

3. Meanwhile, for Tzatziki Sauce, in a small bowl combine Paleo Mayo, cucumber, lemon juice, and garlic. Cover and chill until serving.

4. For a charcoal or gas grill, place lamb kabobs on grill rack directly over medium heat. Cover and grill about 8 minutes for medium (160°F), turning once halfway through grilling.

5. Serve lamb kabobs with Tzatziki Sauce.

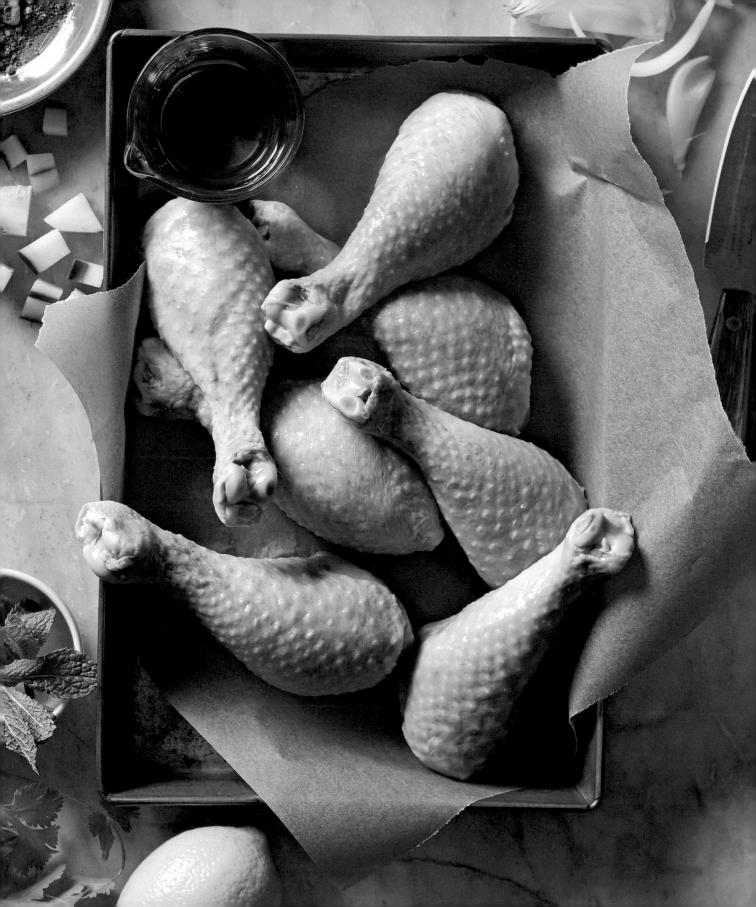

POULTRY

For many novice Paleo dieters, poultry dishes usually mean chicken, turkey, and maybe game hens. Other slightly more exotic poultry possibilities exist—particularly if you want to branch out a bit from the mainstream. Don't forget that ducks, geese, pheasant, quail, dove, partridges, ostrich, and emu fall into this appetizing meat category and that these items can sometimes be found in the frozen food sections of grocery stores, ordered through your local butcher, and via online specialty stores—but also know that they are pricey.

Two national suppliers specializing in exotic poultry are Exotic Meats (www.exoticmeatsandmore.com) and D'Artagnan, LLC (www.dartagnan.com).

Don't feel obligated to utilize exotic poultry in your day-to-day recipes and dishes, but realize that for special occasions, you may want to replace chicken or turkey with pheasant, quail, or duck. You can save money by finding local farmers who produce free-ranging birds that have access to grass fields, ponds, insects, and bugs. Look into Jo Robinson's website (www.eatwild.com) to find a farmer or producer of grass-fed chickens, turkeys, and birds in your vicinity.

Since poultry is comparatively inexpensive, chicken and turkey make some of the best high-protein, low-cost staples you can include in your Paleo diet. From a culinary perspective, chicken, with its tender white meat and savory dark legs, is a mealtime favorite that almost every diner—from refined epicureans to fussy youngsters—enjoys. The recipes in this chapter will quickly help you to learn how to skillfully prepare delicious poultry dishes that are fully Paleo.

Chicken can be included into a vast assortment of dishes because it doesn't overpower the flavors of vegetables and other ingredients. Sample some of these delectable Paleo recipes and you will begin to immediately understand that salt-free, additive-free, and cereal-free poultry dishes can easily be prepared and incorporated into meals that don't put you and your family at risk for heart disease, diabetes, or any other chronic disease.

As a child growing up in the 1950s and early 1960s, it was customary for our family to have chicken for Sunday dinners. I'm not exactly sure why we did this, but Sunday chicken dinners were my parents' norm. From my earliest memories, Mom baked chicken breasts, legs, and wings—all breading-free and with skins intact—for Sunday dinner. We loved them. Fifty years later, this simple cooking method tastes best to me, and I now know simulates Stone Age cooking done over glowing coals. As a contemporary Paleo cook, follow your culinary instincts but make sure that you prepare poultry—and any other dish—in a manner that deemphasizes added salt, sugars, grains, or any other non-Paleo ingredient. By following these simple guidelines, you will make lifelong nutritional choices that are consistent with the evolutionary heritage of our hunter-gatherer ancestors.

ROAST CHICKEN WITH SAFFRON AND LEMON

PREP: 15 minutes   CHILL: 8 hours   ROAST: 1 hour 15 minutes   STAND: 10 minutes   MAKES: 4 servings

SAFFRON IS THE DRIED STAMENS OF A TYPE OF CROCUS FLOWER. IT IS PRICEY, BUT A LITTLE GOES A LONG WAY. IT ADDS ITS EARTHY, DISTINCTIVE FLAVOR AND GORGEOUS YELLOW HUE TO THIS CRISP-SKINNED ROAST CHICKEN.

1   4- to 5-pound whole chicken
3   tablespoons olive oil
6   cloves garlic, crushed and peeled
1½   tablespoons finely shredded lemon peel
1   tablespoon fresh thyme
1½   teaspoons cracked black pepper
½   teaspoon saffron threads
2   bay leaves
1   lemon, quartered

1. Remove neck and giblets from chicken; discard or save for another use. Rinse chicken body cavity; pat dry with paper towels. Snip any excess skin or fat from chicken.

2. In a food processor combine olive oil, garlic, lemon peel, thyme, pepper, and saffron. Process to form a smooth paste.

3. Using fingers, rub paste over the outside surface of the chicken and the inside cavity. Transfer chicken to a large bowl; cover and refrigerate for at least 8 hours or overnight.

4. Preheat oven to 425°F. Place lemon quarters and bay leaves in chicken cavity. Tie legs together with 100%-cotton kitchen string. Tuck wings under chicken. Insert an oven-going meat thermometer into the inside thigh muscle without touching bone. Place chicken on a rack in a large roasting pan.

5. Roast for 15 minutes. Reduce oven temperature to 375°F. Roast about 1 hour more or until juices run clear and thermometer registers 175°F. Tent chicken with foil. Let stand for 10 minutes before carving.

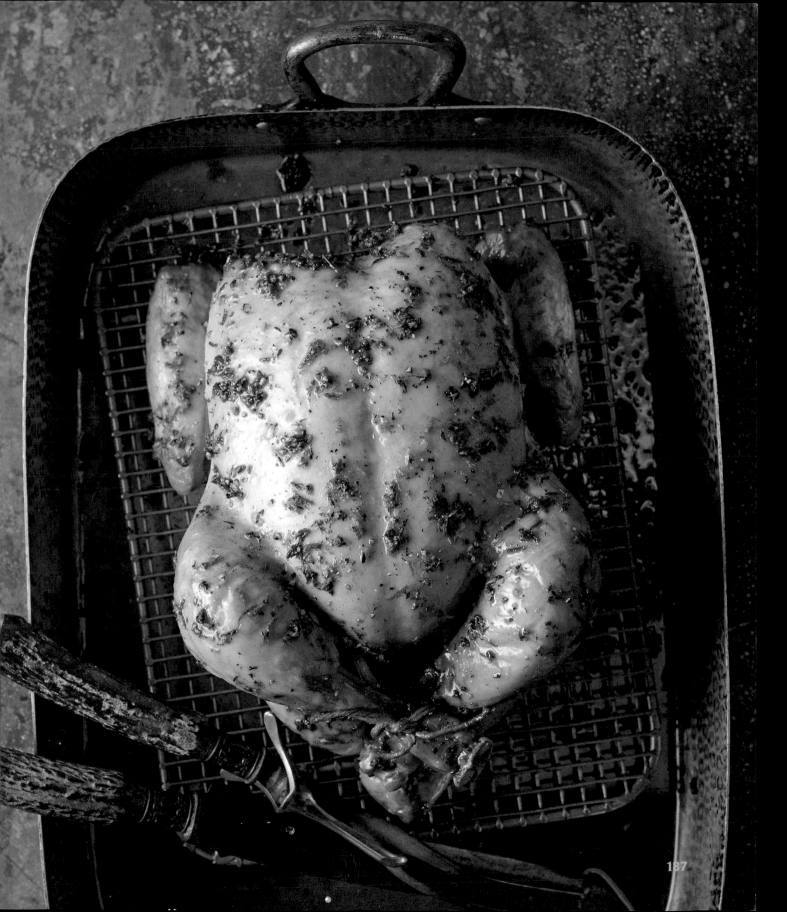

SPATCHCOCKED CHICKEN WITH JICAMA SLAW

PREP: 40 minutes   GRILL: 1 hour 5 minutes   STAND: 10 minutes   MAKES: 4 servings

"SPATCHCOCK" IS AN OLD COOKING TERM THAT'S RECENTLY COME BACK INTO USE TO DESCRIBE THE PROCESS OF SPLITTING A SMALL BIRD—SUCH AS A CHICKEN OR CORNISH HEN— DOWN THE BACK AND THEN OPENING IT AND FLATTENING IT LIKE A BOOK TO HELP IT COOK QUICKLY AND MORE EVENLY. IT'S SIMILAR TO BUTTERFLYING BUT REFERS ONLY TO POULTRY.

CHICKEN

- 1 poblano chile
- 1 tablespoon finely chopped shallot
- 3 cloves garlic, minced
- 1 teaspoon finely shredded lemon peel
- 1 teaspoon finely shredded lime peel
- 1 teaspoon Smoky Seasoning (see recipe, page 324)
- ½ teaspoon dried oregano, crushed
- ½ teaspoon ground cumin
- 1 tablespoon olive oil
- 1 3- to 3½–pound whole chicken

SLAW

- ½ of a medium jicama, peeled and cut into julienne strips (about 3 cups)
- ½ cup thinly sliced scallions (4)
- 1 Granny Smith apple, peeled, cored, and cut into julienne strips
- ⅓ cup snipped fresh cilantro
- 3 tablespoons fresh orange juice
- 3 tablespoons olive oil
- 1 teaspoon Lemon-Herb Seasoning (see recipe, page 324)

1. For a charcoal grill, arrange medium hot coals on one side of the grill. Place a drip pan under the empty side of the grill. Place poblano on the grill rack directly over medium coals. Cover and grill for 15 minutes or until the poblano is charred on all sides, turning occasionally. Immediately wrap poblano in foil; let stand for 10 minutes. Open foil and cut poblano in half lengthwise; remove stems and seeds (see tip, page 56). Using a sharp knife, gently peel off skin and discard. Finely chop the poblano. (For a gas grill, preheat grill; reduce heat to medium. Adjust for indirect cooking. Grill as above over burner that is turned on.)

2. For the rub, in a small bowl combine poblano, shallot, garlic, lemon peel, lime peel, Smoky Seasoning, oregano, and cumin. Stir in oil; mix well to make a paste.

3. To spatchcock the chicken, remove the neck and giblets from chicken (save for another use). Place the chicken, breast side down, on a cutting board. Use kitchen shears to make a lengthwise cut down one side of the backbone, starting from the neck end. Repeat the lengthwise cut to opposite side of the backbone. Remove and discard the backbone. Turn chicken skin side up. Press down between the breasts to break the breast bone so the chicken lies flat.

4. Starting at the neck on one side of the breast, slip your fingers between skin and meat, loosening skin as you work toward the thigh. Free the skin around the thigh. Repeat on the other side. Use your fingers to spread rub over the meat under the skin of the chicken.

5. Place chicken, breast side down, on grill rack over drip pan. Weight with two foil-wrapped bricks or a large cast-iron skillet. Cover and grill for 30 minutes. Turn chicken, bone side down, on rack, weighting again with bricks or skillet. Grill, covered, about 30 minutes more or until chicken is no longer pink (175°F in thigh muscle). Remove chicken from grill; let stand for 10 minutes. (For a gas grill, place chicken on grill rack away from heat. Grill as above.)

6. Meanwhile, for the slaw, in a large bowl combine jicama, scallions, apple, and cilantro. In a small bowl whisk together orange juice, oil, and Lemon-Herb Seasoning. Pour over the jicama mixture and toss to coat. Serve chicken with the slaw.

ROASTED CHICKEN HINDQUARTERS WITH VODKA, CARROT, AND TOMATO SAUCE

PREP: 15 minutes   COOK: 15 minutes   ROAST: 30 minutes   MAKES: 4 servings

VODKA CAN BE MADE FROM SEVERAL DIFFERENT FOODSTUFFS, INCLUDING POTATOES, CORN, RYE, WHEAT, AND BARLEY—EVEN GRAPES. ALTHOUGH THERE ISN'T MUCH VODKA IN THIS SAUCE WHEN YOU DIVIDE IT AMONG FOUR SERVINGS, LOOK FOR VOKDA MADE FROM EITHER POTATOES OR GRAPES TO BE PALEO COMPLIANT.

3 tablespoons olive oil

4 bone-in chicken hindquarters or meaty chicken pieces, skinned

1 28-ounce can no-salt-added plum tomatoes, drained

½ cup finely chopped onion

½ cup finely chopped carrot

3 cloves garlic, minced

1 teaspoon Mediterranean Seasoning (see recipe, page 324)

⅛ teaspoon cayenne pepper

1 sprig fresh rosemary

2 tablespoons vodka

1 tablespoon snipped fresh basil (optional)

1. Preheat oven to 375°F. In an extra-large skillet heat 2 tablespoons of the oil over medium-high heat. Add chicken; cook about 12 minutes or until browned, turning to brown evenly. Place skillet in the preheated oven. Roast, uncovered, for 20 minutes.

2. Meanwhile, for sauce, use kitchen scissors to cut up the tomatoes. In a medium saucepan heat the remaining 1 tablespoon oil over medium heat. Add onion, carrot, and garlic; cook for 3 minutes or until tender, stirring frequently. Stir in snipped tomatoes, Mediterranean Seasoning, cayenne pepper, and rosemary sprig. Bring to boiling over medium-high heat; reduce heat. Simmer, uncovered, for 10 minutes, stirring occasionally. Stir in vodka; cook 1 minute more; remove and discard rosemary sprig.

3. Ladle sauce over chicken in skillet. Return skillet to oven. Roast, covered, about 10 minutes more or until chicken is tender and no longer pink (175°F). If desired, sprinkle with basil.

POULET RÔTI AND RUTABAGA FRITES

PREP: 40 minutes   BAKE: 40 minutes   MAKES: 4 servings

THE CRISP RUTABAGA FRITES ARE DELICIOUS SERVED WITH THE ROASTED CHICKEN AND ITS ATTENDANT COOKING JUICES—BUT THEY ARE EQUALLY TASTY MADE ON THEIR OWN AND SERVED WITH PALEO KETCHUP (PAGE 322) OR SERVED BELGIAN-STYLE WITH PALEO AÏOLI (GARLIC MAYO, PAGE 323).

6   tablespoons olive oil
1   tablespoon Mediterranean Seasoning (see recipe, page 324)
4   bone-in chicken thighs, skinned (about 1 ¼ pounds total)
4   chicken drumsticks, skinned (about 1 pound total)
1   cup dry white wine
1   cup Chicken Bone Broth (see recipe, page 235) or no-salt-added chicken broth
1   small onion, quartered
     Olive oil
1½   to 2 pounds rutabagas
2   tablespoons snipped fresh chives
     Black pepper

1. Preheat oven to 400°F. In a small bowl combine 1 tablespoon of the olive oil and the Mediterranean Seasoning; rub onto chicken pieces. In an extra-large oven-going skillet heat 2 tablespoons of the oil. Add chicken pieces, meaty sides down. Cook, uncovered, about 5 minutes or until browned. Remove skillet from heat. Turn chicken pieces, browned sides up. Add wine, Chicken Bone Broth, and onion.

2. Place skillet in oven on middle rack. Bake, uncovered, for 10 minutes.

3. Meanwhile, for frites, lightly brush a large baking sheet with olive oil; set aside. Peel rutabagas. Using a sharp knife, cut rutabagas into ½-inch slices. Cut slices lengthwise into ½-inch strips. In a large bowl toss rutabaga strips with the remaining 3 tablespoons oil. Spread rutabaga strips in a single layer on prepared baking sheet; place in oven on top rack. Bake for 15 minutes; turn frites over. Bake chicken for 10 minutes more or until no longer pink (175°F). Remove chicken from oven. Bake frites 5 to 10 minutes or until browned and tender.

4. Remove chicken and onion from skillet, reserving juices. Cover chicken and onion to keep warm. Bring juices to boiling over medium heat; reduce heat. Simmer, uncovered, about 5 minutes more or until juices are slightly reduced.

5. To serve, toss frites with chives and season with pepper. Serve chicken with cooking juices and frites.

TRIPLE-MUSHROOM COQ AU VIN WITH CHIVE MASHED RUTABAGAS

PREP: 15 minutes   COOK: 1 hour 15 minutes   MAKES: 4 to 6 servings

IF THERE IS ANY GRIT IN THE BOWL AFTER SOAKING THE DRIED MUSHROOMS—AND IT IS LIKELY THAT THERE WILL BE—STRAIN THE LIQUID THROUGH A DOUBLE THICKNESS OF CHEESECLOTH SET IN A FINE-MESH STRAINER.

1   ounce dried porcini or morel
    mushrooms
1   cup boiling water
2   to 2½ pounds chicken thighs
    and drumsticks, skinned
    Black pepper
2   tablespoons olive oil
2   medium leeks, halved
    lengthwise, rinsed, and thinly
    sliced
2   portobello mushrooms, sliced
8   ounces fresh oyster
    mushrooms, stemmed and
    sliced, or sliced fresh button
    mushrooms
¼   cup no-salt-added tomato paste
1   teaspoon dried marjoram,
    crushed
½   teaspoon dried thyme, crushed
½   cup dry red wine
6   cups Chicken Bone Broth (see
    recipe, page 235) or no-salt-
    added chicken broth
2   bay leaves
2   to 2½ pounds rutabagas, peeled
    and chopped
2   tablespoons snipped fresh
    chives
½   teaspoon black pepper
    Snipped fresh thyme (optional)

1. In a small bowl combine the porcini mushrooms and the boiling water; let stand for 15 minutes. Remove mushrooms, reserving the soaking liquid. Chop the mushrooms. Set the mushrooms and soaking liquid aside.

2. Sprinkle chicken with pepper. In an extra-large skillet with a tight-fitting lid heat 1 tablespoon of the olive oil over medium-high heat. Cook chicken pieces, in two batches, in hot oil about 15 minutes until lightly browned, turning once. Remove chicken from the skillet. Stir in leeks, portobello mushrooms, and oyster mushrooms. Cook for 4 to 5 minutes or just until mushrooms start to brown, stirring occasionally. Stir in tomato paste, marjoram, and thyme; cook and stir for 1 minute. Stir in wine; cook and stir for 1 minute. Stir in 3 cups of the Chicken Bone Broth, bay leaves, ½ cup of the reserved mushroom soaking liquid, and rehydrated chopped mushrooms. Return chicken to skillet. Bring to boiling; reduce heat. Simmer, covered, about 45 minutes or until chicken is tender, turning the chicken once halfway through cooking.

3. Meanwhile, in a large saucepan combine rutabagas and the remaining 3 cups broth. If necessary, add water to just cover rutabagas. Bring to boiling; reduce heat. Simmer, uncovered, for 25 to 30 minutes or until rutabagas are tender, stirring occasionally. Drain rutabagas, reserving liquid. Return rutabagas to the saucepan. Add the remaining 1 tablespoon olive oil, the chives, and the ½ teaspoon pepper. Using a potato masher, mash the rutabaga mixture, adding cooking liquid as needed to make desired consistency.

4. Remove bay leaves from chicken mixture; discard. Serve chicken and sauce over mashed rutabagas. If desired, sprinkle with fresh thyme.

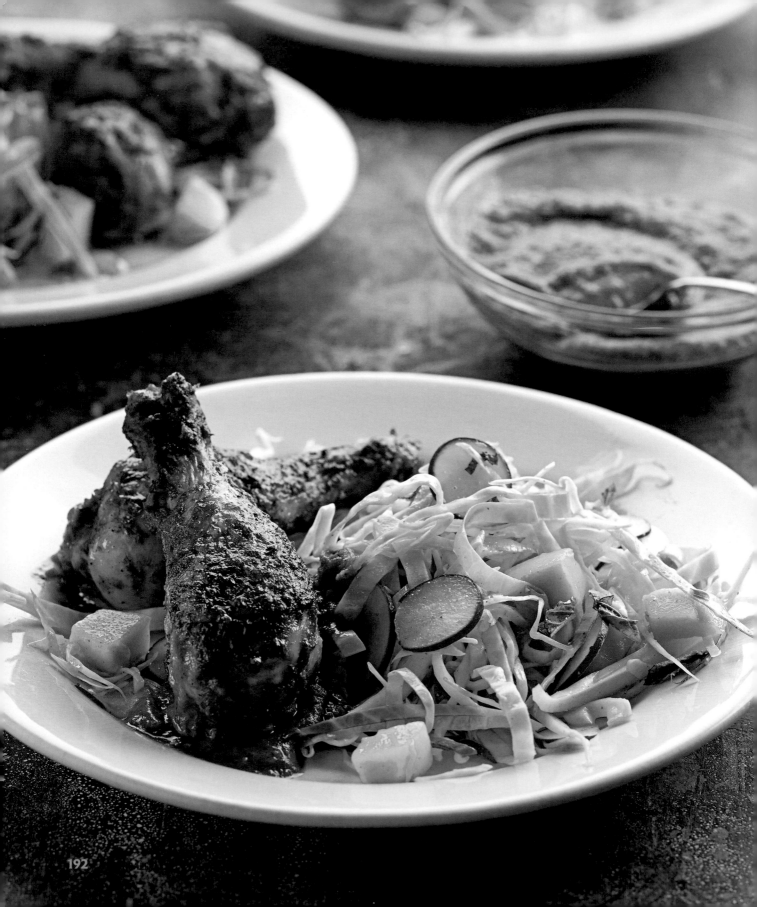

PEACH-BRANDY-GLAZED DRUMSTICKS

PREP: 30 minutes   GRILL: 40 minutes   MAKES: 4 servings

THESE CHICKEN LEGS ARE PERFECT WITH A CRISPY SLAW AND THE SPICY OVEN-BAKED SWEET POTATO FRIES FROM THE RECIPE FOR TUNISIAN SPICE-RUBBED PORK SHOULDER (PAGE 136). THEY'RE SHOWN HERE WITH CRUNCHY CABBAGE SLAW WITH RADISHES, MANGO, AND MINT (PAGE 292).

PEACH-BRANDY GLAZE

- 1 tablespoon olive oil
- ½ cup chopped onion
- 2 fresh medium peaches, halved, pitted, and chopped
- 2 tablespoons brandy
- 1 cup BBQ Sauce (see recipe, page 323)

- 8 chicken drumsticks (2 to 2½ pounds total), skinned if desired

1. For glaze, in a medium saucepan heat olive oil over medium heat. Add onion; cook about 5 minutes or until tender, stirring occasionally. Add peaches. Cover and cook for 4 to 6 minutes or until peaches are tender, stirring occasionally. Add brandy; cook, uncovered, for 2 minutes, stirring occasionally. Cool slightly. Transfer peach mixture to a blender or food processor. Cover and blend or process until smooth. Add BBQ Sauce. Cover and blend or process until smooth. Return sauce to the saucepan. Cook over medium-low heat just until heated through. Transfer ¾ cup of the sauce to a small bowl for brushing on the chicken. Keep remaining sauce warm for serving with grilled chicken.

2. For a charcoal grill, arrange medium-hot coals around a drip pan. Test for medium heat above drip pan. Place chicken drumsticks on grill rack over drip pan. Cover and grill for 40 to 50 minutes or until chicken is no longer pink (175°F), turning once halfway through grilling and brushing with ¾ cup of the Peach-Brandy Glaze for the last 5 to 10 minutes of grilling. (For a gas grill, preheat grill. Reduce heat to medium. Adjust heat for indirect cooking. Add chicken drumsticks to grill rack that is not over the heat. Cover and grill as directed.)

CHILE-MARINATED CHICKEN WITH MANGO-MELON SALAD

PREP: 40 minutes   CHILL/MARINATE: 2 to 4 hours   GRILL: 50 minutes   MAKES: 6 to 8 servings

AN ANCHO CHILE IS A DRIED POBLANO—A GLOSSY, DEEP-GREEN CHILE WITH AN INTENSELY FRESH FLAVOR. ANCHO CHILES HAVE A SLIGHTLY FRUITY FLAVOR WITH A HINT OF PLUM OR RAISIN AND JUST A TOUCH OF BITTERNESS. NEW MEXICO CHILES CAN BE MODERATELY HOT. THEY'RE THE DEEP-RED CHILES YOU SEE BUNCHED AND HANGING IN RISTRAS—COLORFUL ARRANGEMENTS OF DRYING CHILES—IN PARTS OF THE SOUTHWEST.

CHICKEN
- 2 dried New Mexico chiles
- 2 dried ancho chiles
- 1 cup boiling water
- 3 tablespoons olive oil
- 1 large sweet onion, peeled and cut into thick slices
- 4 roma tomatoes, cored
- 1 tablespoon minced garlic (6 cloves)
- 2 teaspoons ground cumin
- 1 teaspoon dried oregano, crushed
- 16 chicken drumsticks

SALAD
- 2 cups cubed cantaloupe
- 2 cups cubed honeydew
- 2 cups cubed mango
- ¼ cup fresh lime juice
- 1 teaspoon chili powder
- ½ teaspoon ground cumin
- ¼ cup snipped fresh cilantro

1. For chicken, remove stems and seeds from dried New Mexico and ancho chiles. Heat a large skillet over medium heat. Toast chiles in the skillet for 1 to 2 minutes or until fragrant and lightly toasted. Place toasted chiles in a small bowl; add the boiling water to the bowl. Let stand at least 10 minutes or until ready to use.

2. Preheat the broiler. Line a baking sheet with foil; brush 1 tablespoon of the olive oil over foil. Place onion slices and tomatoes on pan. Broil about 4 inches from heat for 6 to 8 minutes or until softened and charred. Drain chiles, reserving the water.

3. For marinade, in a blender or food processor combine chiles, onion, tomatoes, garlic, cumin, and oregano. Cover and blend or process until smooth, adding reserved water as needed to puree and reach desired consistency.

4. Place chicken in a large resealable plastic bag set in a shallow dish. Pour marinade over chicken in bag, turning bag to coat evenly. Marinate in refrigerator for 2 to 4 hours, turning bag occasionally.

5. For salad, in an extra-large bowl combine cantaloupe, honeydew, mango, lime juice, the remaining 2 tablespoons olive oil, chili powder, cumin, and cilantro. Toss to coat. Cover and chill for 1 to 4 hours.

6. For a charcoal grill, arrange medium-hot coals around a drip pan. Test for medium heat above the pan. Drain chicken, reserving the marinade. Place chicken on the grill rack over the drip pan. Brush chicken generously with some of the reserved marinade (discard any extra marinade). Cover and grill for 50 minutes or until chicken is no longer pink (175°F), turning once halfway through grilling. (For a gas grill, preheat grill. Reduce heat to medium. Adjust for indirect cooking. Continue as directed, placing chicken on the burner that is turned off.) Serve chicken drumsticks with salad.

TANDOORI-STYLE CHICKEN LEGS WITH CUCUMBER RAITA

PREP: 20 minutes   MARINATE: 2 to 24 hours   BROIL: 25 minutes   MAKES: 4 servings

THE RAITA IS MADE WITH CASHEW CREAM, LEMON JUICE, MINT, CILANTRO, AND CUCUMBER. IT PROVIDES A COOLING COUNTERPOINT TO THE HOT AND SPICY CHICKEN.

CHICKEN

- 1 onion, cut into thin wedges
- 1 2-inch piece fresh ginger, peeled and quartered
- 4 cloves garlic
- 3 tablespoons olive oil
- 2 tablespoons fresh lemon juice
- 1 teaspoon ground cumin
- 1 teaspoon ground turmeric
- ½ teaspoon ground allspice
- ½ teaspoon ground cinnamon
- ½ teaspoon black pepper
- ¼ teaspoon cayenne pepper
- 8 chicken drumsticks

CUCUMBER RAITA

- 1 cup Cashew Cream (see recipe, page 327)
- 1 tablespoon fresh lemon juice
- 1 tablespoon snipped fresh mint
- 1 tablespoon snipped fresh cilantro
- ½ teaspoon ground cumin
- ⅛ teaspoon black pepper
- 1 medium cucumber, peeled, seeded, and diced (1 cup)

  Lemon wedges

1. In a blender or food processor combine onion, ginger, garlic, olive oil, lemon juice, cumin, turmeric, allspice, cinnamon, black pepper, and cayenne pepper. Cover and blend or process until smooth.

2. Using the tip of a paring knife, pierce each drumstick four or five times. Place drumsticks in a large resealable plastic bag set in a large bowl. Add onion mixture; turn to coat. Marinate in the refrigerator for 2 to 24 hours, turning bag occasionally.

3. Preheat broiler. Remove chicken from marinade. Using paper towels, wipe excess marinade from drumsticks. Arrange drumsticks on the rack of an unheated broiler pan or rimmed baking sheet lined with foil. Broil 6 to 8 inches from heat source for 15 minutes. Turn drumsticks over; broil about 10 minutes or until chicken is no longer pink (175°F).

4. For the raita, in a medium bowl combine Cashew Cream, lemon juice, mint, cilantro, cumin, and black pepper. Gently stir in cucumber.

5. Serve chicken with raita and lemon wedges.

5 WAYS WITH CHICKEN BREAST

ANYONE WHO HAS SPENT ANY TIME ON A WEIGHT-LOSS PROGRAM OR "DIET" OF SOME KIND HAS EATEN HIS OR HER SHARE OF CHICKEN BREAST. IT CAN GET MONOTONOUS—BUT NOT WITH A SPARK OF IMAGINATION AND A WHOLE HOST OF FRESH INGREDIENTS. BONE-IN OR BONELESS, SKIN-ON OR SKINLESS, CHICKEN BREAST IS ENDLESSLY INTERESTING DONE RIGHT.

Grilled Chicken Paillard Salad with Raspberries, Beets, and Roasted Almonds, *recipe page 198*

5 WAYS WITH CHICKEN BREAST

WHEN YOU HAVE CHICKEN BREASTS IN THE REFRIGERATOR OR FREEZER, YOU HAVE THE START OF A GREAT MEAL. IT'S ECONOMICAL AND VERSATILE IN EQUAL MEASURE. CHICKEN BREAST CAN BE GRILLED, ROASTED, STIR-FRIED, PAN-SEARED, POACHED, OR STEWED—AND ITS MILD FLAVOR TAKES BEAUTIFULLY TO ALL KINDS OF FLAVORINGS—FROM INDIAN-STYLE CURRY TO A SICILIAN-STYLE STUFFED ROULADE TO A MIDDLE EASTERN-INSPIRED WRAP DRESSED WITH A LEMONY, GARLICKY PINE NUT DRESSING.

1. CURRIED CHICKEN STEW WITH ROOT VEGETABLES, ASPARAGUS, AND GREEN APPLE-MINT RELISH

PREP: 30 minutes
COOK: 35 minutes
STAND: 5 minutes
MAKES: 4 servings

- 2 tablespoons refined coconut oil or olive oil
- 2 pounds bone-in chicken breasts, skinned if desired
- 1 cup chopped onion
- 2 tablespoons grated fresh ginger
- 2 tablespoons minced garlic
- 2 tablespoons salt-free curry powder
- 2 tablespoons minced, seeded jalapeño (see tip, page 56)
- 4 cups Chicken Bone Broth (see recipe, page 235) or no-salt-added chicken broth
- 2 medium sweet potatoes (about 1 pound), peeled and chopped
- 2 medium turnips (about 6 ounces), peeled and chopped
- 1 cup seeded, diced tomato
- 8 ounces asparagus, trimmed and cut into 1-inch lengths
- 1 13.5-ounce can natural coconut milk (such as Nature's Way)
- ½ cup snipped fresh cilantro
  Apple-Mint Relish (recipe follows)
  Lime wedges

1. In a 6-quart Dutch oven heat oil over medium-high heat. Brown chicken in batches in hot oil, turning to brown evenly, about 10 minutes. Transfer chicken to a plate; set aside.

2. Turn heat to medium. Add onion, ginger, garlic, curry powder, and jalapeño to the pot. Cook and stir 5 minutes or until onion is softened. Stir in Chicken Bone Broth, sweet potatoes, turnips, and tomato. Return the chicken pieces to the pot, arranging to submerge chicken in as much liquid as possible. Reduce heat to medium-low. Cover and simmer 30 minutes or until chicken is no longer pink and vegetables are tender. Stir in asparagus, coconut milk, and cilantro. Remove from heat. Let stand for 5 minutes. Cut chicken from bones, if necessary, to divide evenly among serving bowls. Serve with Apple-Mint Relish and lime wedges.

Apple-Mint Relish: In a food processor chop ½ cup unsweetened coconut flakes until powdery. Add 1 cup fresh cilantro leaves and steams; 1 cup fresh mint leaves; 1 Granny Smith apple, cored and chopped; 2 teaspoons minced, seeded jalapeño (see tip, page 56); and 1 tablespoon fresh lime juice. Pulse until finely minced.

2. GRILLED CHICKEN PAILLARD SALAD WITH RASPBERRIES, BEETS, AND ROASTED ALMONDS

PREP: 30 minutes
ROAST: 45 minutes
MARINATE: 15 minutes
GRILL: 8 minutes
MAKES: 4 servings

- ½ cup whole almonds
- 1½ teaspoons olive oil
- 1 medium red beet
- 1 medium golden beet
- 2 6- to 8-ounce boneless, skinless chicken breast halves
- 2 cups fresh or frozen raspberries, thawed
- 3 tablespoons white or red wine vinegar
- 2 tablespoons snipped fresh tarragon
- 1 tablespoon minced shallot
- 1 teaspoon Dijon-Style Mustard (see recipe, page 322)
- ¼ cup olive oil
  Black pepper
- 8 cups spring mix lettuces

1. For the almonds, preheat the oven to 400°F. Spread almonds on a small baking sheet and toss with ½ teaspoon olive oil. Bake about 5 minutes or until fragrant and golden. Let cool. (Almonds may be toasted 2 days ahead and stored in an airtight container.)

2. For the beets, place each beet on a small piece of foil and drizzle with each with ½ teaspoon olive oil. Loosely wrap the foil around the beets and place on a baking sheet or in a baking dish. Roast the beets in the 400°F oven for 40 to 50 minutes or until tender when pierced with a knife. Remove from oven and let stand until cool enough to handle. Using a paring knife, remove the skin. Cut beets into wedges and set aside. (Avoid mixing the beets together to prevent the red beets from staining the golden beets. Beets may be roasted 1 day ahead and chilled. Bring to room temperature before serving.)

3. For the chicken, cut each chicken breast in half horizontally. Place each piece of chicken between two pieces of plastic wrap. Using a meat mallet, gently pound to about ¾ inch thick. Place chicken in a shallow dish and set aside.

4. For vinaigrette, in a large bowl lightly crush ¾ cup of the raspberries with a whisk (reserve remaining raspberries for the salad). Add the vinegar, tarragon, shallot, and Dijon-Style Mustard; whisk to blend. Add the ¼ cup olive oil in a thin stream, whisking to mix well. Pour ½ cup vinaigrette over the chicken; turn chicken to coat (reserve remaining vinaigrette for the salad). Marinate chicken at room temperature for 15 minutes. Remove chicken from the marinade and sprinkle with pepper; discard marinade remaining in dish.

5. For a charcoal or gas grill, place chicken on a grill rack directly over medium heat. Cover and grill for 8 to 10 minutes or until chicken is no longer pink, turning once halfway through grilling. (Chicken can also be cooked in a stovetop grill pan.)

6. In a large bowl combine lettuce, beets, and the remaining 1¼ cups raspberries. Pour reserved vinaigrette over salad; gently toss to coat. Divide salad among four serving plates; top each with a grilled chicken breast piece. Coarsely chop the roasted almonds and sprinkle over all. Serve immediately.

3. BROCCOLI RABE-STUFFED CHICKEN BREASTS WITH FRESH TOMATO SAUCE AND CAESAR SALAD

PREP: 40 minutes
COOK: 25 minutes
MAKES: 6 servings

- 3 tablespoons olive oil
- 2 teaspoons minced garlic
- ¼ teaspoon crushed red pepper
- 1 pound broccoli raab, trimmed and chopped
- ½ cup unsulfured golden raisins
- ½ cup water
- 4 5- to 6-ounce skinless, boneless chicken breast halves
- 1 cup chopped onion
- 3 cups chopped tomatoes
- ¼ cup snipped fresh basil
- 2 teaspoons red wine vinegar
- 3 tablespoons fresh lemon juice
- 2 tablespoons Paleo Mayo (see recipe, page 323)
- 2 teaspoons Dijon-Style Mustard (see recipe, page 322)
- 1 teaspoon minced garlic
- ½ teaspoon black pepper
- ¼ cup olive oil
- 10 cups chopped romaine lettuce

1. In a large skillet heat 1 tablespoon of the olive oil over medium-high heat. Add the garlic and crushed red pepper; cook and stir for 30 seconds or until fragrant. Add the chopped broccoli rabe, raisins, and the ½ cup water. Cover and cook about 8 minutes or until broccoli raab is wilted and tender. Remove lid from pan; let any excess water evaporate. Set aside.

2. For roulades, halve each chicken breast lengthwise; place each piece between two pieces of plastic wrap. Using the flat side of a meat mallet, pound chicken lightly to about ¼ inch thick. For each roulade, place about ¼ cup of the broccoli raab mixture on one of the short ends; roll up, folding in the sides to completely enclose filling. (Roulades may be made up to 1 day ahead and chilled until ready to cook.)

3. In a large skillet heat 1 tablespoon of the olive oil over medium-high heat. Add the roulades, seam sides down. Cook about 8 minutes or until browned on all sides, turning two or three times during cooking. Transfer roulades to a platter.

4. For sauce, in the skillet heat 1 tablespoon of the remaining olive oil over medium heat. Add the onion; cook about 5 minutes or until translucent. Stir in the tomatoes and basil. Place roulades on top of the sauce in skillet. Bring to boiling over medium-high heat; reduce heat. Cover and simmer about 5 minutes or until tomatoes start to break down but still retain their shape and roulades are heated through.

5. For dressing, in a small bowl whisk together the lemon juice, Paleo Mayo, Dijon-Style Mustard, garlic, and black pepper. Drizzle in the ¼ cup olive oil, whisking until emulsified. In a large bowl toss dressing with the chopped romaine. To serve, divide romaine among six serving plates. Slice roulades and arrange on romaine; drizzle with tomato sauce.

4. GRILLED CHICKEN SHAWARMA WRAPS WITH SPICED VEGETABLES AND PINE NUT DRESSING

PREP: 20 minutes
MARINATE: 30 minutes
GRILL: 10 minutes
MAKES: 8 wraps (4 servings)

1½ pounds skinless, boneless chicken breast halves, cut into 2-inch pieces
5 tablespoons olive oil
2 tablespoons fresh lemon juice
1¾ teaspoons ground cumin
1 teaspoon minced garlic
1 teaspoon paprika
½ teaspoon curry powder
½ teaspoon ground cinnamon
¼ teaspoon cayenne pepper
1 medium zucchini, halved
1 small eggplant cut into ½-inch slices
1 large yellow sweet pepper, halved and seeded
1 medium red onion, quartered
8 cherry tomatoes
8 large butter lettuce leaves
   Toasted Pine Nut Dressing (see recipe, page 321)
   Lemon wedges

1. For marinade, in a small bowl combine 3 tablespoons of the olive oil, lemon juice, 1 teaspoon of the cumin, garlic, ½ teaspoon of the paprika, curry powder, ¼ teaspoon of the cinnamon, and cayenne pepper. Place chicken pieces in a large resealable plastic bag set in a shallow dish. Pour marinade over the chicken. Seal bag; turn bag to coat. Marinate in the refrigerator for 30 minutes, turning bag occasionally.

2. Remove chicken from marinade; discard marinade. Thread chicken on four long skewers.

3. Place zucchini, eggplant, sweet pepper, and onion on a baking sheet. Drizzle with 2 tablespoons

of the olive oil. Sprinkle with the remaining ¾ teaspoon cumin, remaining ½ teaspoon paprika, and the remaining ¼ teaspoon cinnamon; lightly rub over vegetables. Thread tomatoes on two skewers.

3. For a charcoal or gas grill, place chicken and tomato kabobs and vegetables on a grill rack over medium heat. Cover and grill until chicken is no longer pink and vegetables are lightly charred and crisp-tender, turning once. Allow 10 to 12 minutes for chicken, 8 to 10 minutes for vegetables, and 4 minutes for tomatoes.

4. Remove chicken from skewers. Chop chicken and cut zucchini, eggplant, and sweet pepper into bite-size pieces. Remove the tomatoes from skewers (do not chop). Arrange chicken and vegetables on a platter. To serve, spoon some of the chicken and vegetables into a lettuce leaf; drizzle with Toasted Pine Nut Dressing. Serve with lemon wedges.

5. OVEN-BRAISED CHICKEN BREASTS WITH MUSHROOMS, GARLIC-MASHED CAULIFLOWER, AND ROASTED ASPARAGUS

START TO FINISH: 50 minutes
MAKES: 4 servings

4 10- to 12-ounce bone-in chicken breast halves, skinned
3 cups small white button mushrooms
1 cup thinly sliced leeks or yellow onion
2 cups Chicken Bone Broth (see recipe, page 235) or no-salt-added chicken broth
1 cup dry white wine
1 large bunch fresh thyme
   Black pepper

   White wine vinegar (optional)
1 head cauliflower, separated into florets
12 cloves garlic, peeled
2 tablespoons olive oil
   White or cayenne pepper
1 pound asparagus, trimmed
2 teaspoons olive oil

1. Preheat oven to 400°F. Arrange chicken breasts in a 3-quart rectangular baking dish; top with mushrooms and leeks. Pour Chicken Bone Broth and wine over the chicken and vegetables. Scatter thyme over all and sprinkle with black pepper. Cover dish with foil.

2. Bake for 35 to 40 minutes or until an instant-read thermometer inserted in chicken registers 170°F. Remove and discard thyme sprigs. If desired, season braising liquid with a splash of vinegar before serving.

2. Meanwhile, in a large saucepan cook cauliflower and garlic in enough boiling water to cover about 10 minutes or until very tender. Drain cauliflower and garlic, reserving 2 tablespoons of the cooking liquid. In a food processor or a large mixing bowl place cauliflower and reserved cooking liquid. Process until smooth* or mash with a potato masher; stir in 2 tablespoons olive oil and season to taste with white pepper. Keep warm until ready to serve.

3. Arrange asparagus in a single layer on a baking sheet. Drizzle with 2 teaspoons olive oil and toss to coat. Sprinkle with black pepper. Roast in a 400°F oven about 8 minutes or until crisp-tender, stirring once.

4. Divide mashed cauliflower among six serving plates. Top with chicken, mushrooms, and leeks. Drizzle with some of the braising liquid; serve with roasted asparagus.

*Note: If using a food processor, be careful not to overprocess or cauliflower will get too thin.

THAI-STYLE CHICKEN SOUP

PREP: 30 minutes   FREEZE: 20 minutes   COOK: 50 minutes   MAKES: 4 to 6 servings

TAMARIND IS A MUSKY, SOUR FRUIT USED IN INDIAN, THAI, AND MEXICAN COOKING. MANY COMMERCIALLY PREPARED TAMARIND PASTES CONTAIN SUGAR—BE SURE YOU PURCHASE ONE THAT DOES NOT. KAFFIR LIME LEAVES CAN BE FOUND FRESH, FROZEN, AND DRIED AT MOST ASIAN MARKETS. IF YOU CAN'T FIND THEM, SUBSTITUTE 1½ TEASPOONS FINELY SHREDDED LIME PEEL FOR THE LEAVES IN THIS RECIPE.

2 stalks lemongrass, trimmed

2 tablespoons unrefined coconut oil

½ cup thinly sliced scallions

3 large cloves garlic, thinly sliced

8 cups Chicken Bone Broth (see recipe, page 235) or no-salt-added chicken broth

¼ cup no-sugar-added tamarind paste (such as Tamicon brand)

2 tablespoons nori flakes

3 fresh Thai chiles, thinly sliced with seeds intact (see tip, page 56)

3 kaffir lime leaves

1 3-inch piece ginger, thinly sliced

4 6-ounce skinless, boneless chicken breast halves

1 14.5-ounce can no-salt-added fire-roasted diced tomatoes, undrained

6 ounces thin asparagus spears, trimmed and thinly sliced diagonally into ½-inch pieces

½ cup packed Thai basil leaves (see page 99)

1. Using the back of a knife with firm pressure, bruise the lemongrass stalks. Finely chop bruised stalks.

2. In a Dutch oven heat coconut oil over medium heat. Add lemongrass and scallions; cook for 8 to 10 minutes, stirring often. Add garlic; cook and stir for 2 to 3 minutes or until very fragrant.

3. Add Chicken Bone Broth, tamarind paste, nori flakes, chiles, lime leaves, and ginger. Bring to boiling; reduce heat. Cover and simmer for 40 minutes.

4. Meanwhile, freeze chicken for 20 to 30 minutes or until firm. Thinly slice chicken.

5. Strain soup through a fine-mesh sieve into a large saucepan, pressing with the back of a large spoon to extract flavors. Discard solids. Bring soup to boiling. Stir in chicken, undrained tomatoes, asparagus, and basil. Reduce heat; simmer, uncovered, for 2 to 3 minutes or until chicken is cooked through. Serve immediately.

LEMON AND SAGE ROASTED CHICKEN WITH ENDIVE

PREP: 15 minutes   ROAST: 55 minutes   STAND: 5 minutes   MAKES: 4 servings

THE LEMON SLICES AND SAGE LEAF PLACED UNDER THE SKIN OF THE CHICKEN FLAVOR THE MEAT AS IT COOKS—AND MAKE AN EYE-CATCHING DESIGN UNDER THE CRISP, OPAQUE SKIN AFTER IT COMES OUT OF THE OVEN.

4   bone-in chicken breast halves (with skin)
1   lemon, very thinly sliced
4   large sage leaves
2   teaspoons olive oil
2   teaspoons Mediterranean Seasoning (see recipe, page 324)
½   teaspoon black pepper
2   tablespoons extra virgin olive oil
2   shallots, sliced
2   cloves garlic, minced
4   heads endive, halved lengthwise

1. Preheat oven to 400°F. Using a paring knife, very carefully loosen the skin from each breast half, leaving it attached on one side. Place 2 lemon slices and 1 sage leaf on the meat of each breast. Gently pull skin back into place and press gently to secure it.

2. Arrange chicken in a shallow roasting pan. Brush chicken with 2 teaspoons olive oil; sprinkle with Mediterranean Seasoning and ¼ teaspoon of the pepper. Roast, uncovered, about 55 minutes or until skin is browned and crisp and an instant-read thermometer inserted into chicken registers 170°F. Let chicken stand for 10 minutes before serving.

3. Meanwhile, in a large skillet heat the 2 tablespoons olive oil over medium heat. Add shallots; cook about 2 minutes or until translucent. Sprinkle endive with the remaining ¼ teaspoon pepper. Add garlic to skillet. Place endive in skillet, cut sides down. Cook about 5 minutes or until browned. Carefully turn endive over; cook for 2 to 3 minutes more or until tender. Serve with chicken.

CHICKEN WITH SCALLIONS, WATERCRESS, AND RADISHES

PREP: 20 minutes   COOK: 8 minutes   BAKE: 30 minutes   MAKES: 4 servings

ALTHOUGH IT MIGHT SOUND ODD TO COOK RADISHES, THEY ARE BARELY COOKED HERE—JUST ENOUGH TO MELLOW THEIR PEPPERY BITE AND TENDERIZE THEM A BIT.

3 tablespoons olive oil

4 10- to 12-ounce bone-in chicken breast halves (with skin)

1 tablespoon Lemon-Herb Seasoning (see recipe, page 324)

¾ cup sliced scallions

6 radishes, thinly sliced

¼ teaspoon black pepper

½ cup dry white vermouth or dry white wine

⅓ cup Cashew Cream (see recipe, page 327)

1 bunch watercress, stems trimmed, roughly chopped

1 tablespoon snipped fresh dill

1. Preheat oven to 350°F. In a large skillet heat olive oil over medium-high heat. Pat chicken dry with a paper towel. Cook chicken, skin sides down, for 4 to 5 minutes or until skin is golden and crisp. Turn chicken over; cook about 4 minutes or until browned. Arrange chicken, skin sides up, in a shallow baking dish. Sprinkle chicken with Lemon-Herb Seasoning. Bake about 30 minutes or until an instant-read thermometer inserted into chicken registers 170°F.

2. Meanwhile, pour all but 1 tablespoon drippings from skillet; return skillet to heat. Add scallions and radishes; cook about 3 minutes or just until scallions wilt. Sprinkle with pepper. Add vermouth, stirring to scrape up browned bits. Bring to boiling; cook until reduced and slightly thickened. Stir in Cashew Cream; bring to boiling. Remove skillet from heat; add watercress and dill, stirring gently just until watercress wilts. Stir in any chicken juices that have accumulated in the baking dish.

3. Divide scallion mixture among four serving plates; top with chicken.

CHICKEN TIKKA MASALA

PREP: 30 minutes   MARINATE: 4 to 6 hours   COOK: 15 minutes   BROIL: 8 minutes   MAKES: 4 servings

THIS WAS INSPIRED BY A VERY POPULAR INDIAN DISH THAT MAY NOT HAVE BEEN CREATED IN INDIA AT ALL, BUT RATHER AT AN INDIAN RESTAURANT IN THE UNITED KINGDOM. TRADITIONAL CHICKEN TIKKA MASALA CALLS FOR CHICKEN TO BE MARINATED IN YOGURT AND THEN COOKED IN A SPICY TOMATO SAUCE SPLASHED WITH CREAM. WITHOUT ANY DAIRY BLUNTING THE FLAVOR OF THE SAUCE, THIS VERSION IS ESPECIALLY CLEAN-TASTING. INSTEAD OF RICE, IT'S SERVED OVER CRISP ZUCCHINI NOODLES.

1½ pounds skinless, boneless chicken thighs or chicken breast halves
¾ cup natural coconut milk (such as Nature's Way)
6 cloves garlic, minced
1 tablespoon grated fresh ginger
1 teaspoon ground coriander
1 teaspoon paprika
1 teaspoon ground cumin
¼ teaspoon ground cardamom
4 tablespoons refined coconut oil
1 cup chopped carrots
1 thinly sliced celery
½ cup chopped onion
2 jalapeño or serrano chiles, seeded (if desired) and finely chopped (see tip, page 56)
1 14.5-ounce can no-salt-added fire-roasted diced tomatoes, undrained
1 8-ounce can no-salt-added tomato sauce
1 teaspoon no-salt-added garam masala
3 medium zucchini
½ teaspoon black pepper
Fresh cilantro leaves

1. If using chicken thighs, cut each thigh into three pieces. If using chicken breast halves, cut each breast half into 2-inch pieces, cutting any thick portions in half horizontally to make them thinner. Place chicken in a large resealable plastic bag; set aside. For marinade, in a small bowl combine ½ cup of the coconut milk, the garlic, ginger, coriander, paprika, cumin, and cardamom. Pour marinade over chicken in bag. Seal bag and turn to coat chicken. Place bag in a medium bowl; marinate in the refrigerator for 4 to 6 hours, turning bag occasionally.

2. Preheat broiler. In a large skillet heat 2 tablespoons of the coconut oil over medium heat. Add carrots, celery, and onion; cook for 6 to 8 minutes or until vegetables are tender, stirring occasionally. Add jalapeños; cook and stir for 1 minute more. Add undrained tomatoes and tomato sauce. Bring to boiling; reduce heat. Simmer, uncovered, about 5 minutes or until sauce thickens slightly.

3. Drain chicken, discarding marinade. Arrange chicken pieces in a single layer on the unheated rack of a broiler pan. Broil 5 to 6 inches from the heat for 8 to 10 minutes or until chicken is no longer pink, turning once halfway through broiling. Add cooked chicken pieces and the remaining ¼ cup coconut milk to tomato mixture in skillet. Cook for 1 to 2 minutes or until heated through. Remove from the heat; stir in garam masala.

4. Trim ends off zucchini. Using a julienne cutter, cut zucchini into long thin strips. In an extra-large skillet heat the remaining 2 tablespoons coconut oil over medium-high heat. Add zucchini strips and black pepper. Cook and stir for 2 to 3 minutes or until zucchini is crisp-tender.

5. To serve, divide zucchini among four serving plates. Top with chicken mixture. Garnish with cilantro leaves.

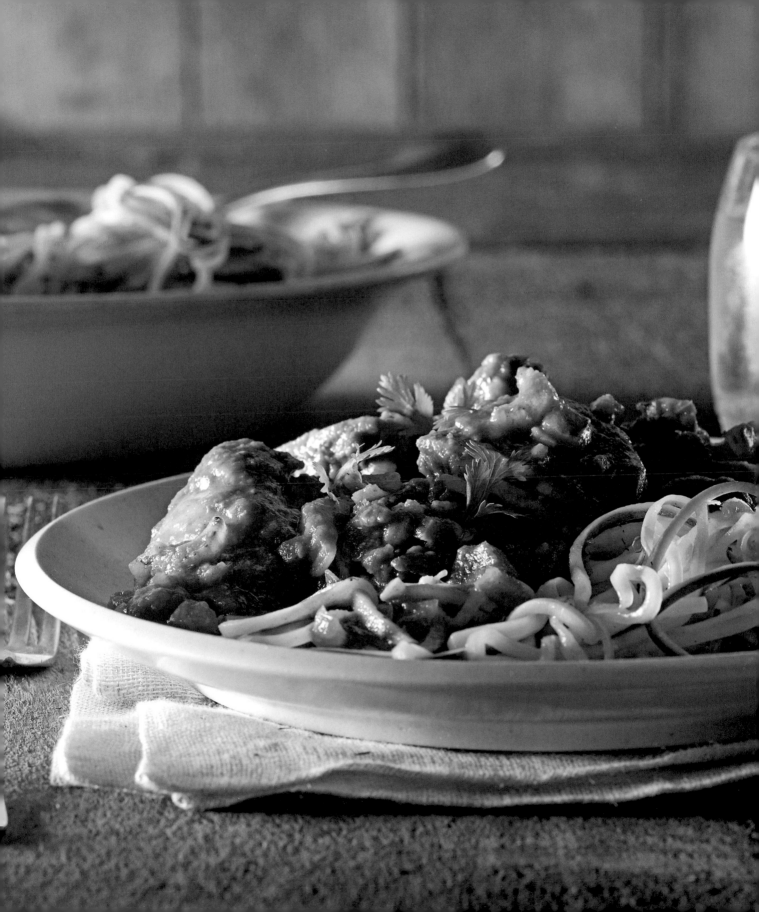

RAS EL HANOUT CHICKEN THIGHS

PREP: 20 minutes   COOK: 40 minutes   MAKES: 4 servings

RAS EL HANOUT IS A COMPLEX AND EXOTIC MORROCAN SPICE MIXTURE. THE PHRASE MEANS "HEAD OF THE SHOP" IN ARABIC, WHICH IMPLIES THAT IT IS A UNIQUE BLEND OF THE BEST SPICES THE SPICE SELLER HAS TO OFFER. THERE'S NO SET RECIPE FOR RAS EL HANOUT, BUT IT OFTEN CONTAINS SOME BLEND OF GINGER, ANISE, CINNAMON, NUTMEG, PEPPERCORNS, CLOVES, CARDAMOM, DRIED FLOWERS (SUCH AS LAVENDER AND ROSE), NIGELLA, MACE, GALANGAL, AND TURMERIC.

1 tablespoon ground cumin
2 teaspoons ground ginger
1½ teaspoons black pepper
1½ teaspoons ground cinnamon
1 teaspoon ground coriander
1 teaspoon cayenne pepper
1 teaspoon ground allspice
½ teaspoon ground cloves
¼ teaspoon ground nutmeg
1 teaspoon saffron threads
  (optional)
4 tablespoons unrefined coconut
  oil
8 bone-in chicken thighs
1 8-ounce package fresh
  mushrooms, sliced
1 cup chopped onion
1 cup chopped red, yellow, or
  green sweet pepper (1 large)
4 roma tomatoes, cored, seeded,
  and chopped
4 cloves garlic, minced
2 13.5-ounce cans natural
  coconut milk (such as
  Nature's Way)
3 to 4 tablespoons fresh lime
  juice
¼ cup finely snipped fresh
  cilantro

1. For the ras el hanout, in medium mortar or small bowl combine the cumin, ginger, black pepper, cinnamon, coriander, cayenne pepper, allspice, cloves, nutmeg, and, if desired, saffron. Grind with a pestle or stir with a spoon to mix well. Set aside.

2. In an extra-large skillet heat 2 tablespoons of the coconut oil over medium heat. Sprinkle chicken thighs with 1 tablespoon of the ras el hanout. Add chicken to skillet; cook for 5 to 6 minutes or until browned, turning once halfway through cooking. Remove chicken from skillet; keep warm.

3. In the same skillet heat the remaining 2 tablespoons coconut oil over medium heat. Add mushrooms, onion, sweet pepper, tomatoes, and garlic. Cook and stir about 5 minutes or until vegetables are tender. Stir in coconut milk, lime juice, and 1 tablespoon of the ras el hanout. Return chicken to skillet. Bring to boiling; reduce heat. Simmer, covered, about 30 minutes or until chicken is tender (175°F).

4. Serve chicken, vegetables, and sauce in bowls. Garnish with cilantro.

Note: Store leftover Ras el Hanout in a covered container for up to 1 month.

STAR FRUIT ADOBO CHICKEN THIGHS OVER BRAISED SPINACH

PREP: 40 minutes   MARINATE: 4 to 8 hours   COOK: 45 minutes   MAKES: 4 servings

IF NECESSARY, PAT THE CHICKEN DRY WITH A PAPER TOWEL AFTER IT COMES OUT OF THE MARINADE BEFORE BROWNING IT IN THE SKILLET. ANY LIQUID LEFT ON THE MEAT WILL SPATTER IN THE HOT OIL.

8 bone-in chicken thighs (1½ to 2 pounds), skinned
¾ cup white or cider vinegar
¾ cup fresh orange juice
½ cup water
¼ cup chopped onion
¼ cup snipped fresh cilantro
4 cloves garlic, minced
½ teaspoon black pepper
1 tablespoon olive oil
1 star fruit (carambola), sliced
1 cup Chicken Bone Broth (see recipe, page 235) or no-salt-added chicken broth
2 9-ounce packages fresh spinach leaves
   Fresh cilantro leaves (optional)

1. Place chicken in a stainless-steel or enamel Dutch oven; set aside. In a medium bowl combine vinegar, orange juice, the water, onion, ¼ cup snipped cilantro, garlic, and pepper; pour over chicken. Cover and marinate in the refrigerator for 4 to 8 hours.

2. Bring chicken mixture in Dutch oven to boiling over medium-high heat; reduce heat. Cover and simmer for 35 to 40 minutes or until chicken is no longer pink (175°F).

3. In an extra-large skillet heat oil over medium-high heat. With tongs, remove chicken from Dutch oven, shaking gently so cooking liquid drips off; reserve cooking liquid. Brown the chicken on all sides, turning frequently to brown evenly.

4. Meanwhile, for sauce, strain cooking liquid; return to Dutch oven. Bring to boiling. Boil about 4 minutes to reduce and thicken slightly; add star fruit; boil for 1 minute more. Return chicken to the sauce in Dutch oven. Remove from heat; cover to keep warm.

5. Wipe out the skillet. Pour Chicken Bone Broth into skillet. Bring to boiling over medium-high heat; stir in spinach. Reduce heat; simmer for 1 to 2 minutes or until spinach is just wilted, stirring constantly. Using a slotted spoon, transfer spinach to a serving platter. Top with chicken and sauce. If desired, sprinkle with cilantro leaves.

CHICKEN-POBLANO CABBAGE TACOS WITH CHIPOTLE MAYO

PREP: 25 minutes   BAKE: 40 minutes   MAKES: 4 servings

SERVE THESE MESSY-BUT-TASTY TACOS WITH A FORK TO RETRIEVE ANY OF THE FILLING THAT HAPPENS TO FALL OUT OF THE CABBAGE LEAF WHILE YOU'RE EATING IT.

 1 tablespoon olive oil
 2 poblano chiles, seeded (if desired) and chopped (see tip, page 56)
 ½ cup chopped onion
 3 cloves garlic, minced
 1 tablespoon salt-free chili powder
 2 teaspoons ground cumin
 ½ teaspoon black pepper
 1 8-ounce can no-salt-added tomato sauce
 ¾ cup Chicken Bone Broth (see recipe, page 235) or no-salt-added chicken broth
 1 teaspoon dried Mexican oregano, crushed
 1 to 1½ pounds skinless, boneless chicken thighs
10 to 12 medium to large cabbage leaves
    Chipotle Paleo Mayo (see recipe, page 323)

1. Preheat oven to 350°F. In a large ovenproof skillet heat oil over medium-high heat. Add poblano chiles, onion, and garlic; cook and stir for 2 minutes. Stir in chili powder, cumin, and black pepper; cook and stir for 1 minute more (if necessary, reduce heat to prevent spices from burning).

2. Add tomato sauce, Chicken Bone Broth, and oregano to skillet. Bring to boiling. Carefully place chicken thighs in the tomato mixture. Cover skillet with lid. Bake about 40 minutes or until chicken is tender (175°F), turning chicken once halfway.

3. Remove chicken from skillet; cool slightly. Using two forks, shred chicken into bite-size pieces. Stir shredded chicken into tomato mixture in skillet.

4. To serve, spoon chicken mixture into cabbage leaves; top with Chipotle Paleo Mayo.

CHICKEN STEW WITH BABY CARROTS AND BOK CHOY

PREP: 15 minutes   COOK: 24 minutes   STAND: 2 minutes   MAKES: 4 servings

BABY BOK CHOY IS VERY DELICATE AND CAN GET OVERCOOKED IN A FLASH. TO KEEP IT CRISP AND FRESH-TASTING— NOT WILTED AND SOGGY—BE SURE IT STEAMS IN THE COVERED HOT POT (OFF THE HEAT) FOR NO MORE THAN 2 MINUTES BEFORE YOU SERVE THE STEW.

2 tablespoons olive oil

1 leek, sliced (white and light green parts)

4 cups Chicken Bone Broth (see recipe, page 235) or no-salt-added chicken broth

1 cup dry white wine

1 tablespoon Dijon-Style Mustard (see recipe, page 322)

½ teaspoon black pepper

1 sprig fresh thyme

1¼ pounds skinless, boneless chicken thighs, cut into 1-inch pieces

8 ounces baby carrots with tops, scrubbed, trimmed, and halved lengthwise, or 2 medium carrots, bias-sliced

2 teaspoons finely shredded lemon peel (set aside)

1 tablespoon fresh lemon juice

2 heads baby bok choy

½ teaspoon snipped fresh thyme

1. In a large saucepan heat 1 tablespoon of the olive oil over medium heat. Cook leek in hot oil for 3 to 4 minutes or until wilted. Add Chicken Bone Broth, wine, Dijon-Style Mustard, ¼ teaspoon of the pepper, and thyme sprig. Bring to boiling; reduce heat. Cook for 10 to 12 minutes or until liquid is reduced by about one-third. Discard thyme sprig.

2. Meanwhile, in a Dutch oven heat the remaining 1 tablespoon olive oil over medium-high heat. Sprinkle chicken with the remaining ¼ teaspoon pepper. Cook in hot oil about 3 minutes or until browned, stirring occasionally. Drain fat if necessary. Carefully add the reduced broth mixture to pot, scraping up any brown bits; add carrots. Bring to boiling; reduce heat. Simmer, uncovered, for 8 to 10 minutes or just until carrots are tender. Stir in lemon juice. Cut bok choy in half lengthwise. (If bok choy heads are large, cut into quarters.) Place bok choy on top of chicken in pot. Cover and remove from heat; let stand for 2 minutes.

3. Ladle stew into shallow bowls. Sprinkle with lemon peel and snipped thyme.

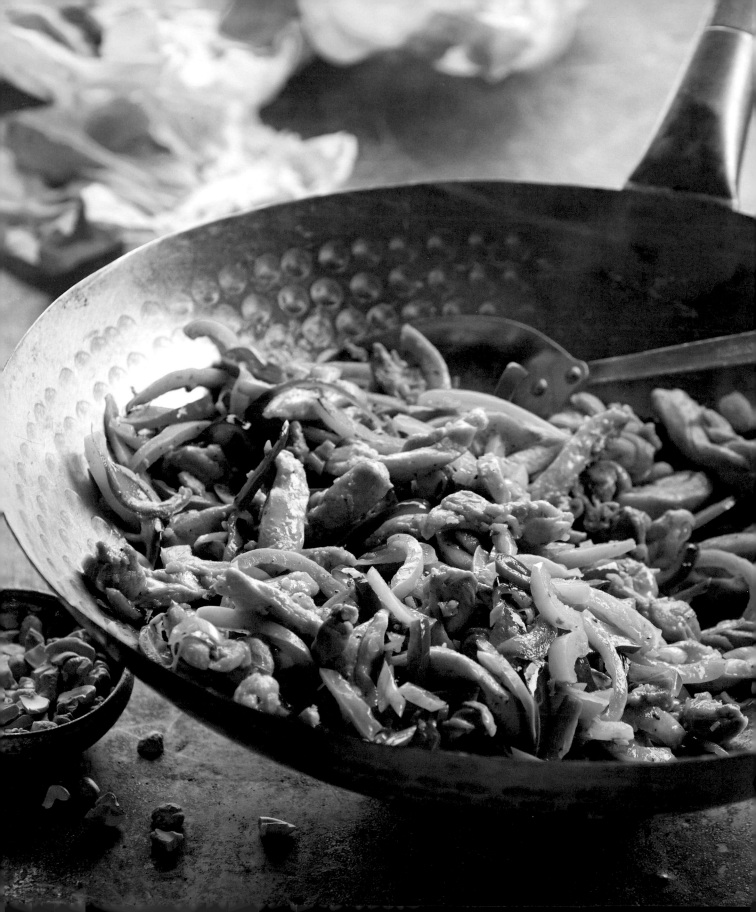

CASHEW-ORANGE CHICKEN AND SWEET PEPPER STIR-FRY IN LETTUCE WRAPS

START TO FINISH: 45 minutes   MAKES: 4 to 6 servings

YOU WILL FIND TWO TYPES OF COCONUT OIL ON THE SHELVES—REFINED AND EXTRA VIRGIN, OR UNREFINED. AS THE NAME IMPLIES, EXTRA VIRGIN COCONUT OIL IS FROM THE FIRST PRESSING OF THE FRESH, RAW COCONUT. IT IS ALWAYS THE BETTER CHOICE WHEN YOU ARE COOKING OVER MEDIUM OR MEDIUM-HIGH HEAT. REFINED COCONUT OIL HAS A HIGHER SMOKE POINT, SO USE IT ONLY WHEN YOU ARE COOKING OVER HIGH HEAT.

1 tablespoon refined coconut oil

1½ to 2 pounds skinless, boneless chicken thighs, cut into thin bite-size strips

3 red, orange, and/or yellow sweet peppers, stemmed, seeded, and thinly sliced into bite-size strips

1 red onion, halved lengthwise and thinly sliced

1 teaspoon finely shredded orange peel (set aside)

½ cup fresh orange juice

1 tablespoon minced fresh ginger

3 cloves garlic, minced

1 cup unsalted raw cashews, toasted and coarsely chopped (see tip, page 57)

½ cup sliced green scallions (4)

8 to 10 butter or iceberg lettuce leaves

1. In a wok or large skillet heat the coconut oil over high heat. Add chicken; cook and stir for 2 minutes. Add peppers and onion; cook and stir for 2 to 3 minutes or until vegetables just start to soften. Remove the chicken and vegetables from the wok; keep warm.

2. Wipe out wok with paper towel. Add the orange juice to the wok. Cook about 3 minutes or until juice boils and reduces slightly. Add ginger and garlic. Cook and stir for 1 minute. Return the chicken and pepper mixture to the wok. Stir in orange peel, cashews, and scallions. Serve stir-fry on lettuce leaves.

VIETNAMESE COCONUT-LEMONGRASS CHICKEN

START TO FINISH: 30 minutes   MAKES: 4 servings

THIS QUICK COCONUT CURRY CAN BE ON THE TABLE IN 30 MINUTES FROM THE TIME YOU START CHOPPING, MAKING IT AN IDEAL MEAL FOR A BUSY WEEKNIGHT.

1 tablespoon unrefined coconut oil

4 stalks lemongrass (pale parts only)

1 3.2-ounce package oyster mushrooms, chopped

1 large onion, thinly sliced, rings halved

1 fresh jalapeño, seeded and finely chopped (see tip, page 56)

2 tablespoons minced fresh ginger

3 cloves garlic minced

1½ pounds skinless, boneless chicken thighs, thinly sliced and cut into bite-size pieces

½ cup natural coconut milk (such as Nature's Way)

½ cup Chicken Bone Broth (see recipe, page 235) or no-salt-added chicken broth

1 tablespoon salt-free red curry powder

½ teaspoon black pepper

½ cup snipped fresh basil leaves

2 tablespoons fresh lime juice
Unsweetened shaved coconut (optional)

1. In an extra-large skillet heat coconut oil over medium heat. Add lemongrass; cook and stir for 1 minute. Add mushrooms, onion, jalapeño, ginger, and garlic; cook and stir for 2 minutes or until onion is just tender. Add chicken; cook about 3 minutes or until chicken is cooked through.

2. In a small bowl combine coconut milk, Chicken Bone Broth, curry powder, and black pepper. Add to chicken mixture in skillet; cook for 1 minute or until the liquid has slightly thickened. Remove from heat; stir in fresh basil and lime juice. If desired, sprinkle servings with coconut.

GRILLED CHICKEN AND APPLE ESCAROLE SALAD

PREP: 30 minutes   GRILL: 12 minutes   MAKES: 4 servings

IF YOU LIKE A SWEETER APPLE, GO WITH HONEYCRISP. IF YOU LIKE A TART APPLE, USE GRANNY SMITH—OR, FOR BALANCE, TRY A MIX OF THE TWO VARIETIES.

3 medium Honeycrisp or Granny Smith apples
4 teaspoons extra virgin olive oil
½ cup finely chopped shallots
2 tablespoons snipped fresh parsley
1 tablespoon poultry seasoning
3 to 4 heads escarole, quartered
1 pound ground chicken or turkey breast
⅓ cup chopped toasted hazelnuts*
⅓ cup Classic French Vinaigrette (see recipe, page 321)

1. Halve and core apples. Peel and finely chop 1 of the apples. In a medium skillet heat 1 teaspoon of the olive oil over medium heat. Add chopped apple and shallots; cook until tender. Stir in parsley and poultry seasoning. Set aside to cool.

2. Meanwhile, core the remaining 2 apples and cut into wedges. Brush cut sides of apple wedges and escarole with the remaining olive oil. In a large bowl combine chicken and the cooled apple mixture. Divide into eight portions; shape each portion into a 2-inch-diameter patty.

3. For a charcoal or gas grill, place chicken patties and apple wedges on a grill rack directly over medium heat. Cover and grill for 10 minutes, turning once halfway through grilling. Add escarole, cut sides down. Cover and grill for 2 to 4 minutes or until escarole is lightly charred, apples are tender, and chicken patties are done (165°F).

4. Coarsely chop escarole. Divide escarole among four serving plates. Top with chicken patties, apple slices, and hazelnuts. Drizzle with Classic French Vinaigrette.

***Tip:** To toast hazelnuts, preheat oven to 350°F. Spread nuts in a single layer in a shallow baking pan. Bake for 8 to 10 minutes or until lightly toasted, stirring once to toast evenly. Cool nuts slightly. Place the warm nuts on a clean kitchen towel; rub with the towel to remove the loose skins.

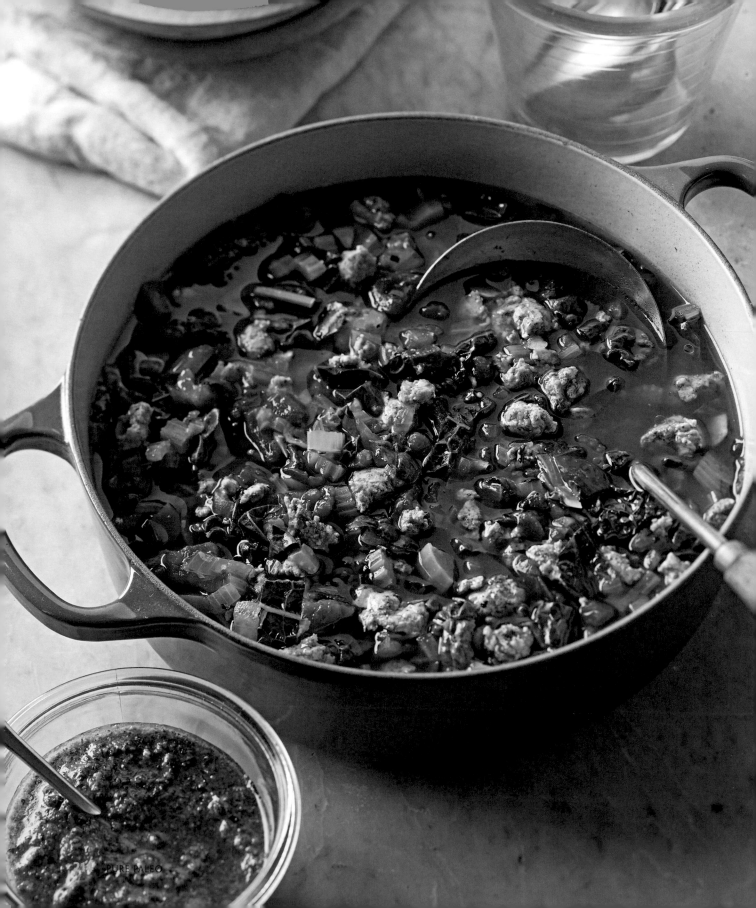

TUSCAN CHICKEN SOUP
WITH KALE RIBBONS

PREP: 15 minutes   COOK: 20 minutes   MAKES: 4 to 6 servings

A SPOONFUL OF PESTO—YOUR CHOICE OF EITHER BASIL OR ARUGULA—ADDS GREAT TASTE TO THIS SAVORY SOUP SEASONED WITH SALT-FREE POULTRY SEASONING. TO KEEP THE KALE RIBBONS BRIGHT GREEN AND AS FULL OF NUTRIENTS AS POSSIBLE, COOK THEM ONLY UNTIL THEY WILT.

1 pound ground chicken
2 tablespoons no-salt-added poultry seasoning
1 teaspoon finely shredded lemon peel
1 tablespoon olive oil
1 cup chopped onion
½ cup chopped carrots
1 cup chopped celery
4 cloves garlic, sliced
4 cups Chicken Bone Broth (see recipe, page 235) or no-salt-added chicken broth
1 14.5-ounce can no-salt-added fire-roasted tomatoes, undrained
1 bunch Lacinato (Tuscan) kale, stems removed, cut into ribbons
2 tablespoons fresh lemon juice
1 teaspoon snipped fresh thyme
   Basil or Arugula Pesto (see recipes, page 320)

1. In a medium bowl combine ground chicken, poultry seasoning, and lemon peel. Mix well.

2. In a Dutch oven heat olive oil over medium heat. Add chicken mixture, onion, carrots, and celery; cook for 5 to 8 minutes or until chicken is no longer pink, stirring with a wooden spoon to break up meat and adding garlic slices the last 1 minute of cooking. Add Chicken Bone Broth and tomatoes. Bring to boiling; reduce heat. Cover and simmer for 15 minutes. Stir in kale, lemon juice, and thyme. Simmer, uncovered, about 5 minutes or until kale is just wilted.

3. To serve, ladle soup into serving bowls and top with Basil or Arugula Pesto.

CHICKEN LARB

THIS VERSION OF THE POPULAR THAI DISH OF HIGHLY SEASONED GROUND CHICKEN AND VEGETABLES SERVED IN LETTUCE LEAVES IS INCREDIBLY LIGHT AND FLAVORFUL—WITHOUT THE ADDITION OF THE SUGAR, SALT, AND FISH SAUCE (WHICH IS VERY HIGH IN SODIUM) THAT ARE TRADITIONALLY PART OF THE INGREDIENTS LIST. WITH GARLIC, THAI CHILES, LEMONGRASS, LIME PEEL, LIME JUICE, MINT, AND CILANTRO, YOU WON'T MISS THEM.

1 tablespoon refined coconut oil

2 pounds ground chicken (95% lean or ground breast)

8 ounces button mushrooms, finely chopped

1 cup finely chopped red onion

1 to 2 Thai chiles, seeded and finely chopped (see tip, page 56)

2 tablespoons minced garlic

2 tablespoons finely chopped lemongrass*

¼ teaspoon ground cloves

¼ teaspoon black pepper

1 tablespoon finely shredded lime peel

½ cup fresh lime juice

⅓ cup tightly packed fresh mint leaves, chopped

⅓ cup tightly packed fresh cilantro, chopped

1 head iceberg lettuce, separated into leaves

1. In an extra-large skillet heat coconut oil over medium-high heat. Add ground chicken, mushrooms, onion, chile(s), garlic, lemongrass, cloves, and black pepper. Cook for 8 to 10 minutes or until chicken is cooked through, stirring with a wooden spoon to break up meat as it cooks. Drain if necessary. Transfer chicken mixture to an extra-large bowl. Let cool about 20 minutes or until slightly warmer than room temperature, stirring occasionally.

2. Stir lime peel, lime juice, mint, and cilantro into chicken mixture. Serve in lettuce leaves.

***Tip:** To prepare the lemongrass, you'll need a sharp knife. Cut the woody stem off of the bottom of the stalk and the tough green blades at the top of the plant. Remove the two tough outer layers. You should have a piece of lemongrass that is about 6 inches long and pale yellow-white. Cut the stalk in half horizontally, then cut each half in half again. Slice each quarter of the stalk very thinly.

CHICKEN BURGERS WITH SZECHWAN CASHEW SAUCE

PREP: 30 minutes   COOK: 5 minutes   GRILL: 14 minutes   MAKES: 4 servings

THE CHILI OIL MADE BY WARMING OLIVE OIL WITH CRUSHED RED PEPPER CAN BE USED IN OTHER WAYS AS WELL. USE IT TO SAUTÉ FRESH VEGETABLES—OR TOSS THEM WITH SOME CHILI OIL BEFORE ROASTING.

2 tablespoons olive oil
¼ teaspoon crushed red pepper
2 cups raw cashew pieces, toasted (see tip, page 57)
¼ cup olive oil
½ cup shredded zucchini
¼ cup finely chopped chives
2 cloves garlic, minced
2 teaspoons finely shredded lemon peel
2 teaspoons grated fresh ginger
1 pound ground chicken or turkey breast

SZECHWAN CASHEW SAUCE
1 tablespoon olive oil
2 tablespoons finely chopped scallions
1 tablespoon grated fresh ginger
1 teaspoon Chinese five-spice powder
1 teaspoon fresh lime juice
4 green leaf or butter lettuce leaves

1. For the chili oil, in a small saucepan combine the olive oil and the crushed red pepper. Warm over low heat for 5 minutes. Remove from heat; let cool.

2. For cashew butter, place cashews and 1 tablespoon of the olive oil in a blender. Cover and blend until creamy, stopping to scrape down the sides as needed and adding additional olive oil, 1 tablespoon at a time, until the entire ¼ cup has been used and the butter is very soft; set aside.

3. In a large bowl combine the zucchini, chives, garlic, lemon peel, and the 2 teaspoons ginger. Add ground chicken; mix well. Shape chicken mixture into four ½-inch-thick patties.

4. For a charcoal or gas grill, place patties on the greased rack directly over medium heat. Cover and grill for 14 to 16 minutes or until done (165°F), turning once halfway through grilling.

5. Meanwhile, for the sauce, in a small skillet heat the olive oil over medium heat. Add the scallions and the 1 tablespoon ginger; cook over medium-low heat for 2 minutes or until scallions soften. Add ½ cup of the cashew butter (refrigerate remaining cashew butter for up to 1 week), chili oil, lime juice, and five-spice powder. Cook for 2 more minutes. Remove from heat.

6. Serve patties on the lettuce leaves. Drizzle with sauce.

TURKISH CHICKEN WRAPS

PREP: 25 minutes   STAND: 15 minutes   COOK: 8 minutes   MAKES: 4 to 6 servings

"BAHARAT" SIMPLY MEANS "SPICE" IN ARABIC. AN ALL-PURPOSE SEASONING IN MIDDLE EASTERN CUISINE, IT IS OFTEN USED AS A RUB ON FISH, POULTRY, AND MEATS OR MIXED WITH OLIVE OIL AND USED AS A VEGETABLE MARINADE. THE COMBINATION OF WARM, SWEET SPICES SUCH AS CINNAMON, CUMIN, CORIANDER, CLOVES, AND PAPRIKA MAKES IT PARTICULARLY AROMATIC. THE ADDITION OF DRIED MINT IS A TURKISH TOUCH.

⅓ cup snipped unsulfured dried apricots

⅓ cup snipped dried figs

1 tablespoon unrefined coconut oil

1½ pounds ground chicken breast

3 cups sliced leeks (white and light green parts only) (3)

⅔ of a medium green and/or red sweet peppers, thinly sliced

2 tablespoons Baharat Seasoning (see recipe, right)

2 cloves garlic, minced

1 cup chopped, seeded tomatoes (2 medium)

1 cup chopped, seeded cucumber (½ of a medium)

½ cup chopped shelled unsalted pistachios, toasted (see tip, page 57)

¼ cup snipped fresh mint

¼ cup snipped fresh parsley

8 to 12 large butterhead or Bibb lettuce leaves

1. Place apricots and figs in a small bowl. Add ⅔ cup boiling water; let stand for 15 minutes. Drain, reserving ½ cup of the liquid.

2. Meanwhile, in an extra-large skillet heat coconut oil over medium heat. Add ground chicken; cook for 3 minutes, stirring with a wooden spoon to break up meat as it cooks. Add leeks, sweet pepper, Baharat Seasoning, and garlic; cook and stir about 3 minutes or until chicken is done and pepper is just tender. Add apricots, figs, reserved liquid, tomatoes, and cucumber. Cook and stir about 2 minutes or until tomatoes and cucumber just start to break down. Stir in pistachios, mint, and parsley.

3. Serve chicken and vegetables in lettuce leaves.

Baharat Seasoning: In a small bowl combine 2 tablespoons sweet paprika; 1 tablespoon black pepper; 2 teaspoons dried mint, finely crushed; 2 teaspoons ground cumin; 2 teaspoons ground coriander; 2 teaspoons ground cinnamon; 2 teaspoons ground cloves; 1 teaspoon ground nutmeg; and 1 teaspoon ground cardamom. Store in a tightly sealed container at room temperature. Makes about ½ cup.

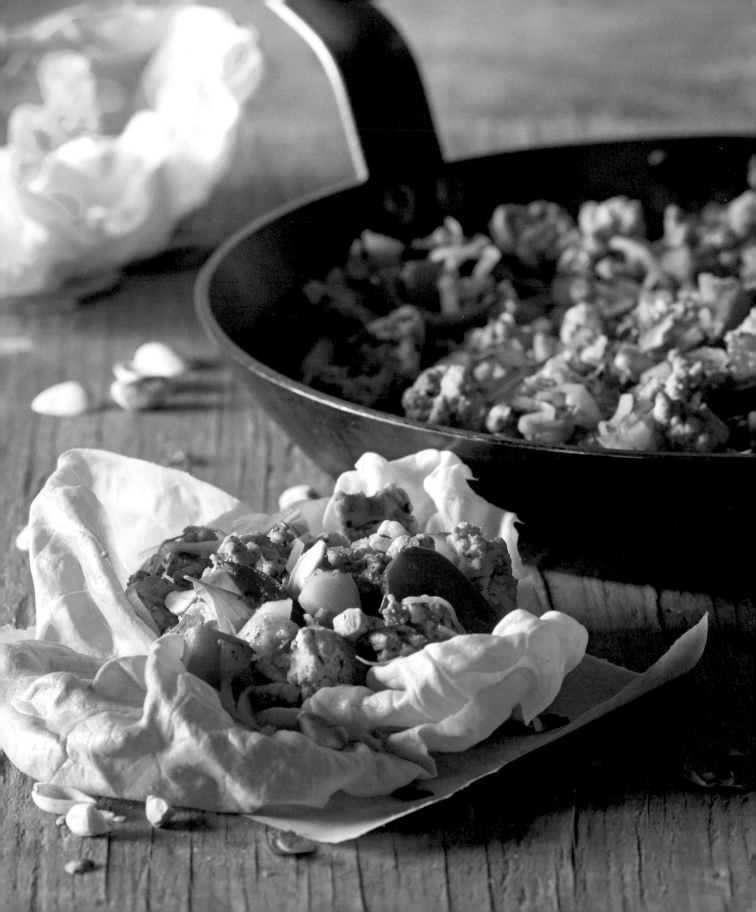

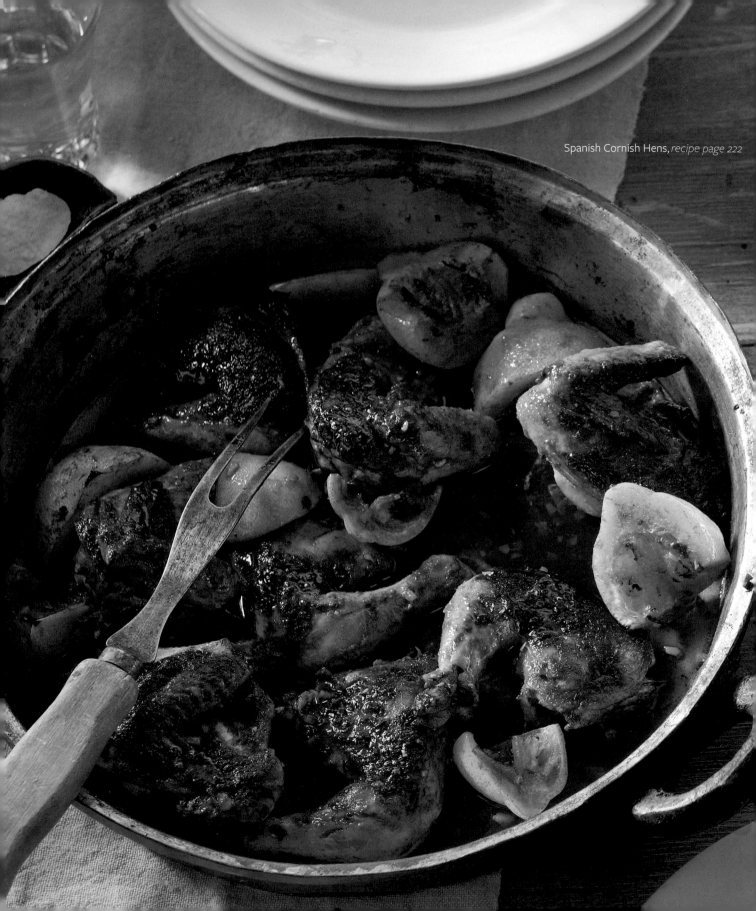

Spanish Cornish Hens, *recipe page 222*

Creamy Celery Root Soup with Herb Oil, *recipe page 295*

SPANISH CORNISH HENS

pictured on page 220

PREP: 10 minutes   BAKE: 30 minutes   BROIL: 6 minutes   MAKES: 2 to 3 servings

THIS RECIPE COULD NOT BE EASIER—AND THE RESULTS ARE ABSOLUTELY AMAZING. COPIOUS AMOUNTS OF SMOKED PAPRIKA, GARLIC, AND LEMON GIVE THESE DIMINUTIVE BIRDS BIG FLAVOR.

2 1½-pound Cornish hens,
   thawed if frozen

1 tablespoon olive oil

6 cloves garlic, chopped

2 to 3 tablespoons smoked sweet
   paprika

¼ to ½ teaspoon cayenne pepper
   (optional)

2 lemons, quartered

2 tablespoons snipped fresh
   parsley (optional)

1. Preheat oven to 375°F. To quarter the game hens, use kitchen shears or a sharp knife to cut along both sides of the narrow backbone. Butterfly the bird open and cut the hen in half through the breastbone. Remove the hindquarters by cutting through the skin and meat that separates the thighs from the breast. Keep the wing and breast intact. Rub olive oil over Cornish hen pieces. Sprinkle with chopped garlic.

2. Place the hen pieces, skin sides up, in an extra-large oven-going skillet. Sprinkle with smoked paprika and cayenne. Squeeze the lemon quarters over the hens; add lemon quarters to the skillet. Turn hen pieces skin sides down in the pan. Cover and bake for 30 minutes. Remove skillet from oven.

3. Preheat broiler. Using tongs, turn the pieces. Adjust oven rack. Broil 4 to 5 inches from the heat for 6 to 8 minutes until skin is browned and hens are done (175°F). Drizzle with pan juices. If desired, sprinkle with parsley.

PISTACHIO-ROASTED CORNISH HENS WITH ARUGULA, APRICOT, AND FENNEL SALAD

PREP: 30 minutes   CHILL: 2 to 12 hours   ROAST: 50 minutes   STAND: 10 minutes   MAKES: 8 servings

A PISTACHIO PESTO MADE WITH PARSLEY, THYME, GARLIC, ORANGE PEEL, ORANGE JUICE, AND OLIVE OIL IS TUCKED UNDER THE SKIN OF EACH BIRD BEFORE MARINATING.

4 20- to 24-ounce Cornish game hens
3 cups raw pistachio nuts
2 tablespoons snipped fresh Italian (flat-leaf) parsley
1 tablespoon snipped thyme
1 large clove garlic, minced
2 teaspoons finely shredded orange peel
2 tablespoons fresh orange juice
¾ cup olive oil
2 large onions, thinly sliced
½ cup fresh orange juice
2 tablespoons fresh lemon juice
¼ teaspoon freshly ground black pepper
¼ teaspoon dry mustard
2 5-ounce packages arugula
1 large bulb fennel, thinly shaved
2 tablespoons snipped fennel fronds
4 apricots, pitted and cut into thin wedges

1. Rinse inside cavities of Cornish game hens. Tie legs together with 100%-cotton kitchen string. Tuck wings under bodies; set aside.

2. In a food processor or blender combine pistachios, parsley, thyme, garlic, orange peel, and orange juice. Process until coarse paste forms. With processor running, add ¼ cup of the olive oil in a slow, steady stream.

3. Using fingers, loosen skin on the breast side of a hen to make a pocket. Spread one-fourth of the pistachio mixture evenly under the skin. Repeat with remaining hens and pistachio mixture. Spread sliced onions over bottom of roasting pan; place hens, breast sides up, on top of onions. Cover and refrigerate for 2 to 12 hours.

4. Preheat oven to 425°F. Roast hens for 30 to 35 minutes or until an instant-read thermometer inserted in an inside thigh muscle registers 175°F.

5. Meanwhile, for dressing, in a small bowl combine orange juice, lemon juice, pepper, and mustard. Mix well. Add the remaining ½ cup olive oil in a slow steady stream, whisking constantly.

6. For salad, in a large bowl combine arugula, fennel, fennel fronds, and apricots. Drizzle lightly with dressing; toss well. Reserve additional dressing for another purpose.

7. Remove hens from oven; tent loosely with foil and let stand 10 minutes. To serve, divide the salad evenly among eight serving plates. Cut hens in half lengthwise; place hen halves on salads. Serve immediately.

DUCK BREAST WITH POMEGRANATE AND JICAMA SALAD

PREP: 15 minutes   COOK: 15 minutes   MAKES: 4 servings

CUTTING A DIAMOND PATTERN INTO THE FAT OF THE DUCK BREASTS ALLOWS THE FAT TO RENDER OUT AS THE GARAM MASALA-SEASONED BREASTS COOK. THE DRIPPINGS ARE COMBINED WITH JICAMA, POMEGRANATE SEEDS, ORANGE JUICE, AND BEEF BROTH AND TOSSED WITH PEPPERY GREENS TO WILT THEM JUST SLIGHTLY.

4 boneless Muscovy duck breasts (about 1½ to 2 pounds total)
1 tablespoon garam masala
1 tablespoon unrefined coconut oil
2 cups diced, peeled jicama
½ cup pomegranate seeds
¼ cup fresh orange juice
¼ cup Beef Bone Broth (see recipe, page 131) or no-salt-added beef broth
3 cups watercress, stems removed
3 cups torn frisée and/or thinly sliced Belgian endive

1. With a sharp knife, make shallow cuts in diamond patterns into the fat of duck breasts at 1-inch intervals. Sprinkle both sides of the breast halves with the garam masala. Heat an extra-large skillet over medium heat. Melt the coconut oil in the hot skillet. Place breast halves, skin sides down, in the skillet. Cook for 8 minutes with the skin sides down, being careful not to brown too quickly (reduce heat if necessary). Turn duck breasts over; cook for 5 to 6 minutes more or until an instant-read thermometer inserted into breast halves registers 145°F for medium. Remove breast halves, reserving drippings in a skillet; cover with foil to keep warm.

2. For dressing, add jicama to drippings in skillet; cook and stir for 2 minutes over medium heat. Add pomegranate seeds, orange juice, and Beef Bone Broth to skillet. Bring to boiling; immediately remove from heat.

3. For salad, in a large bowl combine watercress and frisée. Pour hot dressing over greens; toss to coat.

4. Divide salad among four dinner plates. Thinly slice the duck breasts and arrange on salads.

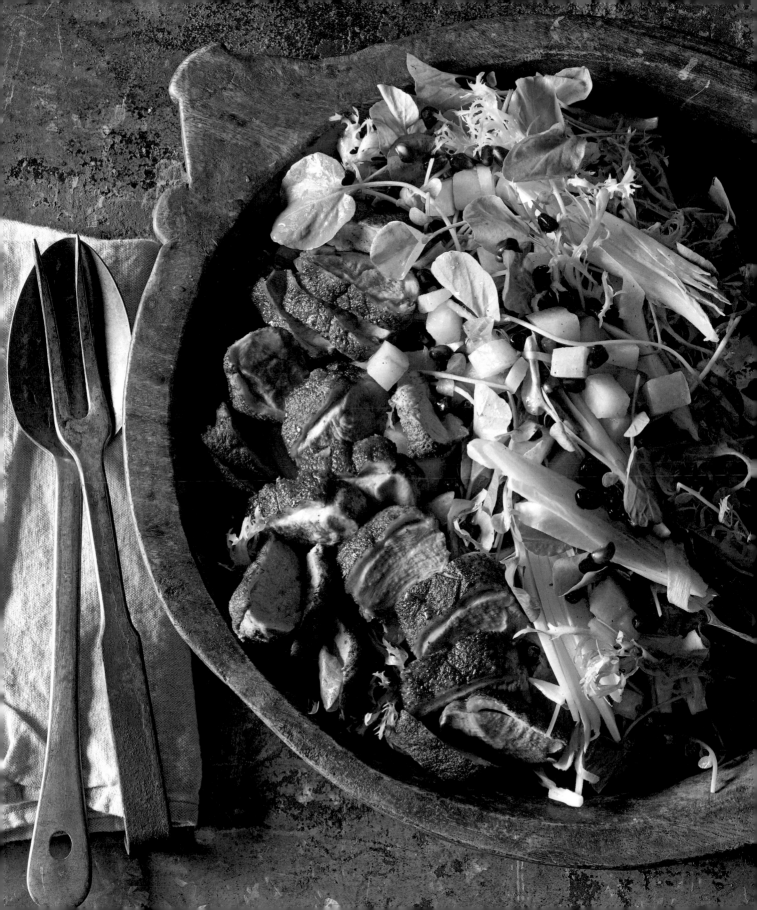

ROASTED TURKEY WITH GARLICKY MASHED ROOTS

PREP: 1 hour   ROAST: 2 hours 45 minutes   STAND: 15 minutes   MAKES: 12 to 14 servings

LOOK FOR A TURKEY THAT HAS NOT BEEN INJECTED WITH A SALT SOLUTION. IF THE LABEL SAYS "ENHANCED" OR "SELF-BASTING," IT LIKELY IS FULL OF SODIUM AND OTHER ADDITIVES.

1 12- to 14–pound turkey
2 tablespoons Mediterranean Seasoning (see recipe, page 324)
¼ cup olive oil
3 pounds medium carrots, peeled, trimmed, and halved or quartered lengthwise
1 recipe Garlicky Mashed Roots (see recipe, right)

1. Preheat oven to 425°F. Remove neck and giblets from turkey; reserve for another use if desired. Carefully loosen skin from the edge of the breast. Run your fingers under the skin to create a pocket on top of the breast and on top of the drumsticks. Spoon 1 tablespoon of the Mediterranean Seasoning under the skin; use your fingers to evenly spread it over the breast and drumsticks. Pull neck skin to the back; fasten with a skewer. Tuck ends of drumsticks under the band of skin across the tail. If there is no band of skin, tie drumsticks securely to the tail with 100%-cotton kitchen string. Twist wing tips under the back.

2. Place turkey, breast side up, on a rack in a shallow extra-large roasting pan. Brush turkey with 2 tablespoons of the oil. Sprinkle turkey with remaining Mediterranean Seasoning. Insert an oven-going meat thermometer into the center of an inside thigh muscle; the thermometer should not touch bone. Cover turkey loosely with foil.

3. Roast for 30 minutes. Reduce oven temperature to 325°F. Roast for 1½ hours. In an extra-large bowl combine carrots and the remaining 2 tablespoons oil; toss to coat. Spread carrots in a large rimmed baking pan. Remove foil from turkey and cut band of skin or string between drumsticks. Roast carrots and turkey for 45 minutes to 1¼ hours more or until the thermometer registers 175°F.

4. Remove turkey from oven. Cover; let stand for 15 to 20 minutes before carving. Serve turkey with carrots and Garlicky Mashed Roots.

Garlicky Mashed Roots: Trim and peel 3 to 3½ pounds rutabagas and 1½ to 2 pounds celery root; cut into 2-inch pieces. In a 6-quart pot cook rutabagas and celery root in enough boiling water to cover for 25 to 30 minutes or until very tender. Meanwhile, in a small saucepan combine 3 tablespoons extra virgin oil and 6 to 8 cloves minced garlic. Cook over low heat for 5 to 10 minutes or until garlic is very fragrant but not browned. Carefully add ¾ cup Chicken Bone Broth (see recipe, page 235) or no-salt-added chicken broth. Bring to boiling; remove from heat. Drain vegetables and return to the pot. Mash vegetables with a potato masher or beat with an electric mixer on low. Add ½ teaspoon black pepper. Gradually mash or beat in broth mixture until vegetables are combined and nearly smooth. If necessary, add an additional ¼ cup Chicken Bone Broth to make desired consistency.

STUFFED TURKEY BREAST WITH PESTO SAUCE AND ARUGULA SALAD

PREP: 30 minutes   ROAST: 1 hour 30 minutes   STAND: 20 minutes   MAKES: 6 servings

THIS IS FOR THE WHITE-MEAT LOVERS OUT THERE—A CRISP-SKINNED BREAST OF TURKEY STUFFED WITH DRIED TOMATOES, BASIL, AND MEDITERRANEAN SPICES. LEFTOVERS MAKE A GREAT LUNCH.

1 cup unsulfured dried tomatoes (not oil-packed)
1 4-pound boneless turkey breast half with skin
3 teaspoons Mediterranean Seasoning (see recipe, page 324)
1 cup loosely packed fresh basil leaves
1 tablespoon olive oil
8 ounces baby arugula
3 large tomatoes, halved and sliced
¼ cup olive oil
2 tablespoons red wine vinegar
Black pepper
1½ cups Basil Pesto (see recipe, page 320)

1. Preheat oven to 375°F. In a small bowl pour enough boiling water over dried tomatoes to cover. Let stand for 5 minutes; drain and finely chop.

2. Place turkey breast, skin side down, on a large sheet of plastic wrap. Place another sheet of plastic wrap over turkey. Using the flat side of a meat mallet, gently pound breast to an even thickness, about ¾ inch thick. Discard plastic wrap. Sprinkle 1½ teaspoons of the Mediterranean Seasoning over the meat. Top with the tomatoes and basil leaves. Carefully roll up turkey breast, keeping skin on the outside. Using 100%-cotton kitchen string, tie roast in four to six places to secure. Brush with 1 tablespoon olive oil. Sprinkle roast with the remaining 1½ teaspoons Mediterranean Seasoning.

3. Place roast on a rack set in a shallow pan with the skin side up. Roast, uncovered, for 1½ hours or until an instant-read thermometer inserted near the center registers 165°F and skin is golden brown and crisp. Remove turkey from oven. Cover loosely with foil; let stand for 20 minutes before slicing.

4. For arugula salad, in a large bowl combine arugula, tomatoes, ¼ cup olive oil, the vinegar, and pepper to taste. Remove strings from roast. Thinly slice turkey. Serve with arugula salad and Basil Pesto.

SPICED TURKEY BREAST WITH CHERRY BBQ SAUCE

PREP: 15 minutes   ROAST: 1 hour 15 minutes   STAND: 45 minutes   MAKES: 6 to 8 servings

THIS IS A NICE RECIPE FOR SERVING A CROWD AT A BACKYARD BARBECUE WHEN YOU WANT TO DO SOMETHING OTHER THAN BURGERS. SERVE IT WITH A CRISP SALAD, SUCH AS CRUNCHY BROCCOLI SALAD (PAGE 299) OR SHAVED BRUSSELS SPROUTS SALAD (PAGE 311).

1 4- to 5-pound whole bone-in turkey breast
3 tablespoons Smoky Seasoning (see recipe, page 324)
2 tablespoons fresh lemon juice
3 tablespoons olive oil
1 cup dry white wine, such as Sauvignon Blanc
1 cup fresh or frozen unsweetened Bing cherries, pitted and chopped
⅓ cup water
1 cup BBQ Sauce (see recipe, page 323)

1. Let turkey breast stand at room temperature for 30 minutes. Preheat oven to 325°F. Place the turkey breast, skin side up, on a rack in a roasting pan.

2. In a small bowl combine the Smoky Seasoning, lemon juice, and olive oil to make a paste. Loosen the skin from the meat; gently spread half of the paste onto the meat under the skin. Spread the remaining paste evenly over the skin. Pour the wine into the bottom of the roasting pan.

3. Roast for 1¼ to 1½ hours or until the skin is golden brown and an instant-read thermometer inserted into center of roast (not touching bone) registers 170°F, turning the roasting pan halfway through cooking time. Let stand for 15 to 30 minutes before carving.

4. Meanwhile, for Cherry BBQ Sauce, in a medium saucepan combine cherries and the water. Bring to boiling; reduce heat. Simmer, uncovered, for 5 minutes. Stir in BBQ Sauce; simmer for 5 minutes. Serve warm or at room temperature with the turkey.

WINE-BRAISED TURKEY TENDERLOIN

PREP: 30 minutes   COOK: 35 minutes   MAKES: 4 servings

COOKING THE PAN-SEARED TURKEY IN A COMBINATION OF WINE, CHOPPED ROMA TOMATOES, CHICKEN BROTH, FRESH HERBS, AND CRUSHED RED PEPPER INFUSES IT WITH GREAT FLAVOR. SERVE THIS STEWLIKE DISH IN SHALLOW BOWLS AND WITH BIG SPOONS TO GET SOME OF THE TASTY BROTH WITH EVERY BITE.

2　8- to 12-ounce turkey tenderloins, cut into 1-inch pieces

2　tablespoons no-salt-added poultry seasoning

2　tablespoons olive oil

6　cloves garlic, minced (1 tablespoon)

1　cup chopped onion

½　cup chopped celery

6　roma tomatoes, seeded and chopped (about 3 cups)

½　cup dry white wine, such as Sauvignon Blanc

½　cup Chicken Bone Broth (see recipe, page 235) or no-salt-added chicken broth

½　teaspoon finely snipped fresh rosemary

¼　to ½ teaspoon crushed red pepper

½　cup fresh basil leaves, chopped

½　cup snipped fresh parsley

1. In a large bowl toss turkey pieces with poultry seasoning to coat. In an extra-large nonstick skillet heat 1 tablespoon of the olive oil over medium heat. Cook turkey in batches in hot oil until browned on all sides. (Turkey does not need to be cooked through.) Transfer to a plate and keep warm.

2. Add the remaining 1 tablespoon olive oil to the pan. Increase heat to medium-high. Add the garlic; cook and stir for 1 minute. Add onion and celery; cook and stir for 5 minutes. Add the turkey and any juices from the plate, tomatoes, wine, Chicken Bone Broth, rosemary, and crushed red pepper. Reduce heat to medium-low. Cover and cook for 20 minutes, stirring occasionally. Add basil and parsley. Uncover and cook for 5 minutes more or until turkey is no longer pink.

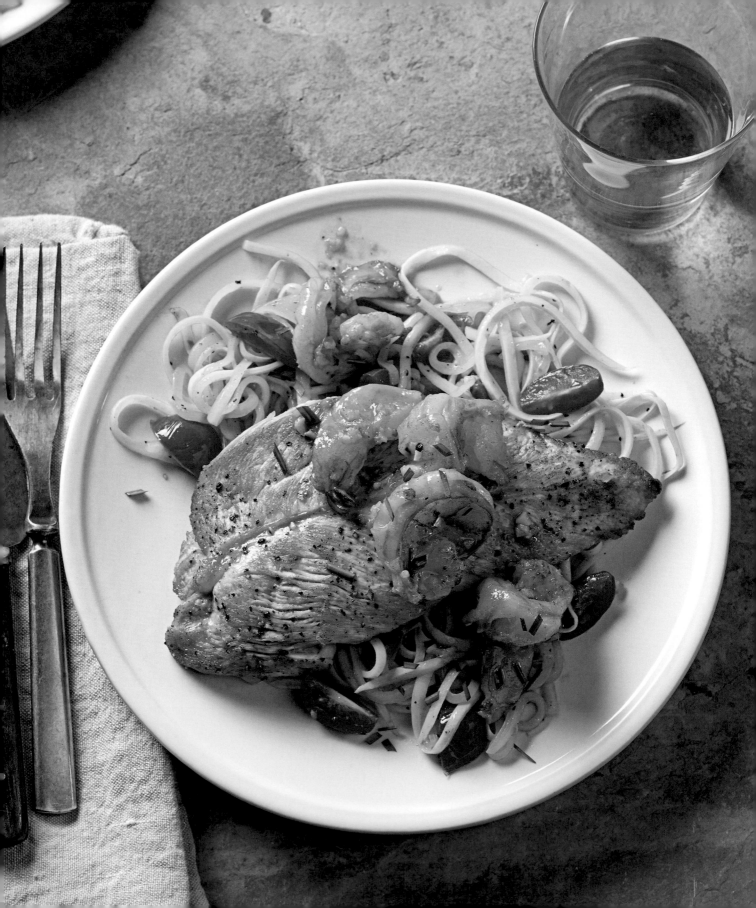

PAN-SAUTÉED TURKEY BREAST WITH CHIVE SCAMPI SAUCE

PREP: 30 minutes   COOK: 15 minutes   MAKES: 4 servings

TO CUT THE TURKEY TENDERLOINS IN HALF HORIZONTALLY AS EVENLY AS POSSIBLE, LIGHTLY PRESS DOWN ON EACH ONE WITH THE PALM OF YOUR HAND, APPLYING CONSISTENT PRESSURE, AS YOU CUT THROUGH THE MEAT.

¼ cup olive oil

2 8- to 12-ounce turkey breast tenderloins, cut in half horizontally

¼ teaspoon freshly ground black pepper

3 tablespoons olive oil

4 cloves garlic, minced

8 ounces peeled and deveined medium shrimp, tails removed and halved lengthwise

¼ cup dry white wine, Chicken Bone Broth (see recipe, page 235), or no-salt-added chicken broth

2 tablespoons snipped fresh chives

½ teaspoon finely shredded lemon peel

1 tablespoon fresh lemon juice
Squash Noodles and Tomatoes (see recipe, right) (optional)

1. In an extra-large skillet heat 1 tablespoon of the olive oil over medium-high heat. Add turkey to skillet; sprinkle with pepper. Reduce heat to medium. Cook for 12 to 15 minutes or until no longer pink and juices run clear (165°F), turning once halfway through cooking time. Remove turkey steaks from skillet. Cover with foil to keep warm.

2. For sauce, in the same skillet heat the 3 tablespoons oil over medium heat. Add garlic; cook for 30 seconds. Stir in shrimp; cook and stir for 1 minute. Stir in wine, chives, and lemon peel; cook and stir for 1 minute more or until shrimp are opaque. Remove from heat; stir in lemon juice. To serve, spoon sauce over turkey steaks. If desired, serve with Squash Noodles and Tomatoes.

Squash Noodles and Tomatoes: Using a mandoline or julienne peeler, slice 2 yellow summer squash into julienne strips. In a large skillet heat 1 tablespoon extra virgin olive oil over medium-high heat. Add squash strips; cook for 2 minutes. Add 1 cup quartered grape tomatoes and ¼ teaspoon freshly ground black pepper; cook for 2 minutes more or until squash is crisp-tender.

BRAISED TURKEY LEGS
WITH ROOT VEGETABLES

PREP: 30 minutes   COOK: 1 hour 45 minutes   MAKES: 4 servings

THIS IS ONE OF THOSE DISHES YOU WANT TO MAKE ON A CRISP FALL AFTERNOON WHEN YOU HAVE TIME TO TAKE A WALK WHILE IT SIMMERS IN THE OVEN. IF THE EXERCISE DOESN'T STIR UP AN APPETITE, THE WONDERFUL AROMA WHEN YOU WALK THROUGH THE DOOR CERTAINLY WILL.

3 tablespoons olive oil

4 20- to 24-ounce turkey legs

½ teaspoon freshly ground black pepper

6 cloves garlic, peeled and crushed

1½ teaspoons fennel seeds, bruised

1 teaspoon whole allspice, bruised*

1½ cups Chicken Bone Broth (see recipe, page 235) or no-salt-added chicken broth

2 sprigs fresh rosemary

2 sprigs fresh thyme

1 bay leaf

2 large onions, peeled and cut into 8 wedges each

6 large carrots, peeled and cut into 1-inch slices

2 large turnips, peeled and cut into 1-inch cubes

2 medium parsnips, peeled and cut into 1-inch slices**

1 celery root, peeled and cut into 1-inch pieces

1. Preheat oven to 350°F. In a large skillet heat the olive oil over medium-high heat until shimmering. Add 2 of the turkey legs. Cook about 8 minutes or until legs are golden brown and crisp on all sides, turning to brown evenly. Transfer turkey legs to a plate; repeat with remaining 2 turkey legs. Set aside.

2. Add pepper, garlic, fennel seeds, and allspice seeds to the skillet. Cook and stir over medium heat for 1 to 2 minutes or until fragrant. Stir in Chicken Bone Broth, rosemary, thyme, and bay leaf. Bring to boiling, stirring to scrape browned bits from the bottom of the skillet. Remove skillet from heat and set aside.

3. In an extra-large Dutch oven with a tight-fitting lid combine onions, carrots, turnips, parsnips, and celery root. Add liquid from skillet; toss to coat. Press turkey legs into the vegetable mixture. Cover with lid.

4. Bake about 1 hour 45 minutes or until vegetables are tender and turkey is cooked through. Serve turkey legs and vegetables in large shallow bowls. Drizzle juices from pan over top.

***Tip:** To bruise allspice and fennel seeds, place seeds on a cutting board. Using a flat side of a chef's knife, press down to lightly crush the seeds.

****Tip:** Cube any large pieces from the tops of the parsnips.

HERBED TURKEY MEAT LOAF WITH CARAMELIZED ONION KETCHUP AND ROASTED CABBAGE WEDGES

PREP: 15 minutes   COOK: 30 minutes   BAKE: 1 hour 10 minutes   STAND: 5 minutes   MAKES: 4 servings

CLASSIC KETCHUP-TOPPED MEAT LOAF IS DEFINITELY ON THE PALEO MENU WHEN THE KETCHUP (PAGE 322) IS FREE OF SALT AND ADDED SUGARS. HERE THE KETCHUP IS STIRRED TOGETHER WITH CARAMELIZED ONIONS, WHICH ARE PILED ON TOP OF THE MEAT LOAF BEFORE BAKING.

1½ pounds ground turkey
2 eggs, lightly beaten
½ cup almond meal
⅓ cup snipped fresh parsley
¼ cup thinly sliced scallions (2)
1 tablespoon snipped fresh sage or 1 teaspoon dried sage, crushed
1 tablespoon snipped fresh thyme or 1 teaspoon dried thyme, crushed
¼ teaspoon black pepper
2 tablespoons olive oil
2 sweet onions, halved and thinly sliced
1 cup Paleo Ketchup (see recipe, page 322)
1 small head cabbage, halved, cored, and cut into 8 wedges
½ to 1 teaspoon crushed red pepper

1. Preheat oven to 350°F. Line a large roasting pan with parchment paper; set aside. In a large bowl combine ground turkey, eggs, almond meal, parsley, scallions, sage, thyme, and black pepper. In the prepared roasting pan shape turkey mixture into an 8×4-inch loaf. Bake for 30 minutes.

2. Meanwhile, for the caramelized onion ketchup, in a large skillet heat 1 tablespoon of the olive oil over medium heat. Add onions; cook about 5 minutes or until onions just start to brown, stirring frequently. Reduce heat to medium-low; cook about 25 minutes or until golden and very soft, stirring occasionally. Remove from heat; stir in Paleo Ketchup.

3. Spoon some of the caramelized onion ketchup over turkey loaf. Arrange cabbage wedges around loaf. Drizzle cabbage with the remaining 1 tablespoon olive oil; sprinkle with crushed red pepper. Bake about 40 minutes or until an instant-read thermometer inserted in center of loaf registers 165°F, topping with additional caramelized onion ketchup and turning the cabbage wedges after 20 minutes. Let turkey loaf stand for 5 to 10 minutes before slicing.

4. Serve turkey loaf with cabbage wedges and any remaining caramelized onion ketchup.

TURKEY POSOLE

PREP: 20 minutes   BROIL: 8 minutes   COOK: 16 minutes   MAKES: 4 servings

THE TOPPINGS ON THIS WARMING, MEXICAN-STYLE SOUP ARE MORE THAN GARNISHES. THE CILANTRO ADDS DISTINCTIVE FLAVOR, AVOCADO CONTRIBUTES CREAMINESS—AND TOASTED PEPITAS PROVIDE A DELIGHTFUL CRUNCH.

8 fresh tomatillos

1¼ to 1½ pounds ground turkey

1 red sweet pepper, seeded and cut into thin bite-size strips

½ cup chopped onion (1 medium)

6 cloves garlic, minced (1 tablespoon)

1 tablespoon Mexican Seasoning (see recipe, page 324)

2 cups Chicken Bone Broth (see recipe, page 235) or no-salt-added chicken broth

1 14.5-ounce can no-salt-added fire-roasted tomatoes, undrained

1 jalapeño or serrano chile pepper, seeded and minced (see tip, page 56)

1 medium avocado, halved, peeled, seeded, and thinly sliced

¼ cup unsalted pepitas, toasted (see tip, page 57)

¼ cup snipped fresh cilantro Lime wedges

1. Preheat the broiler. Remove husks from tomatillos and discard. Wash tomatillos and cut into halves. Place tomatillo halves on the unheated rack of a broiler pan. Broil 4 to 5 inches from the heat for 8 to 10 minutes or until lightly charred, turning once halfway through broiling. Cool slightly on pan on a wire rack.

2. Meanwhile, in a large skillet cook turkey, sweet pepper, and onion over medium-high heat for 5 to 10 minutes or until turkey is browned and vegetables are tender, stirring with a wooden spoon to break up meat as it cooks. Drain off fat if necessary. Add garlic and Mexican Seasoning. Cook and stir for 1 minute more.

3. In a blender combine about two-thirds of the charred tomatillos and 1 cup of the Chicken Bone Broth. Cover and blend until smooth. Add to turkey mixture in skillet. Stir in the remaining 1 cup Chicken Bone Broth, undrained tomatoes, and chile pepper. Coarsely chop the remaining tomatillos; add to the turkey mixture. Bring to boiling; reduce heat. Cover and simmer for 10 minutes.

4. To serve, ladle soup into shallow serving bowls. Top with avocado, pepitas, and cilantro. Pass lime wedges to squeeze over soup.

CHICKEN BONE BROTH

PREP: 15 minutes   ROAST: 30 minutes   COOK: 4 hours   CHILL: overnight   MAKES: about 10 cups

FOR THE FRESHEST, BEST TASTE—AND HIGHEST NUTRIENT CONTENT—USE HOMEMADE CHICKEN BROTH IN YOUR RECIPES. (IT ALSO DOESN'T CONTAIN ANY SALT, PRESERVATIVES, OR ADDITIVES.) ROASTING THE BONES BEFORE SIMMERING ENHANCES FLAVOR. AS THEY SLOWLY COOK IN LIQUID, THE BONES INFUSE THE BROTH WITH MINERALS SUCH AS CALCIUM, PHOSPHORUS, MAGNESIUM, AND POTASSIUM. THE SLOW COOKER VARIATION BELOW MAKES IT ESPECIALLY EASY TO DO. FREEZE IT IN 2- AND 4-CUP CONTAINERS AND THAW ONLY WHAT YOU NEED.

2 pounds chicken wings and backs
4 carrots, chopped
2 large leeks, white and pale green parts only, thinly sliced
2 stalks celery with leaves, coarsely chopped
1 parsnip, coarsely chopped
6 large sprigs Italian (flat-leaf) parsley
6 sprigs fresh thyme
4 cloves garlic, halved
2 teaspoons whole black peppercorns
2 whole cloves
Cold water

1. Preheat oven to 425°F. Arrange chicken wings and backs on a large baking sheet; roast for 30 to 35 minutes or until well browned.

2. Transfer browned chicken pieces and any browned bits accumulated on the baking sheet to a large stockpot. Add carrots, leeks, celery, parsnip, parsley, thyme, garlic, peppercorns, and cloves. Add enough cold water (about 12 cups) to a large stockpot to cover chicken and vegetables. Bring to simmering over medium heat; adjust heat to maintain broth at a very low simmer, with bubbles just breaking the surface. Cover and simmer for 4 hours.

3. Strain hot broth through a large colander lined with two layers of damp 100%-cotton cheesecloth. Discard solids. Cover broth and chill overnight. Before using, remove fat layer from top of broth and discard.

Tip: To clarify stock (optional), in a small bowl combine 1 egg white, 1 crushed eggshell, and ¼ cup cold water. Stir mixture into strained stock in pot. Return to boiling. Remove from heat; let stand for 5 minutes. Strain hot broth through a colander lined with a fresh double layer of 100%-cotton cheesecloth. Chill and skim fat before using.

Slow Cooker Directions: Prepare as directed, except in Step 2 place ingredients in a 5- to 6-quart slow cooker. Cover and cook on low-heat setting for 12 to 14 hours. Continue as directed in Step 3. Makes about 10 cups.

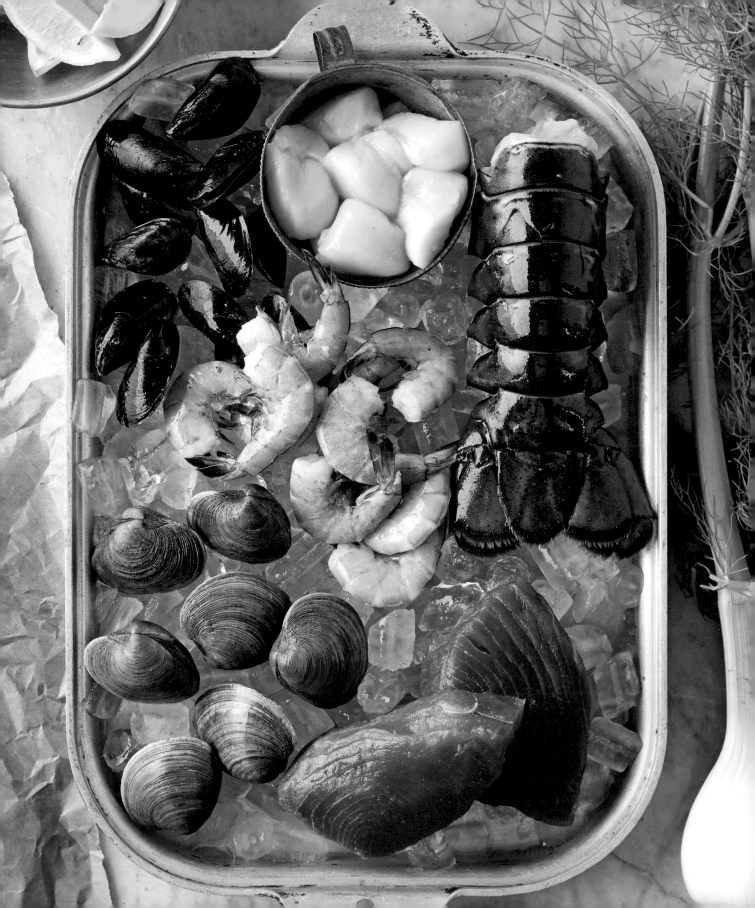

GREEN HARISSA SALMON, **240**

GRILLED SALMON WITH MARINATED ARTICHOKE HEART SALAD, **242**

FLASH-ROASTED CHILE-SAGE SALMON WITH GREEN TOMATO SALSA, **243**

ROASTED SALMON AND ASPARAGUS EN PAPILLOTE WITH LEMON-HAZELNUT PESTO, **244**

SPICE-RUBBED SALMON WITH MUSHROOM-APPLE PAN SAUCE, **245**

SOLE EN PAPILLOTE WITH JULIENNE VEGETABLES, **247**

ARUGULA PESTO FISH TACOS WITH SMOKY LIME CREAM, **248**

ALMOND-CRUSTED SOLE, **249**

RIESLING-POACHED COD WITH PESTO-STUFFED TOMATOES, **252**

GRILLED COD AND ZUCCHINI PACKETS WITH SPICY MANGO-BASIL SAUCE, **252**

BROILED PISTACHIO-CILANTRO-CRUSTED COD OVER SMASHED SWEET POTATOES, **252**

ROSEMARY-AND-TANGERINE COD WITH ROASTED BROCCOLI, **253**

CURRIED COD LETTUCE WRAPS WITH PICKLED RADISHES, **253**

ROASTED HADDOCK WITH LEMON AND FENNEL, **254**

PECAN-CRUSTED SNAPPER WITH REMOULADE AND CAJUN-STYLE OKRA AND TOMATOES, **255**

TARRAGON TUNA PATTIES WITH AVOCADO-LEMON AÏOLI, **256**

STRIPED BASS TAGINE, **258**

HALIBUT IN GARLIC-SHRIMP SAUCE WITH SOFFRITO COLLARD GREENS, **259**

SEAFOOD BOUILLABAISSE, **260**

CLASSIC SHRIMP CEVICHE, **261**

COCONUT-CRUSTED SHRIMP AND SPINACH SALAD, **263**

TROPICAL SHRIMP AND SCALLOP CEVICHE, **264**

JAMAICAN JERK SHRIMP WITH AVOCADO OIL, **265**

SHRIMP SCAMPI WITH WILTED SPINACH AND RADICCHIO, **266**

CRAB SALAD WITH AVOCADO, GRAPEFRUIT, AND JICAMA, **267**

CAJUN LOBSTER TAIL BOIL WITH TARRAGON AÏOLI, **270**

MUSSELS FRITES WITH SAFFRON AÏOLI, **271**

SEARED SCALLOPS WITH BEET RELISH, **272**

GRILLED SCALLOPS WITH CUCUMBER-DILL SALSA, **274**

SEARED SCALLOPS WITH TOMATO, OLIVE OIL, AND HERB SAUCE, **275**

Fish and shellfish are essential elements of contemporary Paleo diets. These foods not only taste good but are also good for us because they are the best source of the healthful omega-3 fatty acids known as EPA and DHA. Fatty fish such as salmon, mackerel, herring, and sardines are particularly enriched in EPA and DHA. A multitude of scientific papers spanning numerous chronic illnesses overwhelmingly demonstrates the therapeutic health benefits of these fatty acids. In large clinical experiments, patients with previously diagnosed heart disease who were given EPA and DHA supplements showed significantly reduced cardiovascular events including deaths, nonfatal heart attacks, and nonfatal strokes.

Because of its omega-3 fatty acid content, fish and seafood are known to be good medicine for inflammatory bowel diseases, mental disorders including depression, certain cancers, macular degeneration, type 2 diabetes, and many other chronic diseases. The tasty fish and shellfish dishes in this chapter will provide you with sufficient EPA and DHA to reduce your risk of heart and other diseases without requiring you to supplement with fish oil capsules.

As with all other Paleo ingredients, use the freshest fish and shellfish you can find. This task can sometimes be challenging, particularly for those of us who don't live close to the oceans. Once fish are caught, they begin to immediately lose their freshness. Most fish and shellfish have a shelf life of about 7 to 12 days once they are out of the water. Frequently, caught fish linger on a boat for a few days, and then it may take a day or two longer to transport them to market. If the fish are not immediately put on ice or if they become warm during any stage of transport, they will spoil even quicker. Spoiled fish release a pungent odor from a chemical called trimethylamine. Any time you notice a strong fishy smell, don't buy the fish or seafood. Fresh fish is practically odorless. If you purchase whole fish, look for moist, bright-red gills, a sign of freshness. Fish with clumped-together brown gills should be avoided. Be cautious when buying fish or seafood that is labeled "previously frozen"; it could be fresh fish that spoiled, was frozen, and then rethawed by the retailer. Obviously, the highest-quality fresh fish comes right off the boat—the day that it is caught. A good second choice is fish caught at sea and then quick-frozen onboard the boat. Freezing entirely stops the bacterial growth that causes spoilage and bad odors. Similarly, if you buy fresh fish and can't eat it within a day or two, freeze it and thaw it when you are ready to cook it.

Besides all of their nutritional and therapeutic health benefits, fish and seafood are simply delicious. In the United States, we think about fish and seafood as lunch and dinner only. Yet in Asian and European countries, fish and shellfish are frequently served for breakfast. One of my favorite breakfasts is steamed cold crab legs or prawns served with a bowl of fresh, seasonal fruit. Check out all of the wonderfully appetizing fish and shellfish recipes in this chapter and don't hesitate to use them as ways to incorporate these high-protein, omega-3-enriched foods into your diet.

GREEN HARISSA SALMON

PREP: 25 minutes   BAKE: 10 minutes   GRILL: 8 minutes   MAKES: 4 servings

A STANDARD VEGETABLE PEELER IS USED TO SHAVE FRESH RAW ASPARAGUS INTO THIN RIBBONS FOR THE SALAD. TOSSED WITH BRIGHT CITRUS VINAIGRETTE (PAGE 320) AND TOPPED WITH SMOKY TOASTED SUNFLOWER SEEDS, IT'S A REFRESHING ACCOMPANIMENT TO THE SALMON AND SPICY GREEN HERB SAUCE.

SALMON
4 6- to 8-ounce fresh or frozen skinless salmon fillets, about 1 inch thick
   Olive oil

HARISSA
1½ teaspoons cumin seeds
1½ teaspoons coriander seeds
1 cup tightly packed fresh parsley leaves
1 cup roughly chopped fresh cilantro (leaves and stems)
2 jalapeños, seeded and coarsely chopped (see tip, page 56)
1 scallion, cut up
2 cloves garlic
1 teaspoon finely shredded lemon peel
2 tablespoons fresh lemon juice
⅓ cup olive oil

SPICED SUNFLOWER SEEDS
⅓ cup raw sunflower seeds
1 teaspoon olive oil
1 teaspoon Smoky Seasoning (see recipe, page 324)

SALAD
12 large asparagus spears, trimmed (about 1 pound)
⅓ cup Bright Citrus Vinaigrette (see recipe, page 320)

1. Thaw fish, if frozen; pat dry with paper towels. Brush both sides of fish lightly with olive oil. Set aside.

2. For harissa, in a small skillet toast cumin seeds and coriander seeds over medium-low heat for 3 to 4 minutes or until lightly toasted and fragrant. In a food processor combine toasted cumin and coriander seeds, the parsley, cilantro, jalapeños, scallion, garlic, lemon peel, lemon juice, and olive oil. Process until smooth. Set aside.

3. For spiced sunflower seeds, preheat oven to 300°F. Line a baking sheet with parchment paper; set aside. In a small bowl combine sunflower seeds and 1 teaspoon olive oil. Sprinkle the Smoky Seasoning over the seeds; stir to coat. Spread sunflower seeds evenly on the parchment paper. Bake about 10 minutes or until lightly toasted.

4. For a charcoal or gas grill, place salmon on a greased grill rack directly over medium heat. Cover and grill for 8 to 12 minutes or until fish begins to flake when tested with a fork, turning once halfway through grilling.

5. Meanwhile, for salad, using a vegetable peeler, shave asparagus spears into long thin ribbons. Transfer to a platter or medium bowl. (The tips will snap off as the spears get thinner; add them to platter or bowl.) Drizzle the Bright Citrus Vinaigrette over shaved spears. Sprinkle with spiced sunflower seeds.

6. To serve, place a fillet on each of four plates; spoon some of the green harissa on each fillet. Serve with shaved asparagus salad.

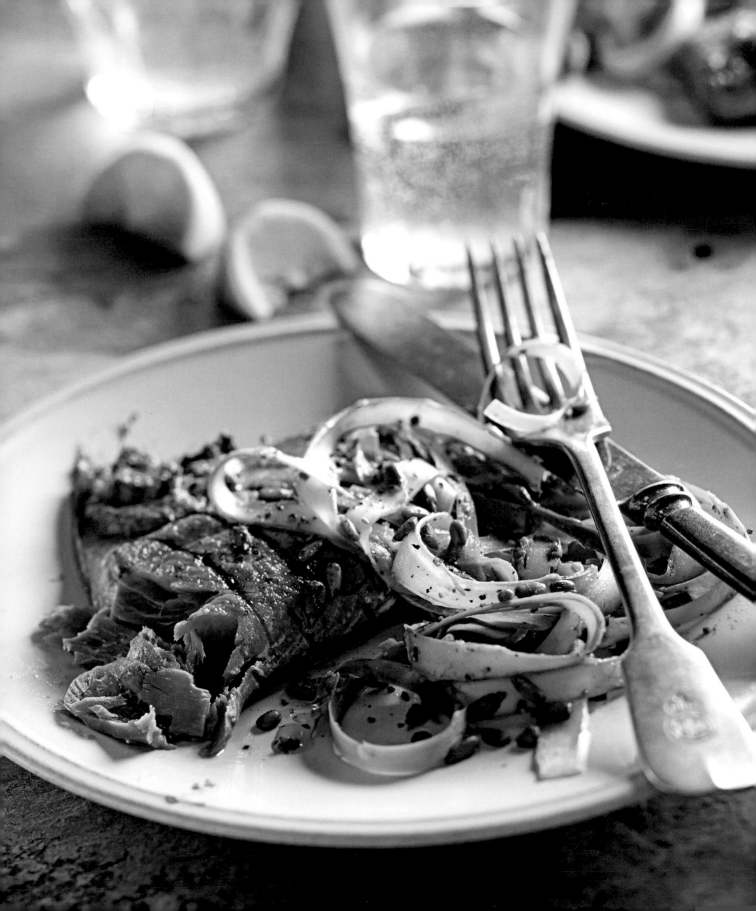

GRILLED SALMON WITH MARINATED ARTICHOKE HEART SALAD

PREP: 20 minutes   GRILL: 12 minutes   MAKES: 4 servings

OFTENTIMES, THE BEST TOOLS FOR TOSSING A SALAD ARE YOUR HANDS. GETTING THE TENDER LETTUCES AND GRILLED ARTICHOKES TO INCORPORATE EVENLY IN THIS SALAD IS BEST DONE WITH CLEAN HANDS.

4 6-ounce fresh or frozen salmon fillets

1 9-ounce package frozen artichoke hearts, thawed and drained

5 tablespoons olive oil

2 tablespoons minced shallots

1 tablespoon finely shredded lemon peel

¼ cup fresh lemon juice

3 tablespoons snipped fresh oregano

½ teaspoon freshly ground black pepper

1 tablespoon Mediterranean seasoning (see recipe, page 324)

1 5-ounce package mixed baby lettuces

1. Thaw fish, if frozen. Rinse fish; pat dry with paper towels. Set fish aside.

2. In a medium bowl toss artichoke hearts with 2 tablespoons of the olive oil; set aside. In a large bowl combine 2 tablespoons of the olive oil, the shallots, lemon peel, lemon juice, and oregano; set aside.

3. For a charcoal or gas grill, place the artichoke hearts in a grill basket and grill directly over medium-high heat. Cover and grill for 6 to 8 minutes or until nicely charred and heated through, stirring frequently. Remove artichokes from grill. Let cool 5 minutes, then add artichokes to shallot mixture. Season with pepper; toss to coat. Set aside.

4. Brush salmon with the remaining 1 tablespoon olive oil; sprinkle with the Mediterranean Seasoning. Place salmon on the grill rack, seasoned sides down, directly over medium-high heat. Cover and grill for 6 to 8 minutes or until fish begins to flake when tested with a fork, carefully turning once halfway through grilling.

5. Add lettuces to bowl with marinated artichokes; toss gently to coat. Serve salad with grilled salmon.

FLASH-ROASTED CHILE-SAGE SALMON WITH GREEN TOMATO SALSA

PREP: 35 minutes   CHILL: 2 to 4 hours   ROAST: 10 minutes   MAKES: 4 servings

"FLASH-ROASTING" REFERS TO THE TECHNIQUE OF HEATING A DRY SKILLET IN THE OVEN AT A HIGH TEMPERATURE, ADDING SOME OIL AND THE FISH, CHICKEN, OR MEAT (IT SIZZLES!), THEN FINISHING THE DISH IN THE OVEN. FLASH-ROASTING CUTS DOWN ON COOKING TIME AND CREATES A DELICIOUSLY CRISP CRUST ON THE EXTERIOR—AND A JUICY, FLAVORFUL INTERIOR.

SALMON

- 4 5- to 6-ounce fresh or frozen salmon fillets
- 3 tablespoons olive oil
- ¼ cup finely chopped onion
- 2 cloves garlic, peeled and sliced
- 1 tablespoon ground coriander
- 1 teaspoon ground cumin
- 2 teaspoons sweet paprika
- 1 teaspoon dried oregano, crushed
- ¼ teaspoon cayenne pepper
- ⅓ cup fresh lime juice
- 1 tablespoon snipped fresh sage

GREEN TOMATO SALSA

- 1½ cups diced firm green tomatoes
- ⅓ cup finely chopped red onion
- 2 tablespoons snipped fresh cilantro
- 1 jalapeño, seeded and minced (see tip, page 56)
- 1 clove garlic, minced
- ½ teaspoon ground cumin
- ¼ teaspoon chili powder
- 2 to 3 tablespoons fresh lime juice

1. Thaw fish, if frozen. Rinse fish; pat dry with paper towels. Set fish aside.

2. For chile-sage paste, in a small saucepan combine 1 tablespoon of the olive oil, onion, and garlic. Cook over low heat for 1 to 2 minutes or until fragrant. Stir in coriander and cumin; cook and stir for 1 minute. Stir in paprika, oregano, and cayenne pepper; cook and stir for 1 minute. Add lime juice and sage; cook and stir about 3 minutes or just until a smooth paste forms; cool.

3. Using your fingers, coat both sides of fillets with chile-sage paste. Place fish in a glass or nonreactive dish; cover tightly with plastic wrap. Refrigerate for 2 to 4 hours.

4. Meanwhile, for salsa, in a medium bowl combine tomatoes, onion, cilantro, jalapeño, garlic, cumin, and chili powder. Toss well to mix. Drizzle with lime juice; toss to coat.

4. Using a rubber spatula, scrape as much paste as you can off of the salmon. Discard paste.

5. Place an extra-large cast-iron skillet in the oven. Turn oven to 500°F. Preheat oven with skillet in it.

6. Remove hot skillet from oven. Pour 1 tablespoon olive oil into the pan. Tip pan to cover the bottom of the skillet with oil. Place fillets in the skillet, skin sides down. Brush tops of fillets with the remaining 1 tablespoon olive oil.

7. Roast salmon about 10 minutes or until fish begins to flake when tested with a fork. Serve fish with salsa.

ROASTED SALMON AND ASPARAGUS EN PAPILLOTE WITH LEMON-HAZELNUT PESTO

PREP: 20 minutes   ROAST: 17 minutes   MAKES: 4 servings

COOKING "EN PAPILLOTE" SIMPLY MEANS COOKING IN PAPER. IT IS A BEAUTIFUL WAY TO COOK FOR MANY REASONS. THE FISH AND VEGETABLES STEAM INSIDE THE PARCHMENT PACKET, SEALING IN JUICES, FLAVOR, AND NUTRIENTS—AND THERE ARE NO POTS AND PANS TO WASH AFTERWARDS.

4 6-ounce fresh or frozen salmon fillets

1 cup lightly packed fresh basil leaves

1 cup lightly packed fresh parsley leaves

½ cup hazelnuts, toasted*

5 tablespoons olive oil

1 teaspoon finely shredded lemon peel

2 tablespoons fresh lemon juice

1 clove garlic, chopped

1 pound slender asparagus, trimmed

4 tablespoons dry white wine

1. Thaw salmon, if frozen. Rinse fish; pat dry with paper towels. Preheat oven to 400°F.

2. For pesto, in a blender or food processor combine basil, parsley, hazelnuts, olive oil, lemon peel, lemon juice, and garlic. Cover and blend or process until smooth; set aside.

3. Cut four 12-inch squares of parchment paper. For each packet, place a salmon fillet in the center of a parchment square. Top with one-fourth of the asparagus and 2 to 3 tablespoons pesto; drizzle with 1 tablespoon wine. Bring up two opposite sides of the parchment paper and fold together several times over fish. Fold ends of parchment to seal. Repeat to make three more packets.

4. Roast for 17 to 19 minutes or until fish begins to flake when tested with a fork (carefully open packet to check doneness).

***Tip:** To toast hazelnuts, preheat oven to 350°F. Spread nuts in a single layer in a shallow baking pan. Bake for 8 to 10 minutes or until lightly toasted, stirring once to toast evenly. Cool nuts slightly. Place warm nuts on a clean kitchen towel; rub with the towel to remove the loose skins.

SPICE-RUBBED SALMON WITH MUSHROOM-APPLE PAN SAUCE

START TO FINISH: **40 minutes**   MAKES: **4 servings**

THIS WHOLE SALMON FILLET TOPPED WITH A MIXTURE OF SAUTÉED MUSHROOMS, SHALLOT, RED-SKINNED APPLE SLICES—AND SERVED ON A BED OF BRIGHT-GREEN SPINACH—MAKES AN IMPRESSIVE DISH TO SERVE TO GUESTS.

1   1½-pound fresh or frozen whole salmon fillet, skin on
1   teaspoon fennel seeds, finely crushed*
½   teaspoon dried sage, crushed
½   teaspoon ground coriander
¼   teaspoon dry mustard
¼   teaspoon black pepper
2   tablespoons olive oil
1½ cups fresh cremini mushrooms, quartered
1   medium shallot, very thinly sliced
1   small cooking apple, quartered, cored, and thinly sliced
¼   cup dry white wine
4   cups fresh spinach
    Small sprigs fresh sage (optional)

1. Thaw salmon, if frozen. Preheat oven to 425°F. Line a large baking sheet with parchment paper; set aside. Rinse fish; pat dry with paper towels. Place salmon, skin side down, on prepared baking sheet. In a small bowl combine fennel seeds, ½ teaspoon dried sage, coriander, mustard, and pepper. Sprinkle evenly over salmon; rub in with your fingers.

2. Measure thickness of fish. Roast salmon for 4 to 6 minutes per ½-inch thickness or until fish begins to flake when tested with a fork.

3. Meanwhile, for pan sauce, in a large skillet heat olive oil over medium heat. Add mushrooms and shallot; cook for 6 to 8 minutes or until mushrooms are tender and starting to brown, stirring occasionally. Add apple; cover and cook and stir for 4 minutes more. Carefully add wine. Cook, uncovered, for 2 to 3 minutes or until apple slices are just tender. Using a slotted spoon, transfer mushroom mixture to a medium bowl; cover to keep warm.

4. In the same skillet cook spinach for 1 minute or until spinach is just wilted, stirring constantly. Divide spinach among four serving plates. Cut salmon fillet into four equal portions, cutting to, but not through, the skin. Use a large spatula to lift salmon portions off of the skin; place one salmon portion on spinach on each plate. Spoon mushroom mixture evenly over salmon. If desired, garnish with fresh sage.

*****Tip:** Use a mortar and pestle or spice grinder to finely crush the fennel seeds.

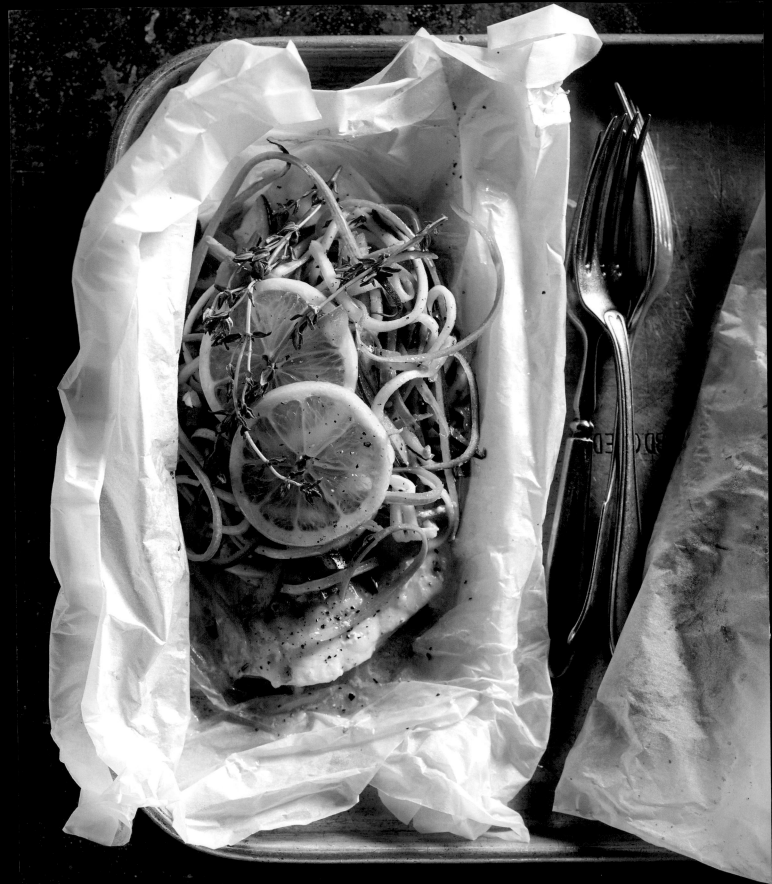

SOLE EN PAPILLOTE WITH JULIENNE VEGETABLES

PREP: 30 minutes   BAKE: 12 minutes   MAKES: 4 servings

YOU CAN CERTAINLY JULIENNE VEGETABLES WITH A GOOD SHARP CHEF'S KNIFE, BUT IT IS VERY TIME-CONSUMING. A JULIENNE PEELER (SEE "EQUIPMENT", PAGE 22) MAKES QUICK WORK OF CREATING LONG, THIN, CONSISENTLY SHAPED STRIPS OF VEGETABLES.

4 6-ounce fresh or frozen sole, flounder, or other firm white fish fillets
1 zucchini, julienne cut
1 large carrot, julienne cut
½ of a red onion, julienne cut
2 roma tomatoes, seeded and finely chopped
2 cloves garlic, minced
1 tablespoon olive oil
½ teaspoon black pepper
1 lemon, cut into 8 thin slices, seeds removed
8 sprigs fresh thyme
4 teaspoons olive oil
¼ cup dry white wine

1. Thaw fish, if frozen. Preheat oven to 375°F. In a large bowl combine zucchini, carrot, onion, tomatoes, and garlic. Add 1 tablespoon olive oil and ¼ teaspoon of the pepper; toss well to combine. Set vegetables aside.

2. Cut four 14-inch squares of parchment paper. Rinse fish; pat dry with paper towels. Place a fillet in the center of each square. Sprinkle with the remaining ¼ teaspoon pepper. Arrange vegetables, lemon slices, and thyme sprigs on top of fillets, dividing evenly. Drizzle each stack with 1 teaspoon olive oil and 1 tablespoon white wine.

3. Working with one packet at a time, bring up two opposite sides of the parchment paper and fold together several times over fish. Fold ends of parchment to seal.

4. Arrange packets on a large baking sheet. Bake about 12 minutes or until fish begins to flake when tested with a fork (carefully open packet to check doneness).

5. To serve, place each packet on a dinner plate; carefully open packets.

ARUGULA PESTO FISH TACOS
WITH SMOKY LIME CREAM

PREP: 30 minutes   GRILL: 4 to 6 minutes per ½-inch thickness   MAKES: 6 servings

YOU CAN SUBSTITUTE COD FOR THE SOLE—JUST NOT TILAPIA. TILAPIA IS UNFORTUNATELY ONE OF THE WORST CHOICES FOR FISH. IT IS ALMOST UNIVERSALLY FARM-RAISED AND FREQUENTLY UNDER HORRIBLE CONDITIONS—SO WHILE TILAPIA IS NEARLY UBIQUITOUS, IT SHOULD BE AVOIDED.

4 4- to 5-ounce fresh or frozen sole fillets, about ½ inch thick
1 recipe Arugula Pesto (see recipe, page 320)
½ cup Cashew Cream (see recipe, page 327)
1 teaspoon Smoky Seasoning (see recipe, page 324)
½ teaspoon finely shredded lime peel
12 butterhead lettuce leaves
1 ripe avocado, halved, seeded, peeled, and cut into thin slices
1 cup chopped tomato
¼ cup snipped fresh cilantro
1 lime, cut into wedges

1. Thaw fish, if frozen. Rinse fish; pat dry with paper towels. Set fish aside.

2. Rub some of the Arugula Pesto on both sides of the fish.

3. For a charcoal or gas grill, place fish on a greased rack directly over medium heat. Cover and grill for 4 to 6 minutes or until fish begins to flake when tested with a fork, turning once halfway through grilling.

4. Meanwhile, for Smoky Lime Cream, in a small bowl stir together the Cashew Cream, Smoky Seasoning, and lime peel.

5. Using a fork, break fish into pieces. Fill butterhead leaves with fish, avocado slices, and tomato; sprinkle with cilantro. Drizzle tacos with Smoky Lime Cream. Serve with lime wedges to squeeze over tacos.

ALMOND-CRUSTED SOLE

PREP: 15 minutes   COOK: 3 minutes   MAKES: 2 servings

JUST A LITTLE BIT OF ALMOND FLOUR CREATES A NICE CRUST ON THIS EXTREMELY QUICK-COOKING PAN-FRIED FISH SERVED WITH CREAMY DILLED MAYONNAISE AND A SQUEEZE OF FRESH LEMON.

12 ounces fresh or frozen sole
    fillets
 1 tablespoon Lemon-Herb
    Seasoning (see recipe, page
    324)
 ¼ to ½ teaspoon black pepper
 ⅓ cup almond flour
 2 to 3 tablespoons olive oil
 ¼ cup Paleo Mayo (see recipe,
    page 323)
 1 teaspoon snipped fresh dill
    Lemon wedges

1. Thaw fish, if frozen. Rinse fish; pat dry with paper towels. In a small bowl stir together the Lemon-Herb Seasoning and pepper. Coat both sides of fillets with seasoning mixture, pressing lightly to adhere. Spread almond flour on a large plate. Dredge one side of each fillet in the almond flour, pressing lightly to adhere.

2. In a large skillet heat enough oil to coat pan over medium-high heat. Add fish, coated sides down. Cook for 2 minutes. Carefully turn fish over; cook about 1 minute more or until the fish begins to flake when tested with a fork.

3. For sauce, in a small bowl stir together the Paleo Mayo and dill. Serve fish with sauce and lemon wedges.

5 WAYS WITH COD

COD IS THE QUINTESSENTIAL FIRM, WHITE FISH. BECAUSE OF ITS MILD FLAVOR, IT IS A VIRTUAL BLANK SLATE FOR A WORLD OF FLAVORS—AND IT HAS OTHER BENEFITS AS WELL. LIKE OTHER COLD-WATER FISH, COD IS A VERY GOOD SOURCE OF OMEGA-3 FATTY ACIDS.

Curried Cod Lettuce Wraps with Pickled Radishes, *recipe page 253*

5 WAYS WITH COD

COD HAS A MEATY, BUTTERY TEXTURE THAT STANDS UP TO A VARIIETY OF COOKING METHODS, INCLUDING GRILLING, BROILING, POACHING, BAKING/ROASTING, AND PAN-FRYING. LIKE MOST FISH, IT FLAKES EASILY WHEN PROPERLY COOKED—BUT STAYS IN SUBSTANTIAL, TOOTHSOME PIECES.

1. GRILLED COD AND ZUCCHINI PACKETS WITH SPICY MANGO-BASIL SAUCE

PREP: 20 minutes
GRILL: 6 minutes
MAKES: 4 servings

- 1 to 1½ pounds fresh or frozen cod, ½ to 1 inch thick
- 4 24-inch-long pieces 12-inch-wide foil
- 1 medium zucchini, cut into julienne strips
  Lemon-Herb Seasoning (see recipe, page 324)
- ¼ cup Chipotle Paleo Mayo (see recipe, page 323)
- 1 to 2 tablespoons pureed ripe mango*
- 1 tablespoon fresh lime or lemon juice or rice wine vinegar
- 2 tablespoons snipped fresh basil

1. Thaw fish, if frozen. Rinse fish; pat dry with paper towels. Cut fish into four serving-size pieces.

2. Fold each piece of foil in half to create a double-thickness 12-inch square. Place one portion of fish in the middle of a foil square. Top with one-fourth of the zucchini. Sprinkle with Lemon-Herb Seasoning. Bring up two opposite sides of foil and fold several times over zucchini and fish. Fold ends of foil. Repeat to make three more packets. For sauce, in a small bowl stir together Chipotle Paleo Mayo, mango, lime juice, and basil; set aside.

3. For a charcoal grill or gas grill, place packets on the oiled grill rack directly over medium heat. Cover and grill for 6 to 9 minutes or until fish begins to flake when tested with a fork and zucchini is crisp-tender (carefully open packet to test doneness). Do not turn packets while grilling. Top each serving with sauce.

* Tip: For mango puree, in a blender combine ¼ cup chopped mango and 1 tablespoon water. Cover and blend until smooth. Add any leftover pureed mango to a smoothie.

2. RIESLING-POACHED COD WITH PESTO-STUFFED TOMATOES

PREP: 30 minutes
COOK: 10 minutes
MAKES: 4 servings

- 1 to 1½ pounds fresh or frozen cod fillets, about 1 inch thick
- 4 roma tomatoes
- 3 tablespoons Basil Pesto (see recipe, page 320)
- ¼ teaspoon cracked black pepper
- 1 cup dry Riesling or Sauvignon Blanc
- 1 sprig fresh thyme or ½ teaspoon dried thyme, crushed
- 1 bay leaf
- ½ cup water
- 2 tablespoons chopped scallion
  Lemon wedges

1. Thaw fish, if frozen. Cut tomatoes in half horizontally. Scoop out the seeds and some of the flesh. (If necessary for tomato to sit flat, cut a very thin slice off the end, being careful not to make a hole in the bottom of the tomato.) Spoon some pesto into each tomato half; sprinkle with cracked pepper; set aside.

2. Rinse fish; pat dry with paper towels. Cut fish into four pieces. Place a steamer basket in a large skillet with a tight-fitting lid. Add about ½ inch water to skillet. Bring to boiling; reduce heat to medium. Add the tomatoes, cut sides up, to the basket. Cover and steam for 2 to 3 minutes or until warmed through.

3. Remove tomatoes to a plate; cover to keep warm. Remove steamer basket from skillet; discard water. Add wine, thyme, bay leaf, and the ½ cup water to skillet. Bring to boiling; reduce heat to medium-low. Add fish and scallion. Simmer, covered, for 8 to 10 minutes or until fish begins to flake when tested with a fork.

4. Drizzle fish with some of the poaching liquid. Serve fish with pesto-stuffed tomatoes and lemon wedges.

3. BROILED PISTACHIO-CILANTRO-CRUSTED COD OVER SMASHED SWEET POTATOES

PREP: 20 minutes
COOK: 10 minutes
BROIL: 4 to 6 minutes per ½-inch thickness
MAKES: 4 servings

- 1 to 1½ pounds fresh or frozen cod
  Olive oil or refined coconut oil
- 2 tablespoons ground pistachios, pecans, or almonds
- 1 egg white
- ½ teaspoon finely shredded lemon peel
- 1½ pounds sweet potatoes, peeled and cut into chunks
- 2 cloves garlic
- 1 tablespoon coconut oil
- 1 tablespoon grated fresh ginger
- ½ teaspoon ground cumin
- ¼ cup coconut milk (such as Nature's Way)

4 teaspoons Cilantro Pesto or Basil Pesto (see recipes, page 320)

1. Thaw fish, if frozen. Preheat broiler. Oil rack of a broiler pan. In a small bowl combine ground nuts, egg white, and lemon peel; set aside.

2. For the smashed sweet potatoes, in a medium saucepan cook sweet potatoes and garlic in enough boiling water to cover for 10 to 15 minutes or until tender. Drain; return sweet potatoes and garlic to the saucepan. Using a potato masher, mash sweet potatoes. Stir in 1 tablespoon coconut oil, ginger, and cumin. Mash in coconut milk until light and fluffy.

3. Rinse fish; pat dry with paper towels. Cut fish into four pieces and place on the prepared unheated rack of a broiler pan. Tuck under any thin edges. Spread each piece with Cilantro Pesto. Spoon nut mixture on pesto and spread gently. Broil fish 4 inches from the heat for 4 to 6 minutes per ½-inch thickness or until fish begins to flake when tested with a fork, covering with foil during broiling if coating starts to burn. Serve fish with sweet potatoes.

4. ROSEMARY-AND-TANGERINE COD WITH ROASTED BROCCOLI

PREP: 15 minutes
MARINATE: up to 30 minutes
BAKE: 12 minutes
MAKES: 4 servings

1 to 1½ pounds fresh or frozen cod
1 teaspoon finely shredded tangerine peel
½ cup fresh tangerine or orange juice
4 tablespoons olive oil
2 teaspoons snipped fresh rosemary
¼ to ½ teaspoon cracked black pepper

1 teaspoon finely shredded tangerine peel
3 cups broccoli florets
¼ teaspoon crushed red pepper Tangerine slices, seeds removed

1. Preheat oven to 450°F. Thaw fish, if frozen. Rinse fish; pat dry with paper towels. Cut fish into four serving-size pieces. Measure thickness of fish. In a shallow dish combine tangerine peel, tangerine juice, 2 tablespoons of the olive oil, rosemary, and black pepper; add fish. Cover and marinate in the refrigerator for up to 30 minutes.

2. In a large bowl toss broccoli with the remaining 2 tablespoons olive oil and the crushed red pepper. Place in a 2-quart baking dish.

3. Brush a shallow baking pan lightly with additional olive oil. Drain fish, reserving marinade. Place fish in the pan, tucking under any thin edges. Place fish and broccoli in the oven. Bake broccoli for 12 to 15 minutes or until crisp-tender, stirring once halfway through cooking. Bake fish for 4 to 6 minutes per ½-inch thickness of fish or until fish begins to flake when tested with a fork.

4. In a small saucepan bring reserved marinade to boiling; cook for 2 minutes. Drizzle the marinade over the cooked fish. Serve fish with broccoli and tangerine slices.

5. CURRIED COD LETTUCE WRAPS WITH PICKLED RADISHES

PREP: 20 minutes
STAND: 20 minutes
COOK: 6 minutes
MAKES: 4 servings

1 pound fresh or frozen cod fillets
6 radishes, coarsely shredded
6 to 7 tablespoons cider vinegar

½ teaspoon crushed red pepper
2 tablespoons unrefined coconut oil
¼ cup almond butter
1 clove garlic, minced
2 teaspoons finely grated ginger
2 tablespoons olive oil
1½ to 2 teaspoons no-salt-added curry powder
4 to 8 butterhead lettuce leaves or leaf lettuce leaves
1 red sweet pepper, cut into julienne strips
2 tablespoons snipped fresh cilantro

1. Thaw fish, if frozen. In a medium bowl combine radishes, 4 tablespoons of the vinegar, and ¼ teaspoon of the crushed red pepper; let stand for 20 minutes, stirring occasionally.

2. For almond butter sauce, in a small saucepan melt the coconut oil over low heat. Stir in almond butter until smooth. Stir in garlic, ginger, and remaining ¼ teaspoon crushed red pepper. Remove from heat. Add the remaining 2 to 3 tablespoons cider vinegar, stirring until smooth; set aside. (Sauce will thicken slightly when vinegar is added.)

3. Rinse fish; pat dry with paper towels. In a large skillet heat the olive oil and curry powder over medium heat. Add fish; cook for 3 to 6 minutes or until fish begins to flake when tested with a fork, turning once halfway through cooking time. Using two forks, coarsely flake fish.

4. Drain radishes; discard marinade. Spoon some of the fish, sweet pepper strips, radish mixture, and almond butter sauce into each lettuce leaf. Sprinkle with cilantro. Wrap leaf around filling. If desired, secure wraps with wooden toothpicks.

ROASTED HADDOCK WITH LEMON AND FENNEL

PREP: 25 minutes   ROAST: 50 minutes   MAKES: 4 servings

HADDOCK, POLLOCK, AND COD ALL HAVE MILDLY FLAVORED FIRM WHITE FLESH. THEY ARE INTERCHANGEABLE IN MOST RECIPES, INCLUDING THIS SIMPLE DISH OF BAKED FISH AND VEGETABLES WITH HERBS AND WINE.

4 6-ounce fresh or frozen haddock, pollock, or cod fillets, about ½ inch thick

1 large bulb fennel, cored and sliced, fronds reserved and chopped

4 medium carrots, cut in half vertically and sliced into 2- to 3-inch-long pieces

1 red onion, halved and sliced

2 cloves garlic, minced

1 lemon, thinly sliced

3 tablespoons olive oil

½ teaspoon black pepper

¾ cup dry white wine

2 tablespoons finely snipped fresh parsley

2 tablespoons snipped fresh fennel fronds

2 teaspoons finely shredded lemon peel

1. Thaw fish, if frozen. Preheat oven to 400°F. In a 3-quart rectangular baking dish combine fennel, carrots, onion, garlic, and lemon slices. Drizzle with 2 tablespoons of the olive oil and sprinkle with ¼ teaspoon of the pepper; toss to coat. Pour wine into dish. Cover dish with foil.

2. Roast for 20 minutes. Uncover; stir vegetable mixture. Roast 15 to 20 minutes more or until vegetables are crisp-tender. Stir vegetable mixture. Sprinkle fish with the remaining ¼ teaspoon pepper; place fish on top of vegetable mixture. Drizzle with the remaining 1 tablespoon olive oil. Roast about 8 to 10 minutes or until fish begins to flake when tested with a fork.

3. In a small bowl combine parsley, fennel fronds, and lemon peel. To serve, divide fish and vegetable mixture among serving plates. Spoon pan juices over fish and vegetables. Sprinkle with parsley mixture.

PECAN-CRUSTED SNAPPER
WITH REMOULADE AND CAJUN-STYLE
OKRA AND TOMATOES

PREP: 1 hour   COOK: 10 minutes   BAKE: 8 minutes   MAKES: 4 servings

THIS COMPANYWORTHY FISH DISH TAKES A BIT OF TIME TO MAKE, BUT THE RICH FLAVORS MAKE IT WELL WORTH IT. THE REMOULADE—A MAYONNAISE-BASED SAUCE SPIKED WITH MUSTARD, LEMON, AND CAJUN SEASONING AND CONFETTIED WITH CHOPPED RED SWEET PEPPER, SCALLIONS, AND PARSLEY—CAN BE MADE A DAY AHEAD AND CHILLED.

4   tablespoons olive oil
½   cup finely chopped pecans
2   tablespoons chopped fresh
    parsley
1   tablespoon chopped fresh
    thyme
2   8-ounce red snapper fillets,
    ½ inch thick
4   teaspoons Cajun Seasoning (see
    recipe, page 324)
½   cup diced onion
½   cup diced green sweet pepper
½   cup diced celery
1   tablespoon minced garlic
1   pound fresh okra pods, cut into
    1-inch-thick slices (or fresh
    asparagus, cut into 1-inch
    lengths)
8   ounces grape or cherry
    tomatoes, halved
2   teaspoons chopped fresh
    thyme
    Black pepper
    Rémoulade (see recipe, right)

1. In a medium skillet heat 1 tablespoon of the olive oil over medium heat. Add the pecans and toast about 5 minutes or until golden and fragrant, stirring frequently. Transfer pecans to a small bowl and let cool. Add parsley and thyme and set aside.

2. Preheat oven to 400°F. Line a baking sheet with parchment paper or foil. Arrange the snapper fillets on the baking sheet, skin sides down, and sprinkle each with 1 teaspoon of the Cajun Seasoning. Using a pastry brush, dab 2 tablespoons of olive oil onto fillets. Divide the pecan mixture evenly among the fillets, pressing the nuts gently onto the surface of the fish so they adhere. Cover all the exposed areas of the fish fillet with nuts if possible. Bake fish for 8 to 10 minutes or until it flakes easily with the tip of a knife.

3. In a large skillet heat the remaining 1 tablespoon olive oil over medium-high heat. Add onion, sweet pepper, celery, and garlic. Cook and stir for 5 minutes or until vegetables are crisp-tender. Add the sliced okra (or asparagus if using) and the tomatoes; cook for 5 to 7 minutes or until okra is crisp-tender and tomatoes begin to split. Remove from heat and season with thyme and black pepper to taste. Serve vegetables with snapper and Rémoulade.

Remoulade: In a food processor pulse ½ cup chopped red sweet pepper, ¼ cup chopped scallions, and 2 tablespoons chopped fresh parsley until fine. Add ¼ cup Paleo Mayo (see recipe, page 323), ¼ cup Dijon-Style Mustard (see recipe, page 322), 1½ teaspoons lemon juice, and ¼ teaspoon Cajun Seasoning (see recipe, page 321). Pulse until combined. Transfer to a serving bowl and refrigerate until ready to serve. (Remoulade may be made 1 day ahead and chilled.)

TARRAGON TUNA PATTIES WITH AVOCADO-LEMON AÏOLI

PREP: 25 minutes   COOK: 6 minutes   MAKES: 4 servings

ALONG WITH SALMON, TUNA IS ONE OF THE RARE KINDS OF FISH THAT CAN BE FINELY CHOPPED AND FORMED INTO BURGERS. BE CAREFUL NOT TO OVERPROCESS THE TUNA IN THE FOOD PROCESSOR—OVERPROCESSING TOUGHENS IT.

1 pound fresh or frozen skinless tuna fillets

1 egg white, lightly beaten

¾ cup ground golden flaxseed meal

1 tablespoon fresh snipped tarragon or dill

2 tablespoons snipped fresh chives

1 teaspoon finely shredded lemon peel

2 tablespoons flaxseed oil, avocado oil, or olive oil

1 medium avocado, seeded

3 tablespoons Paleo Mayo (see recipe, page 323)

1 teaspoon finely shredded lemon peel

2 teaspoons fresh lemon juice

1 clove garlic, minced

4 ounces baby spinach (about 4 cups tightly packed)

⅓ cup Roasted Garlic Vinaigrette (see recipe, page 321)

1 Granny Smith apple, cored and cut into matchstick-size pieces

¼ cup chopped toasted walnuts (see tip, page 57)

1. Thaw fish, if frozen. Rinse fish; pat dry with paper towels. Cut fish into 1½-inch pieces. Place fish in a food processor; process with on/off pulses until finely chopped. (Be careful not to overprocess or you'll toughen the patty.) Set fish aside.

2. In a medium bowl combine egg white, ¼ cup of the flaxseed meal, tarragon, chives, and lemon peel. Add fish; stir gently to combine. Shape fish mixture into four ½-inch-thick patties.

3. Place remaining ½ cup flaxseed meal in a shallow dish. Dip patties into flaxseed mixture, turning to coat evenly.

4. In an extra-large skillet heat oil over medium heat. Cook tuna patties in hot oil for 6 to 8 minutes or until an instant-read thermometer inserted horizontally into patties registers 160°F, turning once halfway through cooking time.

5. Meanwhile, for the aïoli, in a medium bowl use a fork to mash avocado. Add Paleo Mayo, lemon peel, lemon juice, and garlic. Mash until well mixed and almost smooth.

6. Place the spinach in a medium bowl. Drizzle spinach with Roasted Garlic Vinaigrette; toss to coat. For each serving, place a tuna patty and one-fourth of the spinach on a serving plate. Top tuna with some of the aïoli. Top spinach with apple and walnuts. Serve immediately.

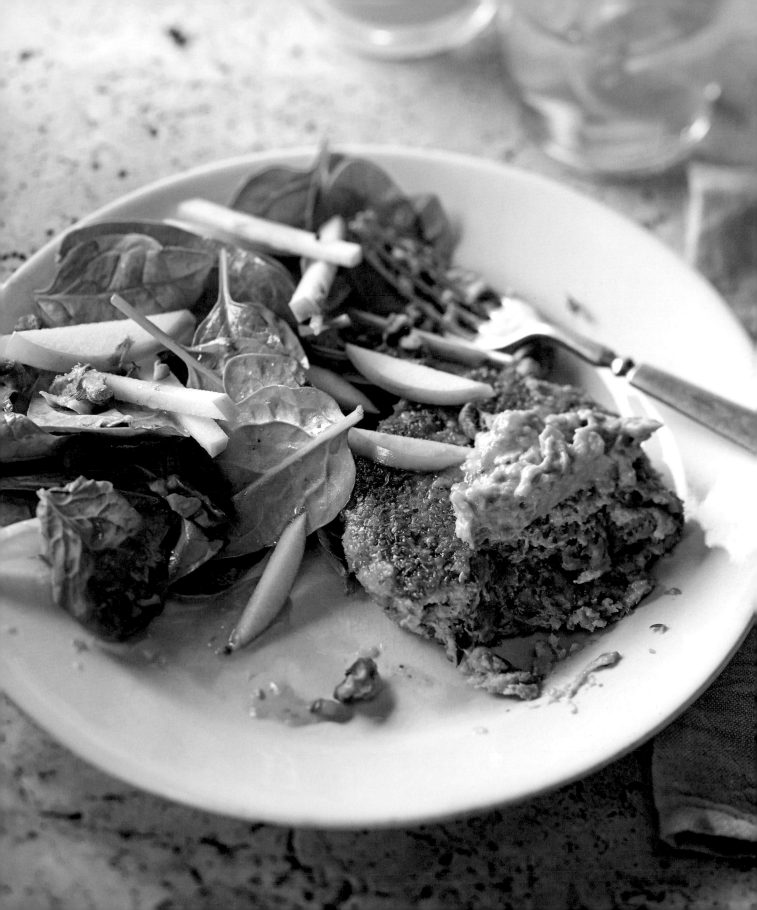

STRIPED BASS TAGINE

PREP: 50 minutes   CHILL: 1 to 2 hours   COOK: 22 minutes   BAKE: 25 minutes   MAKES: 4 servings

A TAGINE IS THE NAME OF BOTH A TYPE OF NORTH AFRICAN DISH (A KIND OF STEW) AND THE CONE-SHAPE POT IT'S COOKED IN. IF YOU DON'T HAVE ONE, A COVERED OVEN-GOING SKILLET WORKS JUST FINE. CHERMOULA IS A THICK NORTH AFRICAN HERB PASTE THAT IS MOST OFTEN USED AS A MARINADE FOR FISH. SERVE THIS COLORFUL FISH DISH WITH A SWEET POTATO OR CAULIFLOWER MASH.

4 6-ounce fresh or frozen striped bass or halibut fillets, skin on
1 bunch cilantro, chopped
1 teaspoon finely shredded lemon peel (set aside)
¼ cup fresh lemon juice
4 tablespoons olive oil
5 cloves garlic, minced
4 teaspoons ground cumin
2 teaspoons sweet paprika
1 teaspoon ground coriander
¼ teaspoon ground anise
1 large onion, peeled, halved, and thinly sliced
1 15-ounce can no-salt-added fire-roasted diced tomatoes, undrained
½ cup Chicken Bone Broth (see recipe, page 235) or no-salt-added chicken broth
1 large yellow sweet pepper, seeded and cut into ½-inch-strips
1 large orange sweet pepper, seeded and cut into ½-inch strips

1. Thaw fish, if frozen. Rinse fish; pat dry with paper towels. Place fish fillets in a shallow, nonmetal baking dish. Set fish aside.

2. For chermoula, in a blender or small food processor combine cilantro, lemon juice, 2 tablespoons of the olive oil, 4 cloves minced garlic, the cumin, paprika, coriander, and anise. Cover and process until smooth.

3. Spoon half of the chermoula over the fish, turning fish to coat both sides. Cover and refrigerate for 1 to 2 hours. Cover remaining chermoula; let stand at room temperature until needed.

4. Preheat oven to 325°F. In a large oven-going skillet heat the remaining 2 tablespoons oil over medium-high heat. Add onion; cook and stir for 4 to 5 minutes or until tender. Stir in the remaining 1 clove minced garlic; cook and stir for 1 minute. Add reserved chermoula, tomatoes, Chicken Bone Broth, sweet pepper strips, and lemon peel. Bring to boiling; reduce heat. Simmer, uncovered, for 15 minutes. If desired, transfer mixture to tagine; top with fish and any remaining chermoula from the dish. Cover; bake for 25 minutes. Serve immediately.

HALIBUT IN GARLIC-SHRIMP SAUCE WITH SOFFRITO COLLARD GREENS

PREP: 30 minutes   COOK: 19 minutes   MAKES: 4 servings

THERE ARE SEVERAL DIFFERENT SOURCES AND TYPES OF HALIBUT, AND THEY CAN BE OF VASTLY DIFFERENT QUALITY—AND FISHED UNDER VERY DIFFERENT CONDITIONS. THE SUSTAINABILITY OF THE FISH, THE ENVIRONMENT IN WHICH IT LIVES, AND THE CONDITIONS UNDER WHICH IT IS RAISED/FISHED ARE ALL FACTORS IN DETERMINING WHICH FISH ARE GOOD CHOICES FOR CONSUMPTION. VISIT THE MONTEREY BAY AQUARIUM WEBSITE (WWW.SEAFOODWATCH .ORG) FOR THE LATEST INFORMATION ON WHICH FISH TO EAT AND WHICH ONES TO AVOID.

4 6-ounce fresh or frozen halibut fillets, about 1 inch thick
Black pepper
6 tablespoons extra virgin olive oil
½ cup finely chopped onion
¼ cup diced red sweet pepper
2 cloves garlic, minced
¾ teaspoon smoked Spanish paprika
½ teaspoon chopped fresh oregano
4 cups collard greens, stemmed, sliced into ¼-inch-thick ribbons (about 12 ounces)
⅓ cup water
8 ounces medium shrimp, peeled, deveined, and coarsely chopped
4 cloves garlic, thinly sliced
¼ to ½ teaspoon crushed red pepper
⅓ cup dry sherry
2 tablespoons lemon juice
¼ cup chopped fresh parsley

1. Thaw fish, if frozen. Rinse fish; pat dry with paper towels. Sprinkle fish with pepper. In a large skillet heat 2 tablespoons of the olive oil over medium heat. Add the fillets; cook for 10 minutes or until golden brown and fish flakes when tested with a fork, turning once halfway through cooking. Transfer the fish to a platter and tent with foil to keep warm.

2. Meanwhile, in another large skillet heat 1 tablespoon of the olive oil over medium heat. Add onion, sweet pepper, 2 cloves minced garlic, paprika, and oregano; cook and stir for 3 to 5 minutes or until tender. Stir in collard greens and the water. Cover and cook for 3 to 4 minutes or until liquid has evaporated and greens are just tender, stirring occasionally. Cover and keep warm until ready to serve.

3. For shrimp sauce, add remaining 3 tablespoons olive oil to the skillet used for cooking the fish. Add the shrimp, 4 cloves sliced garlic, and crushed red pepper. Cook and stir for 2 to 3 minutes or until garlic just begins to turn golden. Add the shrimp; cook for 2 to 3 minutes until shrimp is firm and pink. Stir in the sherry and lemon juice. Cook 1 to 2 minutes or until reduced slightly. Stir in the parsley.

4. Divide shrimp sauce among halibut fillets. Serve with greens.

SEAFOOD BOUILLABAISSE

START TO FINISH: 1¾ hours   MAKES: 4 servings

LIKE ITALIAN CIOPPINO, THIS FRENCH SEAFOOD STEW OF FISH AND SHELLFISH SEEMS TO REPRESENT A SAMPLING OF THE DAY'S CATCH THROWN INTO A POT WITH GARLIC, ONIONS, TOMATOES, AND WINE. THE DISTINGUISHING FLAVOR OF BOUILLABAISSE, HOWEVER, IS THE FLAVOR COMBINATION OF SAFFRON, FENNEL, AND ORANGE ZEST.

1 pound fresh or frozen skinless halibut fillet, cut into 1-inch pieces
4 tablespoons olive oil
2 cups chopped onions
4 cloves garlic, smashed
1 head fennel, cored and chopped
6 roma tomatoes, chopped
¾ cup Chicken Bone Broth (see recipe, page 235) or no-salt-added chicken broth
¼ cup dry white wine
1 cup finely chopped onion
1 head fennel, cored and finely chopped
6 cloves garlic, minced
1 orange
3 roma tomatoes, finely chopped
4 saffron threads
1 tablespoon snipped fresh oregano
1 pound littleneck clams, scrubbed and rinsed
1 pound mussels, beards removed, scrubbed, and rinsed (see tip, page 271)
Snipped fresh oregano (optional)

1. Thaw halibut, if frozen. Rinse fish; pat dry with paper towels. Set fish aside.

2. In a 6- to 8-quart Dutch oven, heat 2 tablespoons of the olive oil over medium heat. Add 2 cups chopped onions , 1 head chopped fennel, and 4 cloves smashed garlic to the pot. Cook for 7 to 9 minutes or until onion is tender, stirring occasionally. Add 6 chopped tomatoes and 1 head chopped fennel; cook for 4 minutes more. Add Chicken Bone Broth and white wine to pot; simmer for 5 minutes; cool slightly. Transfer vegetable mixture to a blender or food processor. Cover and blend or process until smooth; set aside.

3. In the same Dutch oven heat the remaining 1 tablespoon olive oil over medium heat. Add 1 cup finely chopped onion, 1 head finely chopped fennel, and 6 cloves minced garlic. Cook over medium heat 5 to 7 minutes or until nearly tender, stirring frequently.

4. Use a vegetable peeler to remove the zest from the orange in wide strips; set aside. Add the pureed vegetable mixture, 3 chopped tomatoes, saffron, oregano, and orange zest strips to the Dutch oven. Bring to boiling; reduce heat to maintain simmering. Add clams, mussels, and fish; stir gently to coat fish with sauce. Adjust heat as neednd to maintain a simmer. Cover and simmer gently for 3 to 5 minutes until mussels and clams have opened and fish begins to flake when tested with a fork. Ladle into shallow bowls to serve. If desired, sprinkle with additional oregano.

CLASSIC SHRIMP CEVICHE

PREP: 20 minutes   COOK: 2 minutes   CHILL: 1 hour   STAND: 30 minutes   MAKES: 3 to 4 servings

THIS LATIN AMERICAN DISH IS AN EXPLOSION OF TASTES AND TEXTURES. CRUNCHY CUCUMBER AND CELERY, CREAMY AVOCADO, HOT AND SPICY JALAPEÑOS, AND DELICATE, SWEET SHRIMP INTERMINGLE IN LIME JUICE AND OLIVE OIL. IN TRADITIONAL CEVICHE, THE ACID IN THE LIME JUICE "COOKS" THE SHRIMP—BUT A QUICK DIP IN BOILING WATER LEAVES NOTHING TO CHANCE, SAFETYWISE—AND DOESN'T HURT THE FLAVOR OR TEXTURE OF THE SHRIMP.

1 pound fresh or frozen medium shrimp, peeled and deveined, tails removed

½ of a cucumber, peeled, seeded, and chopped

1 cup chopped celery

½ of a small red onion, chopped

1 to 2 jalapeños, seeded and minced (see tip, page 56)

½ cup fresh lime juice

2 roma tomatoes, diced

1 avocado, halved, seeded, peeled, and diced

¼ cup snipped fresh cilantro

3 tablespoons olive oil

½ teaspoon black pepper

1. Thaw shrimp, if frozen. Peel and devein shrimp; remove tails. Rinse shrimp; pat dry with paper towels.

2. Fill a large saucepan half full with water. Bring to boiling. Add shrimp to boiling water. Cook, uncovered, for 1 to 2 minutes or just until shrimp turn opaque; drain. Run shrimp under cool water and drain again. Dice shrimp.

3. In a extra-large nonreactive bowl combine shrimp, cucumber, celery, onion, jalapeños, and lime juice. Cover and refrigerate for 1 hour, stirring once or twice.

4. Stir in tomatoes, avocado, cilantro, olive oil, and black pepper. Cover and let stand at room temperature for 30 minutes. Stir gently before serving.

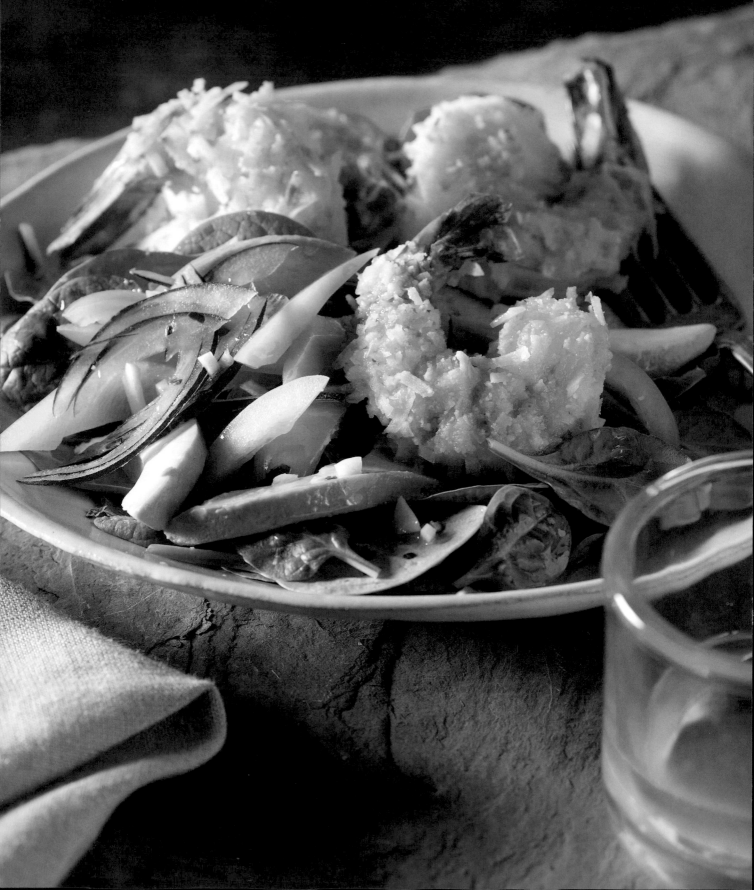

COCONUT-CRUSTED SHRIMP AND SPINACH SALAD

PREP: 25 minutes   BAKE: 8 minutes   MAKES: 4 servings

COMMERCIALLY PRODUCED CANS OF SPRAY OLIVE OIL CAN CONTAIN GRAIN ALCOHOL, LECITHIN, AND PROPELLANT—NOT A TERRIFIC MIX WHEN YOU ARE TRYING TO EAT PURE, REAL FOODS AND AVOID GRAINS, UNHEALTHY FATS, LEGUMES, AND DAIRY. AN OIL MISTER USES ONLY AIR TO PROPEL THE OIL INTO A FINE SPRAY—PERFECT FOR LIGHTLY COATING COCONUT-CRUSTED SHRIMP BEFORE BAKING.

1½   pounds fresh or frozen extra-large shrimp in shells
     Misto spray bottle filled with extra virgin olive oil
2   eggs
¾   cup unsweetened flaked or shredded coconut
¾   cup almond meal
½   cup avocado oil or olive oil
3   tablespoons fresh lemon juice
2   tablespoons fresh lime juice
2   small cloves garlic, minced
⅛   to ¼ teaspoon crushed red pepper
8   cups fresh baby spinach
1   medium avocado, halved, seeded, peeled, and thinly sliced
1   small orange or yellow sweet pepper, cut into thin bite-size strips
½   cup slivered red onion

1. Thaw shrimp, if frozen. Peel and devein shrimp, leaving tails intact. Rinse shrimp; pat dry with paper towels. Preheat oven to 450°F. Line a large baking sheet with foil; lightly coat foil with oil sprayed from the Misto bottle; set aside.

2. In a shallow dish beat eggs with a fork. In another shallow dish combine coconut and almond meal. Dip shrimp into eggs, turning to coat. Dip in coconut mixture, pressing to coat (leave tails uncoated). Arrange shrimp in a single layer on the prepared baking sheet. Coat the tops of the shrimp with oil sprayed from the Misto bottle.

3. Bake for 8 to 10 minutes or until shrimp are opaque and coating is lightly browned.

4. Meanwhile, for dressing, in a small screw-top jar combine avocado oil, lemon juice, lime juice, garlic, and crushed red pepper. Cover and shake well.

5. For salads, divide spinach among four serving plates. Top with avocado, sweet pepper, red onion, and the shrimp. Drizzle with dressing and serve immediately.

TROPICAL SHRIMP AND SCALLOP CEVICHE

PREP: 20 minutes   MARINATE: 30 to 60 minutes   MAKES: 4 to 6 servings

COOL AND LIGHT CEVICHE MAKES A GREAT MEAL FOR A HOT SUMMER NIGHT. WITH MELON, MANGO, SERRANO CHILES, FENNEL, AND MANGO-LIME SALAD DRESSING (PAGE 321), THIS IS A SWEET-HOT TAKE ON THE ORIGINAL.

1   pound fresh or frozen sea scallops

1   pound fresh or frozen large shrimp

2   cups cubed honeydew melon

2   medium mangoes, pitted, peeled, and chopped (about 2 cups)

1   head fennel, trimmed, quartered, cored, and thinly sliced

1   medium red sweet pepper, chopped (about ¾ cup)

1   to 2 serrano chiles, seeded if desired and thinly sliced (see tip, page 56)

½   cup lightly packed fresh cilantro, chopped

1   recipe Mango-Lime Salad Dressing (see recipe, page 321)

1. Thaw scallops and shrimp, if frozen. Split scallops in half horizontally. Peel, devein, and split shrimp in half horizontally. Rinse scallops and shrimp; pat dry with paper towels. Fill a large saucepan three-fourths full with water. Bring to boiling. Add shrimp and scallops; cook for 3 to 4 minutes or until shrimp and scallops are opaque; drain and rinse with cold water to cool quickly. Drain well and set aside.

2. In an extra-large bowl combine melon, mangoes, fennel, sweet pepper, serrano chiles, and cilantro. Add Mango-Lime Salad Dressing; toss gently to coat. Gently stir in cooked shrimp and scallops. Marinate in the refrigerator for 30 to 60 minutes before serving.

JAMAICAN JERK SHRIMP WITH AVOCADO OIL

START TO FINISH: **20 minutes**   MAKES: **4 servings**

WITH A TOTAL TO-THE-TABLE TIME OF 20 MINUTES, THIS DISH OFFERS ONE MORE COMPELLING REASON TO EAT A HEALTHY MEAL AT HOME, EVEN ON THE BUSIEST NIGHTS.

1 pound fresh or frozen medium shrimp
1 cup chopped, peeled mango (1 medium)
⅓ cup thinly sliced red onion sliced
¼ cup snipped fresh cilantro
1 tablespoon fresh lime juice
2 to 3 tablespoons Jamaican Jerk Seasoning (see recipe, page 324)
1 tablespoons extra virgin olive oil
2 tablespoons avocado oil

1. Thaw shrimp, if frozen. In a medium bowl stir together mango, onion, cilantro, and lime juice.

2. Peel and devein shrimp. Rinse shrimp; pat dry with paper towels. Place shrimp in a medium bowl. Sprinkle with Jamaican Jerk Seasoning; toss to coat shrimp on all sides.

3. In a large nonstick skillet heat olive oil over medium-high heat. Add shrimp; cook and stir about 4 minutes or until opaque. Drizzle shrimp with avocado oil and serve with the mango mixture.

SHRIMP SCAMPI WITH WILTED SPINACH AND RADICCHIO

PREP: 15 minutes   COOK: 8 minutes   MAKES: 3 servings

"SCAMPI" REFERS TO A CLASSIC RESTAURANT DISH OF LARGE SHRIMP SAUTÉED OR BROILED WITH BUTTER AND LOTS OF GARLIC AND LEMON. THIS SPICY OLIVE OIL VERSION IS PALEO-APPROVED—AND BUMPED UP NUTRITIONALLY WITH A QUICK SAUTÉ OF RADICCHIO AND SPINACH.

1 pound fresh or frozen large shrimp
4 tablespoons extra virgin olive oil
6 cloves garlic, minced
½ teaspoon black pepper
¼ cup dry white wine
½ cup snipped fresh parsley
½ of a head radicchio, cored and thinly sliced
½ teaspoon crushed red pepper
9 cups baby spinach
Lemon wedges

1. Thaw shrimp, if frozen. Peel and devein shrimp, leaving tails intact. In a large skillet heat 2 tablespoons of the olive oil over medium-high heat. Add shrimp, 4 cloves minced garlic, and black pepper. Cook and stir about 3 minutes or until shrimp are opaque. Transfer shrimp mixture to a bowl.

2. Add white wine to skillet. Cook, stirring to loosen to any browned garlic from bottom of the skillet. Pour wine over shrimp; toss to combine. Stir in parsley. Cover loosely with foil to keep warm; set aside.

3. Add the remaining 2 tablespoons olive oil, the remaining 2 cloves minced garlic, the radicchio, and crushed red pepper to the skillet. Cook and stir over medium heat for 3 minutes or until radicchio just begins to wilt. Carefully stir in the spinach; cook and stir for 1 to 2 minutes more or until spinach is just wilted.

4. To serve, divide spinach mixture among three serving plates; top with shrimp mixture. Serve with lemon wedges for squeezing over shrimp and greens.

CRAB SALAD WITH AVOCADO, GRAPEFRUIT, AND JICAMA

START TO FINISH: **30 minutes**   MAKES: **4 servings**

JUMBO LUMP OR BACKFIN CRABMEAT IS BEST FOR THIS SALAD. JUMBO LUMP CRABMEAT IS MADE UP OF LARGE CHUNKS THAT WORK WELL IN SALADS. BACKFIN IS A BLEND OF BROKEN PIECES OF JUMBO LUMP CRABMEAT AND SMALLER PIECES OF CRABMEAT FROM THE BODY OF THE CRAB. ALTHOUGH SMALLER THAN THE JUMBO LUMP CRAB, BACKFIN WORKS JUST FINE. FRESH IS BEST, OF COURSE, BUT THAWED FROZEN CRAB IS A FINE OPTION.

6 cups baby spinach

½ of a medium jicama, peeled and julienne-cut*

2 pink or ruby red grapefruit, peeled, seeded, and sectioned**

2 small avocados, halved

1 pound jumbo lump or backfin crabmeat

Basil-Grapefruit Dressing (see recipe, right)

1. Divide spinach among four serving plates. Top with jicama, grapefruit sections and any accumulated juice, avocados, and crabmeat. Drizzle with Basil-Grapefruit Dressing.

Basil-Grapefruit Dressing: In a screw-top jar combine ⅓ cup extra virgin olive oil; ¼ cup fresh grapefruit juice; 2 tablespoons fresh orange juice; ½ of a small shallot, minced; 2 tablespoons finely snipped fresh basil; ¼ teaspoon crushed red pepper; and ¼ teaspoon black pepper. Cover and shake well.

*Tip: A julienne peeler makes quick work of cutting the jicama into thin strips.

**Tip: To section grapefruit, cut a slice off the stem end and bottom of the fruit. Set it upright on a work surface. Cut down the fruit in sections from top to bottom, following the rounded shape of the fruit, to remove peel in strips. Hold the fruit over a bowl and, using a paring knife, cut to the center of the fruit on the sides of each segment to release it from the pith. Place segments in bowl with any accumulated juices. Discard pith.

Cajun Lobster Tail Boil with
Tarragon Aïoli, *recipe page 270*

Arugula and Herb Salad with
Poached Eggs, *recipe page 305*

CAJUN LOBSTER TAIL BOIL WITH TARRAGON AÏOLI

pictured on page 268

pictured on page 268

PREP: 20 minutes   COOK: 30 minutes   MAKES: 4 servings

FOR A ROMANTIC DINNER FOR TWO, THIS RECIPE IS EASILY CUT IN HALF. USE VERY SHARP KITCHEN SHEARS TO CUT OPEN THE SHELL OF THE LOBSTER TAILS AND GET AT THE RICHLY FLAVORED MEAT.

2   recipes Cajun Seasoning (see recipe, page 324)
12 cloves garlic, peeled and halved
2   lemons, halved
2   large carrots, peeled
2   celery stalks, peeled
2   fennel bulbs, sliced into thin wedges
1   pound whole button mushrooms
4   7- to 8-ounce Maine lobster tails
4   8-inch bamboo skewers
½   cup Paleo Aïoli (Garlic Mayo) (see recipe, page 323)
¼   cup Dijon-Style Mustard (see recipe, page 322)
2   tablespoons snipped fresh tarragon or parsley

1. In an 8-quart stockpot combine 6 cups water, Cajun Seasoning, garlic, and lemons. Bring to boiling; boil for 5 minutes. Reduce heat to keep liquid at a simmer.

2. Cut the carrots and celery crosswise into four pieces. Add carrots, celery, and fennel to liquid. Cover and cook for 10 minutes. Add mushrooms; cover and cook for 5 minutes. Using a slotted spoon, transfer vegetables to a serving bowl; keep warm.

3. Starting from the body end of each lobster tail, slide a skewer between the meat and the shell, going almost all the way through the tail end. (This will keep the tail from curling as it cooks.) Reduce heat. Cook lobster tails in the barely simmering liquid in pot for 8 to 12 minutes or until shells turn bright red and meat is tender when pierced with a fork. Remove lobster from cooking liquid. Use a kitchen towel to hold the lobster tails and remove and discard the skewers.

4. In a small bowl stir together the Paleo Aïoli, Dijon-Style Mustard, and tarragon. Serve with the lobster and vegetables.

MUSSELS FRITES WITH SAFFRON AÏOLI

START TO FINISH: 1¼ hours   MAKES: 4 servings

THIS IS A PALEO TAKE ON THE FRENCH CLASSIC OF MUSSELS STEAMED IN WHITE WINE AND HERBS AND SERVED WITH THIN AND CRISPY FRITES MADE FROM WHITE POTATOES. DISCARD ANY MUSSELS THAT WON'T CLOSE BEFORE THEY'RE COOKED—AND ANY MUSSELS THAT DON'T OPEN AFTER THEY'RE COOKED.

PARSNIP FRITES

1½   pounds parsnips, peeled and
       cut into 3×¼-inch julienne
3   tablespoons olive oil
2   cloves garlic, minced
¼   teaspoon black pepper
⅛   teaspoon cayenne pepper

SAFFRON AÏOLI

⅓   cup Paleo Aïoli (Garlic Mayo)
       (see recipe, page 323)
⅛   teaspoon saffron threads,
       gently crushed

MUSSELS

4   tablespoons olive oil
½   cup finely chopped shallots
6   cloves garlic, minced
¼   teaspoon black pepper
3   cups dry white wine
3   large sprigs flat-leaf parsley
4   pounds mussels, cleaned and
       debearded*
¼   cup chopped fresh Italian
       (flat-leaf) parsley
2   tablespoons snipped fresh
       tarragon (optional)

1. For parsnip frites, preheat oven to 450°F. Soak cut parsnips in enough cold water to cover in the refrigerator for 30 minutes; drain and pat dry with paper towels.

2. Line a large baking sheet with parchment paper. Place parsnips in an extra-large bowl. In a small bowl combine 3 tablespoons olive oil, 2 cloves minced garlic, ¼ teaspoon black pepper, and cayenne pepper; drizzle over parsnips and toss to coat. Arrange parsnips in an even layer on prepared baking sheet. Bake for 30 to 35 minutes or tender and starting to brown, stirring occasionally.

3. For aïoli, in a small bowl stir together Paleo Aïoli and saffron. Cover and refrigerate until serving time.

4. Meanwhile, in a 6- to 8-quart stockpot or Dutch oven heat the 4 tablespoons olive oil over medium heat. Add shallots, 6 cloves garlic, and ¼ teaspoon black pepper; cook about 2 minutes or until soft and wilted, stirring frequently.

5. Add wine and parsley sprigs to pot; bring to boiling. Add mussels, stirring a few times. Cover tightly and steam for 3 to 5 minutes or until shells open, gently stirring twice. Discard any mussels that do not open.

6. With a large skimmer, transfer mussels into shallow soup dishes. Remove and discard parsley sprigs from cooking liquid; ladle cooking liquid over the mussels. Sprinkle with chopped parsley and, if desired, tarragon. Serve immediately with parsnip frites and saffron aïoli.

*Tip: Cook mussels the day they are purchased. If using wild-harvested mussels, soak in a bowl of cold water for 20 minutes to help flush out grit and sand. (This is not necessary for farm-raised mussels.) Using a stiff brush, scrub mussels, one at a time, under cold running water. Debeard mussels about 10 to 15 minutes before cooking. The beard is the small cluster of fibers that emerge from the shell. To remove the beards, grasp the string between your thumb and forefinger and yank toward the hinge. (This method will not kill the mussel.) You can also use pliers or fish tweezers. Be sure that the shell of each mussel is tightly closed. If any shells are open, tap them gently on the counter. Discard any mussels that don't close within a few minutes. Discard any mussels with cracked or damaged shells.

SEARED SCALLOPS WITH BEET RELISH

START TO FINISH: **30 minutes**   MAKES: **4 servings**

FOR A BEAUTIFUL GOLDEN CRUST, BE SURE THE SURFACE OF THE SCALLOPS IS REALLY DRY—AND THAT THE PAN IS NICE AND HOT—BEFORE ADDING THEM TO THE PAN. ALSO, LET THE SCALLOPS SEAR WITHOUT DISTURBING THEM FOR 2 TO 3 MINUTES, CAREFULLY CHECKING BEFORE TURNING.

1 pound fresh or frozen sea scallops, patted dry with paper towels

3 medium red beets, peeled and cut chopped

½ of a Granny Smith apple, peeled and chopped

2 jalapeños, stemmed, seeded, and minced (see tip, page 56)

¼ cup chopped fresh cilantro

2 tablespoons finely chopped red onion

4 tablespoons olive oil

2 tablespoons fresh lime juice
  White pepper

1. Thaw scallops, if frozen.

2. For beet relish, in a medium bowl combine beets, apple, jalapeños, cilantro, onion, 2 tablespoons of the olive oil, and lime juice. Mix well. Set aside while preparing scallops.

3. Rinse scallops; pat dry with paper towels. In a large skillet heat the remaining 2 tablespoons olive oil over medium-high heat. Add scallops; sauté for 4 to 6 minutes or until golden brown on the exterior and barely opaque. Sprinkle scallops lightly with white pepper.

4. To serve, divide beet relish evenly among serving plates; top with scallops. Serve immediately.

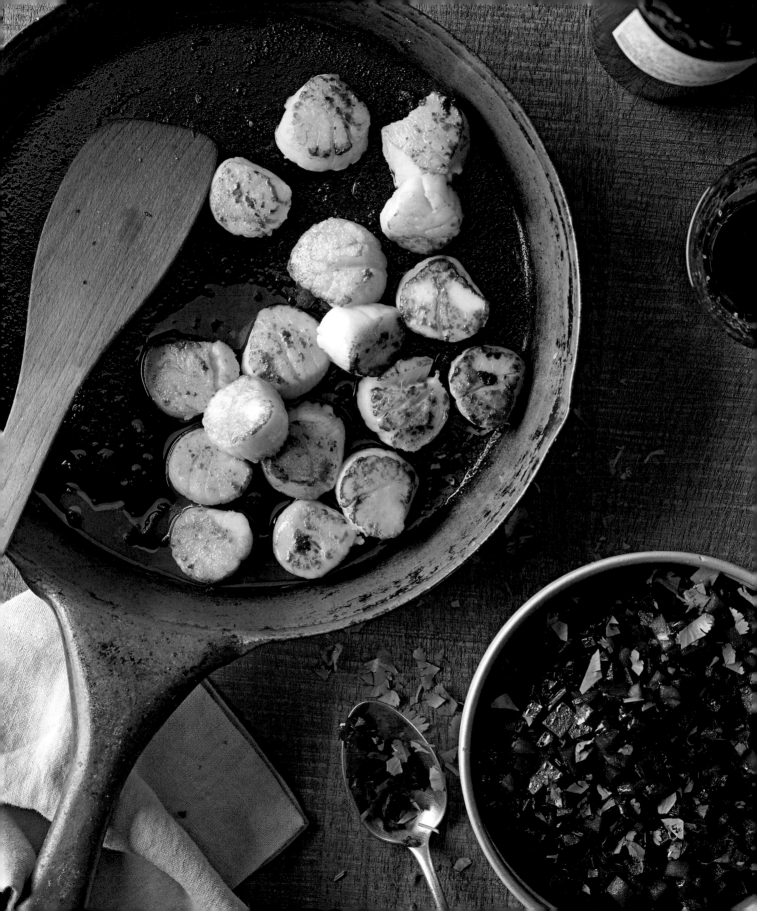

GRILLED SCALLOPS WITH CUCUMBER-DILL SALSA

PREP: 35 minutes   CHILL: 1 to 24 hours   GRILL: 9 minutes   MAKES: 4 servings

HERE'S A TIP FOR GETTING THE MOST FLAWLESS AVOCADOS: BUY THEM WHEN THEY ARE BRIGHT GREEN AND HARD, THEN RIPEN THEM ON THE COUNTER FOR A FEW DAYS—UNTIL THEY GIVE JUST SLIGHTLY WHEN LIGHTLY PRESSED WITH YOUR FINGERS. WHEN HARD AND UNRIPE, THEY WON'T BRUISE IN TRANSIT FROM THE MARKET.

12 or 16 fresh or frozen sea scallops (1¼ to 1¾ pounds total)
¼ cup olive oil
4 cloves garlic, minced
1 teaspoon freshly ground black pepper
2 medium zucchini, trimmed and halved lengthwise
½ of a medium cucumber, halved lengthwise and thinly sliced crosswise
1 medium avocado, halved, seeded, peeled, and chopped
1 medium tomato, cored, seeded, and chopped
2 teaspoons snipped fresh mint
1 teaspoon snipped fresh dill

1. Thaw scallops, if frozen. Rinse scallops with cold water; pat dry with paper towels. In a large bowl combine 3 tablespoons of the oil, the garlic, and ¾ teaspoon of the pepper. Add scallops; toss gently to coat. Cover and chill for at least 1 hour or up to 24 hours, gently stirring occasionally.

2. Brush zucchini halves with the remaining 1 tablespoon oil; sprinkle evenly with remaining ¼ teaspoon pepper.

3. Drain scallops, discarding marinade. Thread two 10- to 12-inch skewers through each scallop, using 3 or 4 scallops for each pair of skewers and leaving a ½-inch space between scallops.* (Threading the scallops on two skewers helps keep them stable when grilling and turning.)

4. For a charcoal or gas grill, place scallop kabobs and zucchini halves on the grill rack directly over medium heat.** Cover and grill until scallops are opaque and zucchini are just tender, turning halfway through grilling. Allow 6 to 8 minutes for scallops and 9 to 11 minutes for zucchini.

5. Meanwhile, for salsa, in a medium bowl combine cucumber, avocado, tomato, mint, and dill. Toss gently to combine. Place 1 scallop kabob on each of four serving plates. Diagonally cut zucchini halves crosswise in half and add to plates with scallops. Spoon cucumber mixture evenly over scallops.

*Tip: If using wooden skewers, soak in enough water to cover for 30 minutes before using.

To broil: Prepare as directed through Step 3. Place scallop kabobs and zucchini halves on the unheated rack of a broiler pan. Broil 4 to 5 inches from the heat until scallops are opaque and zucchini is just tender, turning once halfway through cooking. Allow 6 to 8 minutes for scallops and 10 to 12 minutes for zucchini.

SEARED SCALLOPS WITH TOMATO, OLIVE OIL, AND HERB SAUCE

PREP: 20 minutes   COOK: 4 minutes   MAKES: 4 servings

THE SAUCE IS ALMOST LIKE A WARM VINAIGRETTE. OLIVE OIL, CHOPPED FRESH TOMATO, LEMON JUICE, AND HERBS ARE COMBINED AND VERY GENTLY HEATED—JUST ENOUGH TO MELD THE FLAVORS—AND THEN SERVED WITH THE SEARED SCALLOPS AND A CRUNCHY SUNFLOWER SPROUT SALAD.

SCALLOPS AND SAUCE
- 1 to 1½ pounds large fresh or frozen sea scallops (about 12)
- 2 large roma tomatoes, peeled,* seeded, and chopped
- ½ cup olive oil
- 2 tablespoons fresh lemon juice
- 2 tablespoons snipped fresh basil
- 1 to 2 teaspoons finely chopped chives
- 1 tablespoon olive oil

SALAD
- 4 cups sunflower sprouts
- 1 lemon, cut into wedges
  Extra virgin olive oil

1. Thaw scallops, if frozen. Rinse scallops; pat dry. Set aside.

2. For sauce, in a small saucepan combine tomatoes, ½ cup olive oil, the lemon juice, basil, and chives; set aside.

3. In a large skillet heat the 1 tablespoon olive oil over medium-high heat. Add scallops; cook for 4 to 5 minutes or until browned and opaque, turning once halfway through cooking.

4. For the salad, place the sprouts in a serving bowl. Squeeze lemon wedges over sprouts and drizzle with a little olive oil. Toss to combine.

5. Heat the sauce over low heat until warm; do not boil. To serve, spoon some of the sauce in the center of the plate; top with 3 of the scallops. Serve with the sprouts salad.

*Tip: To easily peel a tomato, drop the tomato into a pot of boiling water for 30 seconds to 1 minute or until the skin starts to split. Remove tomato from the boiling water and immediately plunge into a bowl of ice water to stop the cooking process. When tomato is cool enough to handle, slip the skin off.

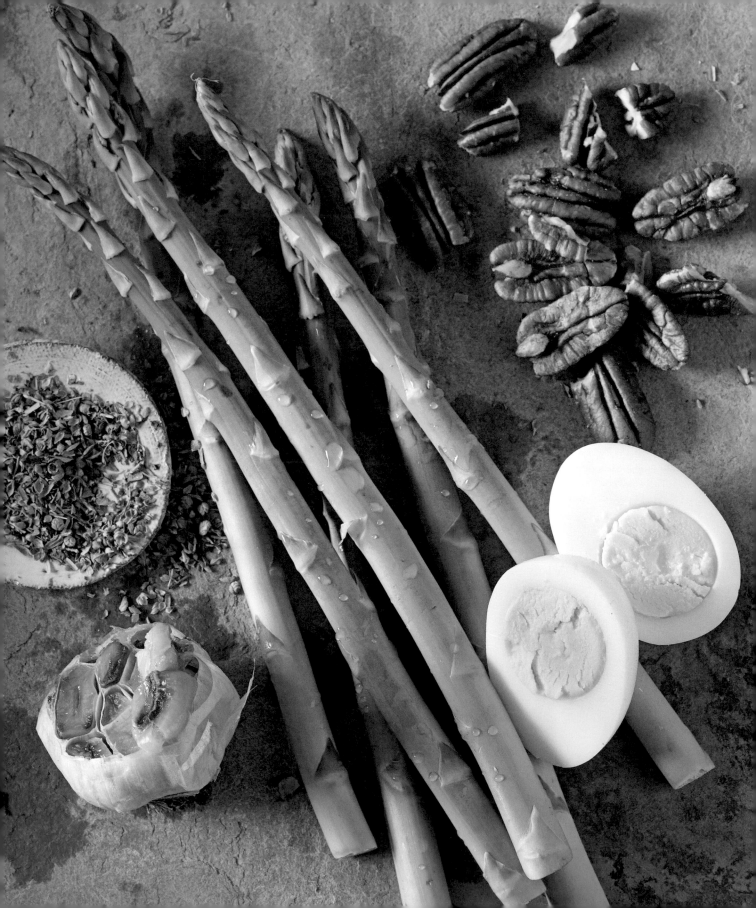

SALADS, SLAWS & VEGETABLE SIDES

Side dishes of all kinds are absolutely essential components of contemporary Paleo diets. These zesty combinations of vegetables and fruits created and tested by our team of chefs and cooks are pure Paleo. Virtually all of the fruits and vegetables in these dishes are fresh, often raw, taste good, and are good for us. The beauty of Paleo Diet cuisine is the unbelievable assortment of luscious produce that can be turned into a salad, crunchy slaw, or vegetable side dish by an inventive cook.

Fresh, raw, or lightly cooked veggies are not only flavorful and appetizing morsels for our palates, but they also serve as excellent medicine for our bodies, particularly when these foods are not adulterated with added salt, refined sugars, or bad fats. As you become accustomed to The Paleo Diet®, make a point of trying to eat about 30% to 35% of your normal food intake as vegetables in one form or another. By doing so, you will ensure that your diet is net alkaline-forming. Diets such as The Paleo Diet®—which contain more alkaline-producing foods (fruits and veggies) than acid-producing foods (cereal grains, cheese, processed foods, and salted foods)—help ward off osteoporosis, stroke, high blood pressure, and kidney stones, as well as other diseases of acid-base imbalance.

Just as important, vegetables—with their dense supply of vitamins, minerals, phytochemicals, and fiber—play a vital role in warding off heart disease and cancer. Almost all Paleo-approved veggies are also nonstarchy, low glycemic-index carbohydrates that help stabilize blood glucose and insulin concentrations, which—if you are overweight or obese—encourages weight loss.

Although it's not a requirement or necessity for The Paleo Diet., many people prefer organic produce over its conventionally grown equivalent. Organic produce is more expensive, but it also typically contains fewer pesticides and nitrates than conventional produce. Both of these compounds may slightly increase the lifetime risk of certain cancers. Personally, I prefer to buy my produce in farmer's markets directly from the farmers because it is normally less expensive, and it is locally grown and locally purchased, which makes more sense from a global-sustainability perspective.

Getting healthy vegetables into your diet, in conjunction with doing away with grains and legumes, permits your body to assimilate all the rich nutrients that veggies have to offer. The slow-release carbohydrate contained in all Paleo-approved veggies (see "Paleo Principles," page 14) will prevent blood sugar and insulin surges, and in turn your energy levels will become normalized throughout the day. Vegetables help you feel satisfied without feeling overly full. The multiplicity of fresh vegetables that you may choose from in The Paleo Diet. is enormous. If you have never tasted fennel or celeriac, try Fennel Slaw or perhaps Creamy Celery Root Soup with Herb Oil. You may want to discover ethnic markets and explore their produce sections for vegetables that you can rarely find at your local grocery store or supermarket. The only vegetables that are forbidden on The Paleo Diet. are white potatoes, peas, green beans, and all legumes, as explained in "Paleo Principles."

CUMIN-ROASTED CAULIFLOWER WITH FENNEL AND PEARL ONIONS

PREP: 15 minutes   COOK: 25 minutes   MAKES: 4 servings

THERE IS SOMETHING PARTICULARLY ENTICING ABOUT THE COMBINATION OF ROASTED CAULIFLOWER AND THE TOASTY, EARTHY TASTE OF CUMIN. THIS DISH HAS THE ADDITIONAL ELEMENT OF SWEETNESS FROM DRIED CURRANTS. IF YOU LIKE, YOU COULD ADD A LITTLE HEAT WITH ¼ TO ½ TEASPOON OF CRUSHED RED PEPPER ALONG WITH THE CUMIN AND CURRANTS IN STEP 2.

3 tablespoons unrefined coconut oil

1 medium head cauliflower, cut into florets (4 to 5 cups)

2 heads fennel, coarsely chopped

1½ cups frozen pearl onions, thawed and drained

¼ cup dried currants

2 teaspoons ground cumin
   Snipped fresh dill (optional)

1. In an extra-large skillet heat coconut oil over medium heat. Add cauliflower, fennel, and pearl onions. Cover and cook for 15 minutes, stirring occasionally.

2. Reduce heat to medium-low. Add currants and cumin to skillet; cook, uncovered, about 10 minutes or until cauliflower and fennel are tender and golden brown. If desired, garnish with dill.

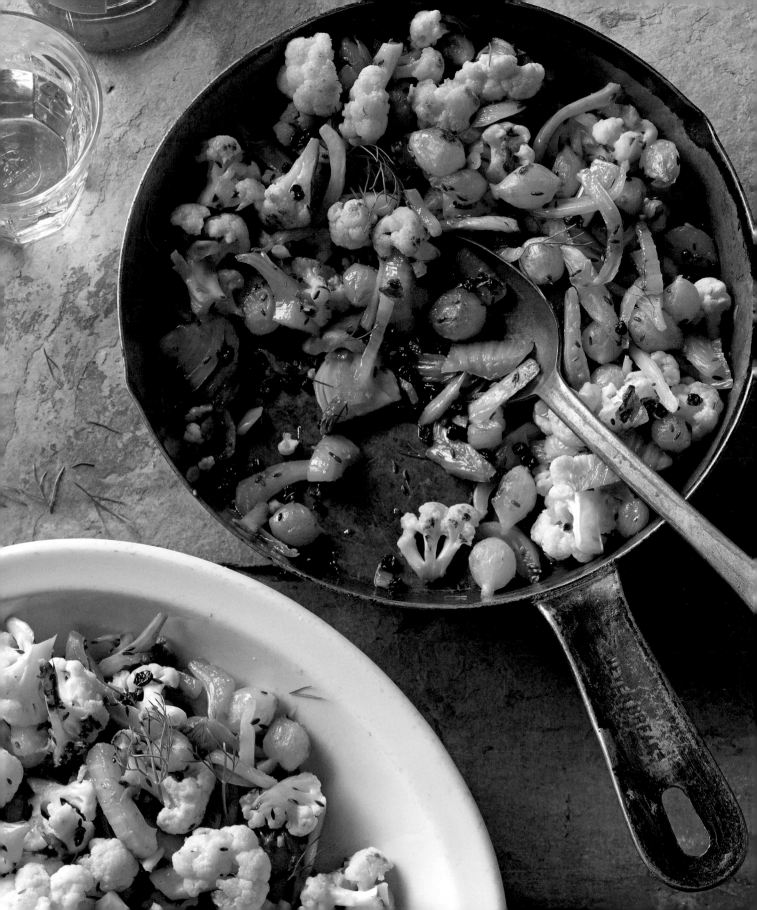

CHUNKY TOMATO-EGGPLANT SAUCE WITH SPAGHETTI SQUASH

PREP: 30 minutes   BAKE: 50 minutes   COOL: 10 minutes   COOK: 10 minutes   MAKES: 4 servings

THIS SAUCY SIDE DISH IS EASILY TURNED INTO A MAIN DISH. ADD ABOUT 1 POUND OF COOKED GROUND BEEF OR BISON TO THE EGGPLANT-TOMATO MIXTURE AFTER YOU MASH IT LIGHTLY WITH A POTATO MASHER.

1 2- to 2½-pound spaghetti squash
2 tablespoons olive oil
1 cup chopped, peeled eggplant
¾ cup chopped onion
1 small red sweet pepper, chopped (½ cup)
4 cloves garlic, minced
4 medium red ripe tomatoes, peeled if desired and coarsely chopped (about 2 cups)
½ cup torn fresh basil

1. Preheat oven to 375°F. Line a small baking pan with parchment paper. Cut spaghetti squash in half crosswise. Use a large spoon to scrape out any seeds and strings. Place squash halves, cut sides down, on prepared baking sheet. Bake, uncovered, for 50 to 60 minutes or until squash is tender. Cool on a wire rack about 10 minutes.

2. Meanwhile, in a large skillet heat olive oil over medium heat. Add onion, eggplant and pepper; cook for 5 to 7 minutes or until vegetables are tender, stirring occasionally. Add garlic; cook and stir 30 seconds more. Add tomatoes; cook for 3 to 5 minutes or until tomatoes are softened, stirring occasionally. Using a potato masher, mash the mixture lightly. Stir in half the basil. Cover and cook for 2 minutes.

3. Use a pot holder or towel to hold squash halves. Use a fork to scrape the squash pulp into a medium bowl. Divide squash among four serving plates. Top evenly with sauce. Sprinkle with remaining basil.

STUFFED PORTOBELLO MUSHROOMS

PREP: 35 minutes   BAKE: 20 minutes   COOK: 7 minutes   MAKES: 4 servings

TO GET THE FRESHEST PORTOBELLOS, LOOK FOR MUSHROOMS THAT STILL HAVE THEIR STEMS INTACT. THE GILLS SHOULD LOOK MOIST BUT NOT WET OR BLACK AND SHOULD HAVE GOOD SEPARATION BETWEEN THEM. TO PREPARE ANY KIND OF MUSHROOMS FOR COOKING, WIPE WITH A SLIGHTLY DAMP PAPER TOWEL. NEVER RUN MUSHROOMS UNDER WATER OR SOAK THEM IN WATER—THEY ARE HIGHLY ABSORBENT AND WILL GET MUSHY AND WATERLOGGED.

4   large portobello mushrooms (about 1 pound total)
¼   cup olive oil
1   tablespoon Smoky Seasoning (see recipe, page 324)
2   tablespoons olive oil
½   cup chopped shallots
1   tablespoon minced garlic
1   pound Swiss chard, stemmed and chopped (about 10 cups)
2   teaspoons Mediterranean Seasoning (see recipe, page 324)
½   cup chopped radishes

1. Preheat oven to 400°F. Remove stems from mushrooms and reserve for Step 2. Use the tip of a spoon to scrape the gills out of the caps; discard gills. Place mushroom caps in a 3-quart rectangular baking dish; brush both sides of mushrooms with the ¼ cup olive oil. Turn mushroom caps so the stemmed sides are up; sprinkle with Smoky Seasoning. Cover baking dish with foil. Bake, covered, about 20 minutes or until tender.

2. Meanwhile, chop reserved mushroom stems; set aside. To prepare chard, remove thick ribs from leaves and discard. Coarsely chop the chard leaves.

3. In an extra-large skillet heat the 2 tablespoons olive oil over medium heat. Add shallots and garlic; cook and stir for 30 seconds. Add chopped mushroom stems, chopped chard, and Mediterranean Seasoning. Cook, uncovered, for 6 to 8 minutes or until chard is tender, stirring occasionally.

4. Divide chard mixture among the mushroom caps. Drizzle any liquid remaining in baking dish over stuffed mushrooms. Top with chopped radishes.

ROASTED RADICCHIO

PREP: 20 minutes   COOK: 15 minutes   MAKES: 4 servings

RADICCHIO IS MOST OFTEN EATEN AS PART OF A SALAD TO PROVIDE A PLEASANT BITTERNESS AMONG THE MIX OF GREENS—BUT IT CAN BE ROASTED OR GRILLED ON ITS OWN AS WELL. A SLIGHT BITTERNESS IS INHERENT TO RADICCHIO, BUT YOU DON'T WANT IT TO BE OVERWHELMING. LOOK FOR SMALLER HEADS WHOSE LEAVES LOOK FRESH AND CRISP—NOT WILTED. THE CUT END MAY BE A LITTLE BROWN BUT SHOULD BE MOSTLY WHITE. IN THIS RECIPE, A SPLASH OF BALSAMIC VINEGAR BEFORE SERVING ADDS A HINT OF SWEETNESS.

2 large heads radicchio
¼ cup olive oil
1 teaspoon Mediterranean Seasoning (see recipe, page 324)
¼ cup balsamic vinegar

1. Preheat oven to 400°F. Quarter the radicchio, leaving some of the core attached (you should have 8 wedges). Brush cut sides of radicchio wedges with olive oil. Place wedges, cut sides down, on a baking sheet; sprinkle with Mediterranean Seasoning.

2. Roast about 15 minutes or until radicchio wilts, turning once halfway through roasting. Arrange radicchio on a serving platter. Drizzle balsamic vinegar; serve immediately.

ROASTED FENNEL WITH ORANGE VINAIGRETTE

PREP: 25 minutes   ROAST: 25 minutes   MAKES: 4 servings

SAVE ANY LEFTOVER VINAIGRETTE TO TOSS WITH SALAD GREENS—OR SERVE WITH GRILLED PORK, POULTRY, OR FISH. STORE LEFTOVER VINAIGRETTE IN A TIGHTLY COVERED CONTAINER IN THE REFRIGERATOR FOR UP TO 3 DAYS.

6 tablespoons extra virgin olive oil, plus more for brushing
1 large fennel bulb, trimmed, cored, and cut into wedges (reserve fronds for garnish if desired)
1 red onion, cut into wedges
½ of an orange, thinly sliced into rounds
½ cup orange juice
2 tablespoons white wine vinegar or champagne vinegar
2 tablespoons apple cider
1 teaspoon ground fennel seeds
1 teaspoon finely shredded orange peel
½ teaspoon Dijon-Style Mustard (see recipe, page 322)
   Black pepper

1. Preheat oven to 425°F. Brush a large baking sheet lightly with olive oil. Arrange the fennel, onion, and orange slices on the baking sheet; drizzle with 2 tablespoons of the olive oil. Gently toss vegetable to coat with oil.

2. Roast vegetables for 25 to 30 minutes or until vegetables are tender and light golden, turning once halfway through roasting.

3. Meanwhile, for orange vinaigrette, in a blender combine orange juice, vinegar, apple cider, fennel seeds, orange peel, Dijon-Style Mustard, and pepper to taste. With the blender running, slowly add the remaining 4 tablespoons olive oil in a thin stream. Continue blending until vinaigrette thickens.

4. Transfer vegetables to a serving platter. Drizzle vegetables with some of the vinaigrette. If desired, garnish with reserved fennel fronds.

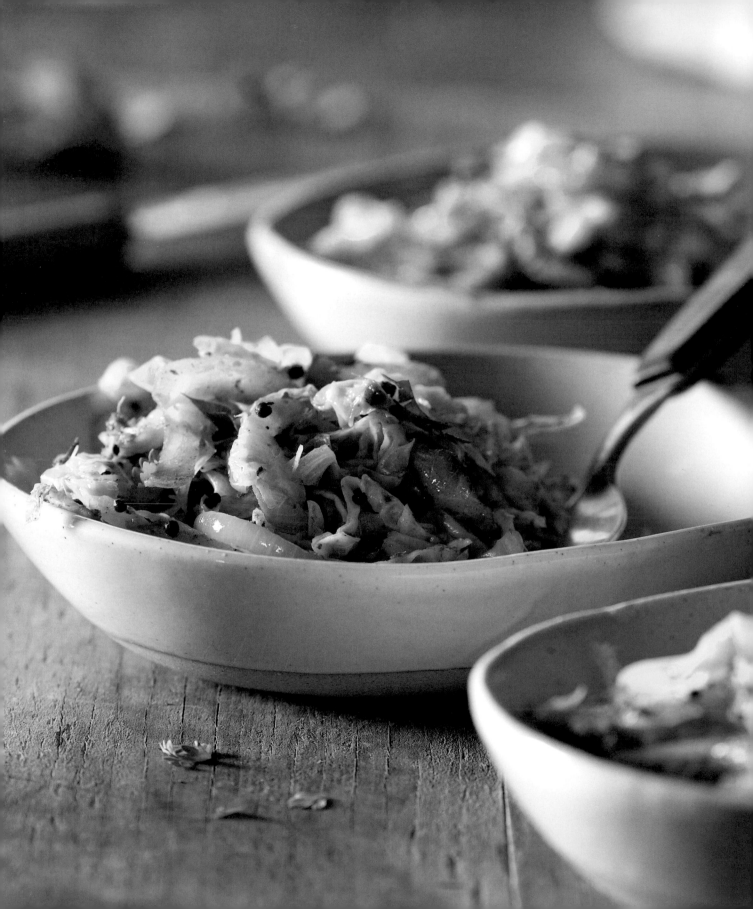

PUNJABI-STYLE SAVOY CABBAGE

PREP: 20 minutes   COOK: 25 minutes   MAKES: 4 servings

IT'S AMAZING WHAT HAPPENS TO A MILDLY-FLAVORED, UNASSUMING CABBAGE WHEN IT'S COOKED WITH GINGER, GARLIC, CHILES, AND INDIAN SPICES. TOASTED MUSTARD, CORIANDER, AND CUMIN SEEDS GIVE THIS DISH BOTH FLAVOR AND CRUNCH. BE FOREWARNED: IT IS HOT! BIRD'S BEAK CHILES ARE SMALL BUT VERY POTENT—AND THE DISH INCLUDES JALAPEÑO TOO. IF YOU PREFER LESS HEAT, JUST USE THE JALAPEÑO.

1 2-inch knob fresh ginger, peeled and cut into ⅓-inch slices
5 cloves garlic
1 large jalapeño, stemmed, seeded, and halved (see tip, page 56)
2 teaspoons no-salt-added garam masala
1 teaspoon ground turmeric
½ cup Chicken Bone Broth (see recipe, page 235) or no-salt-added chicken broth
3 tablespoons refined coconut oil
1 tablespoon black mustard seeds
1 teaspoon coriander seeds
1 teaspoon cumin seeds
1 whole bird's beak chile (chile de arbol) (see tip, page 56)
1 3-inch cinnamon stick
2 cups thinly sliced yellow onions (about 2 medium)
12 cups thinly sliced, cored savoy cabbage (about 1½ pounds)
½ cup snipped fresh cilantro (optional)

1. In a food processor or blender combine ginger, garlic, jalapeño, garam masala, turmeric, and ¼ cup of the Chicken Bone Broth. Cover and process or blend until smooth; set aside.

2. In an extra-large skillet combine coconut oil, mustard seeds, coriander seeds, cumin seeds, chile, and cinnamon stick. Cook over medium-high heat, shaking pan frequently, for 2 to 3 minutes or until the cinnamon stick unfurls. (Be careful—mustard seeds will pop and spatter as they cook.) Add onions; cook and stir for 5 to 6 minutes or until onions are lightly browned. Add ginger mixture. Cook, for 6 to 8 minutes or until mixture is nicely caramelized, stirring often.

3. Add cabbage and the remaining Chicken Bone Broth; mix well. Cover and cook about 15 minutes or until cabbage is tender, stirring twice. Uncover skillet. Cook and stir for 6 to 7 minutes or until cabbage is lightly browned and excess Chicken Bone Broth evaporates.

4. Remove and discard cinnamon stick and chile. If desired, sprinkle with cilantro.

CINNAMON-ROASTED BUTTERNUT SQUASH

PREP: 20 minutes   ROAST: 30 minutes   MAKES: 4 to 6 servings

A DASH OF CAYENNE PEPPER GIVES THESE SWEET ROASTED CUBES OF SQUASH JUST A HINT OF HEAT. IT'S EASILY LEFT OUT IF YOU PREFER. SERVE THIS SIMPLE SIDE WITH ROAST PORK OR PORK CHOPS.

1 butternut squash (about 2 pounds), peeled, seeded, and cut into ¾-inch cubes
2 tablespoons olive oil
½ teaspoon ground cinnamon
¼ teaspoon black pepper
⅛ teaspoon cayenne pepper

1. Preheat oven to 400°F. In a large bowl toss squash with olive oil, cinnamon, black pepper, and cayenne pepper. Line a large rimmed baking sheet with parchment paper. Spread squash in a single layer on the baking sheet.

2. Roast for 30 to 35 minutes or until squash is tender and browned on edges, stirring once or twice.

BROILED ASPARAGUS WITH SIEVED EGG AND PECANS

START TO FINISH: 15 minutes   MAKES: 4 servings

THIS IS A TAKE ON A CLASSIC FRENCH VEGETABLE DISH CALLED ASPARAGUS MIMOSA—SO CALLED BECAUSE THE GREEN, WHITE, AND YELLOW OF THE FINISHED DISH LOOKS LIKE A FLOWER OF THE SAME NAME.

1 pound fresh asparagus, trimmed
5 tablespoons Roasted Garlic Vinaigrette (see recipe, page 321)
1 hard-cooked egg, peeled
3 tablespoons chopped pecans, toasted (see tip, page 57)
  Freshly ground black pepper

1. Position oven rack 4 inches from heating element; preheat broiler to high.

2. Spread asparagus spears on a baking sheet. Drizzle with 2 tablespoons of the Roasted Garlic Vinaigrette. Using your hands, roll asparagus to coat with vinaigrette. Broil for 3 to 5 minutes or until blistered and tender, turning asparagus after every minute. Transfer to a serving platter.

3. Cut the egg in half; press egg through a sieve over the asparagus. (You can also grate the egg using the large holes of a box grater.) Drizzle asparagus and egg with the remaining 3 tablespoons Roasted Garlic Vinaigrette. Top with pecans and sprinkle with pepper.

5 WAYS WITH CABBAGE

PLAIN GREEN HEAD CABBAGE IS AN UNDERESTIMATED, UNDERUTILIZED VEGETABLE. WHILE MOST VEGETABLES CAN BE EATEN RAW OR COOKED, CABBAGE CAN BE SHREDDED, CUT INTO WEDGES, SLICED INTO ROUNDS, AND STUFFED AND ROLLED—AS WELL AS EATEN RAW, COOKED, FERMENTED, AND PICKLED. CABBAGE IS HIGH IN FIBER AND VITAMINS K AND C.

Crunchy Cabbage Slaw with Radishes, Mango, and Mint, *recipe on page 292*

5 WAYS WITH CABBAGE

WHATEVER SHAPE YOUR CABBAGE DISH TAKES, YOU ARE IN GOOD COMPANY AROUND THE WORLD IN MAKING USE OF THIS CRUCIFEROUS VEGETABLE. CABBAGE IS POPULAR IN MANY CUISINES BECAUSE IT IS VERSATILE, INEXPENSIVE, AND STORES WELL. THE ONLY CAVEAT TO COOKING CABBAGE IS TO NOT OVERDO IT. OVERCOOKING ROBS CABBAGE OF ITS NUTRIENTS AND DESTROYS ITS TOOTHSOME TEXTURE AS WELL.

1. CRUNCHY CABBAGE SLAW WITH RADISHES, MANGO, AND MINT

START TO FINISH: 20 minutes
MAKES: 6 servings

- 3 tablespoons fresh lemon juice
- ¼ teaspoon cayenne pepper
- ¼ teaspoon ground cumin
- ¼ cup olive oil
- 4 cups shredded cabbage
- 1½ cups very thinly sliced radishes
- 1 cup cubed ripe mango
- ½ cup bias-sliced scallions
- ⅓ cup chopped fresh mint

1. For dressing, in a large bowl combine lemon juice, cayenne pepper, and ground cumin. Whisk in olive oil in a thin stream.

2. Add cabbage, radishes, mango, scallions, and mint to dressing in bowl. Toss well to combine.

2. ROASTED CABBAGE ROUNDS WITH CARAWAY AND LEMON

PREP: 10 minutes
ROAST: 30 minutes
MAKES: 4 to 6 servings

- 3 tablespoons olive oil
- 1 medium head cabbage, cut into 1-inch-thick rounds
- 2 teaspoons Dijon-Style Mustard (see recipe, page 322)
- 1 teaspoon finely shredded lemon peel
- ¼ teaspoon black pepper
- 1 teaspoon caraway seeds
  Lemon wedges

1. Preheat oven to 400°F. Brush a large rimmed baking sheet with 1 tablespoon of the olive oil. Arrange cabbage rounds on the baking sheet; set aside.

2. In a small bowl whisk together the remaining 2 tablespoons olive oil, Dijon-Style Mustard, and lemon peel. Brush over cabbage rounds on baking sheet, making sure mustard and lemon peel are evenly distributed. Sprinkle with pepper and caraway seeds.

3. Roast for 30 to 35 minutes or until cabbage is tender and edges are golden brown. Serve with lemon wedges to squeeze over cabbage.

3. ROASTED CABBAGE WITH ORANGE-BALSAMIC DRIZZLE

PREP: 15 minutes
ROAST: 30 minutes
MAKES: 4 servings

- 3 tablespoons olive oil
- 1 small head cabbage, cored and cut into 8 wedges
- ½ teaspoon black pepper
- ⅓ cup balsamic vinegar
- 2 teaspoons finely shredded orange peel

1. Preheat oven to 450°F. Brush a large rimmed baking sheet with 1 tablespoon of the olive oil. Arrange cabbage wedges on the baking sheet. Brush cabbage with the remaining 2 tablespoons olive oil and sprinkle with pepper.

2. Roast cabbage for 15 minutes. Turn cabbage wedges over; roast about 15 minutes more or until cabbage is tender and edges are golden brown.

3. In a small saucepan combine the balsamic vinegar and orange peel. Bring to boiling over medium heat; reduce. Simmer, uncovered, about 4 minutes or until reduced by half. Drizzle over roasted cabbage wedges; serve immediately.

4. BRAISED CABBAGE WITH CREAMY DILL SAUCE AND TOASTED WALNUTS

PREP: 20 minutes
COOK: 40 minutes
MAKES: 6 servings

- 3 tablespoons olive oil
- 1 shallot, finely chopped
- 1 small head green cabbage, cut into 6 wedges
- ½ teaspoon black pepper
- 1 cup Chicken Bone Broth (see recipe, page 235) or no-salt-added chicken broth
- ¾ cup Cashew Cream (see recipe, page 327)
- 4 teaspoons finely shredded lemon peel
- 4 teaspoons snipped fresh dill
- 1 tablespoon finely chopped scallions
- ¼ cup chopped walnuts, toasted (see tip, page 57)

1. In an extra-large skillet heat olive oil over medium-high heat. Add shallot; cook for 2 to 3 minutes or until tender and lightly browned. Add cabbage wedges to skillet. Cook, uncovered, for 10 minutes or until lightly browned on each side, turning once halfway through cooking. Sprinkle with pepper.

2. Add Chicken Bone Broth to skillet. Bring to boiling; reduce heat. Cover and simmer for 25 to 30 minutes or until cabbage is tender.

3. Meanwhile, for Creamy Dill Sauce, in a small bowl stir together Cashew Cream, lemon peel, dill, and scallions.

4. To serve, transfer cabbage wedges to serving plates; drizzle with pan juices. Top with dill sauce and sprinkle with toasted walnuts.

5. SAUTÉED GREEN CABBAGE WITH TOASTED SESAME SEEDS

PREP: 20 minutes
COOK: 19 minutes
MAKES: 4 servings

2 tablespoons sesame seeds
2 tablespoons refined coconut oil
1 medium onion, thinly sliced
1 medium tomato, chopped
1 tablespoon minced fresh ginger
3 cloves garlic, minced
¼ teaspoon crushed red pepper
½ of a 3- to 3½-pound head green cabbage, cored and very thinly sliced

1. In an extra-large dry skillet toast sesame seeds over medium heat for 3 to 4 minutes or until golden brown, stirring almost constantly. Transfer seeds to a smal bowl and cool completely. Transfer seeds to a clean spice or coffee grinder; pulse to grind coarsely. Set ground sesame seeds aside.

2. Meanwhile, in the same extra-large skillet heat coconut oil over medium-high heat. Add onion; cook about 2 minutes or just until slightly soft. Stir in tomato, ginger, garlic, and crushed red pepper. Cook and stir for 2 minutes more.

3. Add sliced cabbage to tomato mixture in skillet. Toss with tongs to combine. Cook for 12 to 14 minutes or until cabbage is tender and just begins to brown, stirring occasionally. Add ground sesame seeds; stir well to combine. Serve immediately.

ROASTED CARROT-PARSNIP SOUP WITH GARAM MASALA NUT "CROUTONS"

PREP: 30 minutes   ROAST: 30 minutes   COOK: 10 minutes   MAKES: 8 servings

IF YOUR CARROTS ARE SLENDER AND FRESH AND THE SKIN IS RELATIVELY THIN, THERE IS REALLY NO NEED TO PEEL THEM. A VIGOROUS SCRUB WITH A VEGETABLE BRUSH IS ALL THAT'S NEEDED. EITHER WAY, THOUGH, YOU'RE GETTING VALUABLE NUTRIENTS SUCH AS BETA-CAROTENE.

Olive oil

1½ pounds carrots, peeled, if desired, and cut into 1½-inch pieces

1½ pounds parsnips, peeled and cut into 1½-inch pieces

2 Granny Smith apples, peeled and cut into 1½-inch pieces

2 yellow onions, cut into 1½-inch pieces

2 tablespoons olive oil

1 teaspoon curry powder

¼ teaspoon black pepper

1 tablespoon grated fresh ginger

6 cups Chicken Bone Broth (see recipe, page 235), or no-salt-added chicken broth

1 teaspoon ground cumin

Chicken Bone Broth, no-salt-added chicken broth, water, or unsweetened coconut milk (optional)

Garam Masala Nut "Croutons" (see recipe, right)

1. Preheat the oven to 400°F. Brush an extra-large rimmed baking sheet with olive oil. In an extra-large bowl combine carrots, parsnips, apples, and onions. In a small bowl combine the 2 tablespoons olive oil, ½ teaspoon of the curry powder, and pepper. Pour over vegetables and apples; toss to coat. Spread vegetables and apples in a single layer on the prepared baking sheet. Roast for 30 to 40 minutes or until vegetables and apples are very tender.

2. Working in three batches, place one third of the vegetable-apple mixture and all of the ginger in a food processor or blender; add 2 cups of the Chicken Bone Broth. Cover and process until smooth; transfer to a large saucepan. Repeat with remaining vegetable-apple mixture and 4 more cups of the broth. Add the remaining ½ teaspoon curry powder and the cumin to the pureed mixture. Bring to boiling; reduce heat. Simmer, uncovered, for 10 minutes to meld the flavors. If the soup is too thick, thin with additional broth, water, or coconut milk. Garnish each serving with 1 tablespoon of the Garam Masala Nut "Croutons."

Garam Masala Nut "Croutons": Preheat oven to 300°F. Lightly brush a rimmed baking sheet with olive oil. In a medium bowl whisk together 1 egg white, ½ teaspoon vanilla, ½ teaspoon garam masala or apple pie spice, and a pinch cayenne pepper. Stir in 1 cup sliced almonds. Spread onto prepared pan. Bake for 15 to 25 minutes or until nuts are golden, stirring every 5 minutes. Cool completely. Break up any large chunks. Store in a covered container for up to 1 week. Makes 1 cup.

CREAMY CELERY ROOT SOUP WITH HERB OIL

pictured on page 221

PREP: 15 minutes   COOK: 30 minutes   MAKES: 4 servings

THE HUMBLE CELERY ROOT—SOMETIMES CALLED CELERIAC—IS KNOBBY AND GNARLY AND QUITE HONESTLY A LITTLE FUNKY LOOKING. BUT UNDERNEATH THE WOODY PEEL IS A CRISP, NUTTY-FLAVORED ROOT THAT—WHEN COOKED WITH CHICKEN BROTH AND PUREED—MAKES A CREAMY, CLEAN-TASTING, SILKY SOUP. A DRIZZLE OF HERBED OLIVE OIL ENHANCES BUT DOESN'T OVERWHELM ITS LOVELY FLAVOR.

1 tablespoon olive oil

1 leek, sliced (white and light green parts only)

4 cups Chicken Bone Broth (see recipe, page 235) or no-salt-added chicken broth

½ of a medium celery root (about 10 ounces), peeled and cut into 1-inch cubes

½ of a head cauliflower, cored and broken into florets

¼ cup packed Italian (flat-leaf) parsley

¼ cup packed basil leaves

¼ cup olive oil

1 tablespoon fresh lemon juice

¼ teaspoon black pepper

1. In a large saucepan heat the 1 tablespoon olive oil over medium heat. Add leek; cook for 4 to 5 minutes or until tender. Add Chicken Bone Broth, celery root, and cauliflower. Bring to boiling; reduce heat. Cover and simmer for 20 to 25 minutes or until vegetables are tender. Remove from heat; cool slightly.

2. Meanwhile, for herb oil, in a food processor or blender combine the parsley, basil, and the ¼ cup olive oil. Cover and process or blend until well combined and herbs are in very small pieces. Pour oil through a fine-mesh strainer into a small bowl, pressing herbs with the back of a spoon to extract as much oil as possible. Discard herbs; set herb oil aside.

3. Transfer half of the celery root mixture to the food processor or blender. Cover and process or blend until smooth. Pour into a large bowl. Repeat with remaining celery root mixture. Return all of the mixture back to the saucepan. Stir in lemon juice and pepper; heat through.

4. Ladle soup into bowls. Drizzle with herb oil.

BLUEBERRY AND ROASTED BEET KALE SALAD

PREP: 25 minutes   ROAST: 30 minutes   MAKES: 4 servings

THIS SALAD IS A NUTRITIONAL POWERHOUSE. WITH BEETS, KALE, AND BLUEBERRIES, IT'S LOADED WITH ANTIOXIDANTS, IRON, CALCIUM, VITAMINS, MINERALS, AND ANTI-INFLAMMATORY COMPOUNDS. IT'S EASILY CONVERTED FROM A SIDE INTO A MAIN DISH—JUST ADD 4 OUNCES OF COOKED SALMON, CHICKEN, PORK, OR BEEF TO EACH SALAD.

3 medium beets (about 12 ounces total), trimmed, peeled, and cut into quarters

1 tablespoon olive oil

1 small onion, cut into thin wedges

6 tablespoons balsamic vinegar

6 tablespoons olive oil or flaxseed oil

½ teaspoon snipped fresh rosemary or thyme

3 cups torn fresh romaine lettuce

2 cups torn fresh kale

½ cup fresh blueberries

¼ cup hazelnuts, toasted and coarsely chopped*

1. Preheat oven to 425°F. In a 15×10×1-inch baking pan toss beet wedges with the 1 tablespoon olive oil. Cover with foil. Roast for 10 minutes. Remove foil; add onions, tossing to combine. Roast, uncovered, about 20 minutes more or until beets and onion are tender.

2. For dressing, in a blender combine 2 of the roasted beet wedges, the vinegar, 6 tablespoons olive oil, and the rosemary. Cover and blend until very smooth, scraping sides of bowl as necessary.

3. Divide romaine and kale among four serving plates. Top with the remaining roasted beets and the onion. Drizzle evenly with dressing. Sprinkle with blueberries and hazelnuts.

*Tip: To toast hazelnuts, preheat oven to 350°F. Spread nuts in a single layer in a shallow baking pan. Bake for 8 to 10 minutes or until lightly toasted, stirring once to toast evenly. Cool nuts slightly. Place the warm nuts on a clean kitchen towel; rub with the towel to remove the loose skins.

CRUNCHY BROCCOLI SALAD

PREP: 15 minutes   CHILL: 1 hour   MAKES: 4 to 6 servings

THIS RESEMBLES A VERY POPULAR BROCCOLI SALAD THAT POPS UP AT SUMMER BARBECUES AND POTLUCKS—AND DISAPPEARS JUST AS QUICKLY. THIS VERSION IS PURE PALEO. ALL OF THE ELEMENTS ARE THERE—CRUNCHY, CREAMY, AND SWEET—BUT THERE IS NO PROCESSED SUGAR IN THE DRESSING AND THE SMOKINESS COMES FROM SALT-FREE SMOKY SEASONING INSTEAD OF BACON, WHICH IS LOADED WITH SODIUM.

¾ cup Paleo Mayo (see recipe, page 323)
1½ teaspoons Smoky Seasoning (see recipe, page 324)
3 teaspoons finely shredded orange peel
5 teaspoons fresh orange juice
5 teaspoons white wine vinegar
1 bunch broccoli, cut into small florets (about 5 cups)
⅓ cup unsulfured raisins
¼ cup chopped red onion
¼ cup unsalted roasted sunflower seeds or sliced almonds

1. For dressing, in a small bowl stir together Paleo Mayo, Smoky Seasoning, orange peel, orange juice, and vinegar; set aside.

2. In a large bowl toss together broccoli, raisins, onion, and sunflower seeds. Pour dressing over broccoli mixture; toss well to combine. Cover and refrigerate for at least 1 hour before serving.

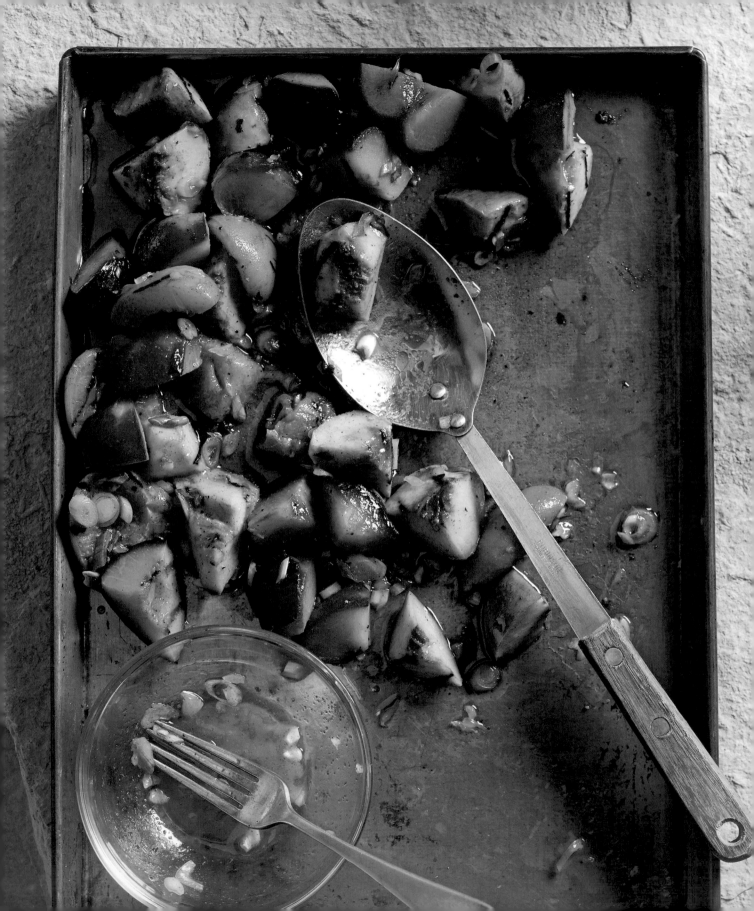

GRILLED FRUIT SALAD WITH SCALLION VINAIGRETTE

PREP: 15 minutes   GRILL: 6 minutes   COOL: 30 minutes   MAKES: 6 servings

IN CREATING INTERESTING FLAVOR, IT'S THE LITTLE THINGS THAT COUNT. THE SCALLION VINAIGRETTE FOR THIS STONE-FRUITS SALAD IS MADE WITH OLIVE OIL, CAYENNE, SCALLIONS, AND THE JUICE OF A TANGERINE THAT'S GRILLED BEFORE SQUEEZING—WHICH GIVES IT A HINT OF SMOKE AND INTENSIFIES THE TANGERINE FLAVOR.

2   peaches, halved lengthwise and pitted
2   plums, halved lengthwise and pitted
3   apricots, halved lengthwise and pitted
1   tangerine or orange, halved crosswise
½   teaspoon black pepper
½   teaspoon paprika
3   to 4 tablespoons olive oil
2   scallions, thinly sliced
¼   to ½ teaspoon cayenne pepper or paprika

1. On a large baking sheet place peaches, plums, apricots, and the tangerine, cut sides up. Sprinkle with black pepper and the ½ teaspoon paprika. Drizzle with 1 to 2 tablespoons of the olive oil, coating the fruit evenly.

2. For a charcoal or gas grill, place fruit, cut sides down, on a grill rack directly over medium heat. Cover and grill for 6 minutes or until charred and slightly softened, turning once halfway through grilling. Let fruit cool until easy to handle. Coarsely chop the peaches, plums, and apricots; set aside.

3. For the dressing, squeeze the juice from the tangerine halves into a small bowl (discard any seeds). Add the scallions, the remaining 2 tablespoons olive oil, and cayenne pepper to the tangerine juice; whisk to combine. Just before serving, toss the grilled fruit with the dressing.

CRUNCHY CURRY CAULIFLOWER

START TO FINISH: **30 minutes**   MAKES: **8 to 10 servings**

MADE FROM RAW CAULIFLOWER, THIS IS A GREAT DISH TO BRING TO A POTLUCK. IT'S INEXPENSIVE, MAKES A GENEROUS NUMBER OF SERVINGS, AND PEOPLE RAVE ABOUT IT (WE KNOW THIS FROM OUR OWN RECIPE TESTING). EVEN BETTER, IT CAN BE MADE UP TO A DAY AHEAD. JUST HOLD OFF ON STIRRING IN THE CILANTRO, PEPITAS, AND RAISINS UNTIL RIGHT BEFORE SERVING.

1 head cauliflower (about 2 pounds)*

⅓ cup olive oil

⅓ cup fresh lemon juice (from 2 lemons)

⅓ cup minced shallots

1 tablespoon yellow curry powder

1 teaspoon cumin seeds, toasted (see tip, page 57)

½ cup snipped fresh cilantro

½ cup pepitas (pumpkin seeds) or sliced almonds, toasted (see tip, page 57)

½ cup unsulfured golden raisins

1. Remove outer leaves from cauliflower and cut off the stem. Place, stem side down, on a cutting board. Slice very thinly, cutting from top to bottom. (Some of the pieces will crumble.) Place cauliflower in a large mixing bowl; break up any large pieces. (You should have about 6 cups cauliflower.)

2. In a small mixing bowl whisk together the olive oil, lemon juice, shallots, curry powder, and cumin seeds. Pour mixture over cauliflower; toss to coat. Let stand for 10 to 15 minutes, stirring occasionally.

3. Just before serving, stir in cilantro, pepitas, and raisins.

***Note:** Romanesco cauliflower can be used here, although it's not as widely available as conventional cauliflower.

Make-Ahead Directions: Prepare salad through Step 2. Cover and chill up to 24 hours, stirring occasionally. Just before serving, stir in cilantro, pepitas, and raisins.

NEO-CLASSIC WALDORF SALAD

PREP: 20 minutes   COOL: 1 hour   MAKES: 4 to 6 servings

CLASSIC WALDORF SALAD WAS CREATED AT THE WALD0RF ASTORIA HOTEL IN NEW YORK. IN ITS PUREST FORM IT IS A COMBINATION OF APPLES, CELERY, AND MAYONNAISE. WALNUTS—AND SOMETIMES RAISINS—WERE ADDED LATER. THIS FRESHENED-UP VERSION IS MADE WITH PEARS AND ASIAN PEARS—WHICH HAVE A TEXTURE SIMILAR TO APPLES— AND EMBELLISHED WITH DRIED CHERRIES, HERBS, AND TOASTED PECANS.

2 ripe firm pears (such as Bosc or Anjou), cored and diced

2 Asian pears cored and diced

2 tablespoons lime juice

2 stalks celery sliced

¾ cup dried unsweetened tart cherries or cranberries

1 tablespoon snipped fresh tarragon

1 tablespoon snipped fresh Italian (flat-leaf) parsley

¼ cup Cashew Cream (see recipe, page 327)

2 tablespoons Paleo Mayo (see recipe, page 323)

½ cup chopped toasted pecans (see tip, page 57)

1. In a large mixing bowl toss the pears and Asian pears with the lime juice, celery, cherries, and herbs to combine.

2. In a small bowl whisk together the Cashew Cream and Paleo Mayo; pour over the pear mixture and gently stir to coat. Refrigerate for 1 hour to allow flavors to blend. Sprinkle the salad with pecans before serving.

GRILLED ROMAINE HEARTS WITH BASIL GREEN GODDESS DRESSING

pictured on page 109

PREP: 15 minutes   GRILL: 6 minutes   MAKES: 6 servings

THIS IS A STEAK KNIFE-AND-FORK SALAD. ROMAINE HEARTS ARE STURDY ENOUGH TO STAND UP TO GRILLING, AND THE COMBINATION OF CRISP, LIGHTLY CHARRED LETTUCE AND CREAMY HERB DRESSING IS JUST OUTSTANDING. IT'S THE PERFECT ACCOMPANIMENT TO A GRILLED STEAK.

½ cup Paleo Mayo (see recipe, page 323)
½ cup snipped fresh basil
¼ cup snipped fresh parsley
2 tablespoons snipped fresh chives
3 tablespoons olive oil
2 tablespoons fresh lemon juice
1 tablespoon white wine vinegar
3 romaine lettuce hearts, halved lengthwise
1 cup grape or cherry tomatoes, halved
   Cracked black pepper
   Snipped fresh basil (optional)

1. For dressing, in a food processor or blender combine Paleo Mayo, the ½ cup basil, the parsley, chives, 2 tablespoons of the olive oil, the lemon juice, and vinegar. Cover and process or blend until smooth and light green. Cover and chill until needed.

2. Drizzle the remaining 1 tablespoon olive oil over the halved romaine hearts. Use your hands to rub the oil evenly over all sides.

3. For a charcoal or gas grill, place the romaine, cut sides down, on a grill rack directly over medium heat. Cover and grill about 6 minutes or until romaine is lightly charred, turning once halfway through grilling.

4. To serve, spoon dressing over grilled romaine. Top with cherry tomatoes, cracked pepper, and, if desired, additional snipped basil.

ARUGULA AND HERB SALAD WITH POACHED EGGS

pictured on page 269

START TO FINISH: **20 minutes**   MAKES: **4 servings**

THE VINEGAR ADDED TO THE POACHING WATER FOR THE EGGS HELPS THE EDGES OF THE WHITES QUICKLY COAGULATE SO THAT THEY KEEP THEIR SHAPE BETTER DURING COOKING.

6 cups arugula
2 tablespoons snipped fresh tarragon
2 teaspoons snipped fresh thyme
3 to 4 tablespoons Classic French Vinaigrette (see recipe, page 321)
1 cup quartered grape or cherry tomatoes
3 large radishes
4 cups water
1 tablespoon cider vinegar
4 eggs
   Cracked black pepper

1. For salad, in a large salad bowl combine arugula, tarragon, and thyme. Drizzle with 2 to 3 tablespoons of the Classic French Vinaigrette; toss to coat. Divide salad among four serving plates. Top with tomatoes; set salads aside.

2. Remove and discard radish tops and roots; grate the radishes. Set radishes aside.

3. In a large skillet combine the water and vinegar. Bring to boiling. Reduce heat to simmering (small bubbles will break the surface). Break an egg into a custard cup and gently slide it into the water mixture. Repeat with the remaining eggs, spacing so that they do not touch. Simmer, uncovered, about 3 minutes or until the whites are set and yolks are just starting to thicken. Remove each egg with a slotted spoon and place on top of a salad. Drizzle salads with the remaining 1 tablespoon vinaigrette. Garnish with grated radish and sprinkle with pepper. Serve immediately.

HEIRLOOM TOMATO AND WATERMELON SALAD WITH PINK PEPPERCORN DRIZZLE

START TO FINISH: **30 minutes**   MAKES: **6 servings**

THIS IS SUMMER IN A BOWL—JUICY RIPE HEIRLOOM TOMATOES AND WATERMELON. USING A MIX OF HEIRLOOM TOMATOES—WHATEVER YOU'RE GROWING IN YOUR GARDEN, GET IN YOUR CSA BOX, OR BUY AT THE FARMER'S MARKET—WILL MAKE A BEAUTIFUL PRESENTATION.

1	miniature seedless watermelon (4 to 4½ pounds)
4	large heirloom tomatoes
¼	of a red onion, cut into paper-thin slivers
¼	cup loosely packed fresh mint leaves
¼	cup basil chiffonade*
¼	cup olive oil
2	tablespoons fresh lemon juice
1½	teaspoons pink peppercorns

1. Remove rind from watermelon; cut melon into 1-inch chunks. Stem and core tomatoes; cut into wedges. On a large serving platter or in a large serving bowl combine watermelon chunks and tomato wedges; toss to combine. Sprinkle with onion, mint, and basil chiffonade.

2. For dressing, in a small jar with a tight-fitting lid combine olive oil, lemon juice, and peppercorns. Cover and shake vigorously to combine. Drizzle over tomato-watermelon salad. Serve at room temperature.

*Note: For a chiffonade, stack the basil leaves on top of one another and roll up tightly. Thinly slice the roll, then separate the basil into thin ribbons.

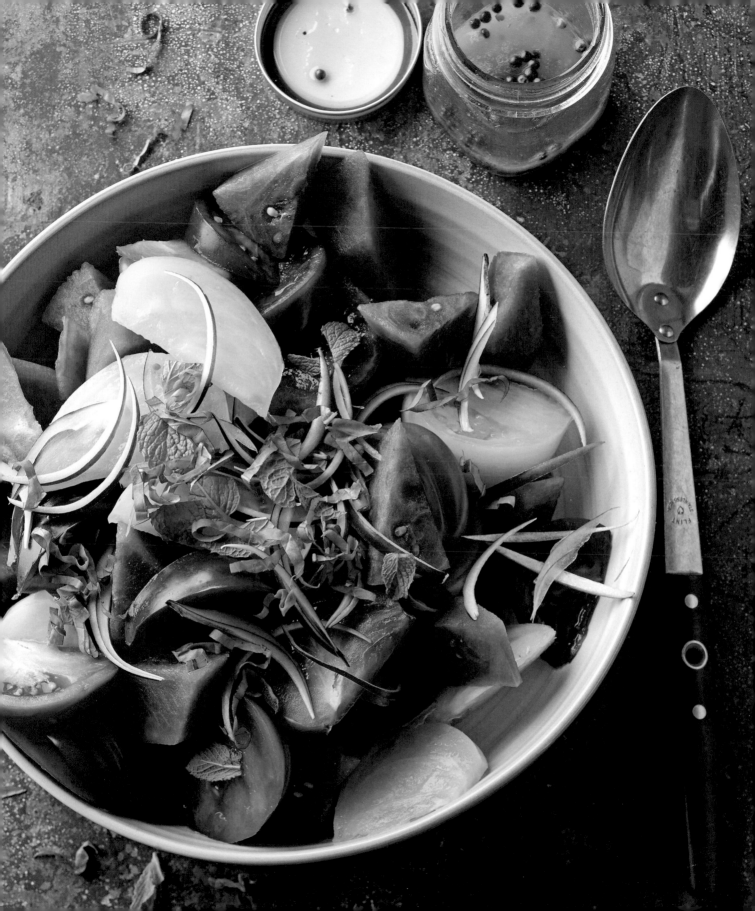

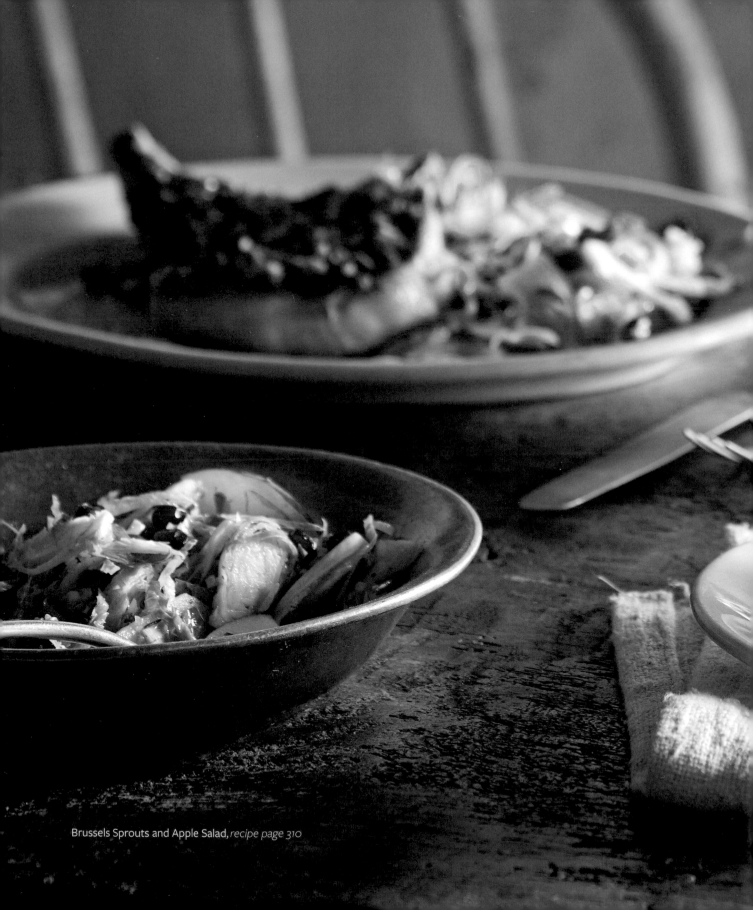

Brussels Sprouts and Apple Salad, *recipe page 310*

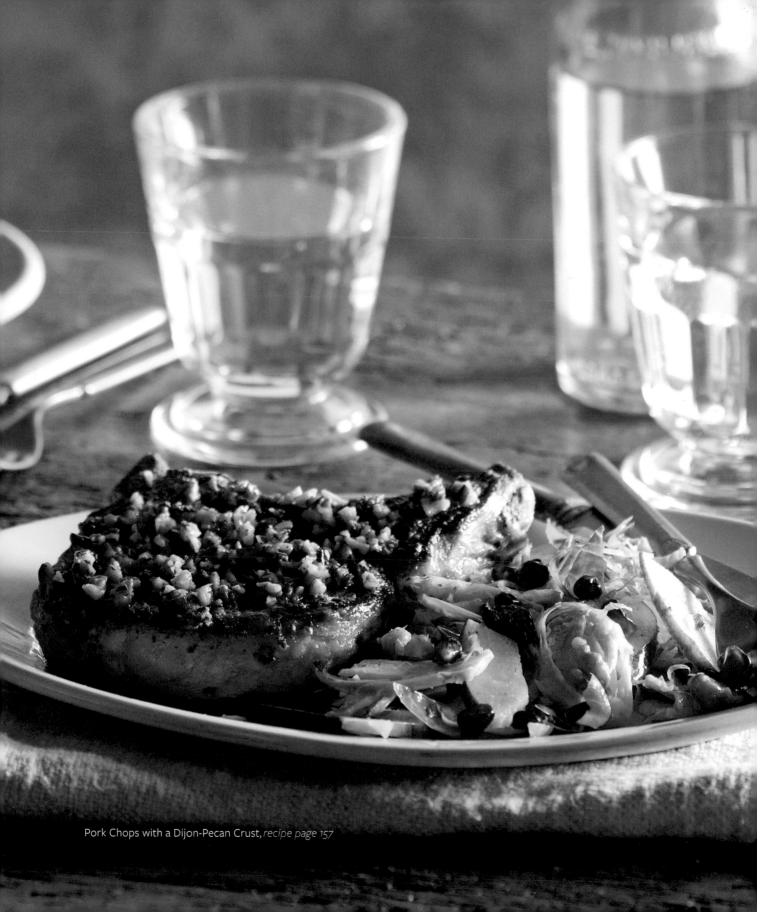

Pork Chops with a Dijon-Pecan Crust, *recipe page 157*

BRUSSELS SPROUTS AND APPLE SALAD

pictured on page 308

PREP: **10 minutes**   STAND: **10 minutes**   MAKES: **6 servings**

POMEGRANATES ARE IN SEASON IN FALL AND WINTER. YOU CAN BUY THE FRUIT WHOLE AND EXTRACT THE SEEDS. OR LOOK FOR JUST THE SEEDS—ALSO CALLED ARILS—IN SMALL TUBS IN THE PRODUCE SECTION. IF POMEGRANATES ARE NOT IN SEASON, LOOK FOR UNSWEETENED FREEZE-DRIED SEEDS TO ADD CRUNCH AND COLOR TO THIS SALAD.

12 ounces Brussels sprouts, trimmed and discolored leaves removed

1 Fuji or Pink Lady apple, cored and quartered

½ cup Bright Citrus Vinaigrette (see recipe, page 320)

⅓ cup pomegranate seeds

⅓ cup no-sugar-added dried cranberries, currants, or cherries

⅓ cup chopped walnuts, toasted (see tip, page 57)

1. Slice the Brussels sprouts and apple in a food processor fitted with a slicing blade.

2. Transfer Brussels sprouts and apple to a large mixing bowl. Drizzle with Bright Citrus Vinaigrette; toss to mix. Let stand for 10 minutes, stirring occasionally. Stir in the pomegranate seeds and cranberries. Top with walnuts; serve immediately.

SHAVED BRUSSELS SPROUTS SALAD

START TO FINISH: **15 minutes**   MAKES: **6 servings**

MEYER LEMONS ARE A CROSS BETWEEN A LEMON AND AN ORANGE. THEY ARE SMALLER THAN REGULAR LEMONS AND THEIR JUICE IS SWEETER AND NOT AS ACIDIC. THEY HAVE BECOME MUCH EASIER TO FIND IN RECENT YEARS, BUT IF YOU CAN'T FIND THEM, REGULAR LEMONS WORK JUST FINE.

1   pound Brussels sprouts, trimmed and discolored leaves removed
1   cup coarsely chopped walnuts, toasted (see tip, page 57)
⅓   cup fresh Meyer lemon juice or regular lemon juice
⅓   cup walnut oil or olive oil
1   clove garlic, minced
¼   teaspoon freshly ground black pepper

1. Very thinly slice the Brussels sprouts in a food processor fitted with a slicing blade. Transfer sprouts to a large bowl; add toasted walnuts.

2. For dressing in a small bowl whisk together lemon juice, oil, garlic, and pepper. Pour over salad and toss to combine.

MEXICAN SLAW

PREP: 20 minutes   STAND: 2 to 4 hours   MAKES: 4 servings

THERE ARE A FEW CONVENIENCE PRODUCTS THAT CAN BE INTEGRATED INTO THE PALEO DIET®—AND PACKAGED BROCCOLI SLAW IS ONE OF THEM. THE MOST COMMON TYPE IS A BLEND OF SHREDDED BROCCOLI, CARROTS, AND RED CABBAGE. IF THOSE ARE THE ONLY INGREDIENTS ON THE LABEL, FEEL FREE TO USE IT. IT CAN SAVE YOU TIME—AND WE CAN ALL USE MORE OF THAT.

1 small red onion, halved and thinly sliced
¼ cup cider vinegar
1½ cups shredded broccoli (packaged broccoli slaw)
½ cup very thin bite-size strips peeled jicama
½ cup cherry or grape tomatoes, halved
2 tablespoons snipped fresh cilantro
2 tablespoons avocado oil
1 teaspoon Mexican Seasoning (see recipe, page 324)
1 medium avocado, halved, seeded, peeled, and chopped

1. In a small bowl combine red onion and vinegar. Toss to coat. Press down on the onion slices with the back of a fork. Cover and let stand at room temperature for 2 to 4 hours, stirring occasionally.

2. In a large bowl combine broccoli, jicama, and tomatoes. Using a slotted spoon, transfer onion to the bowl with the broccoli mixture, reserving vinegar. Stir to combine.

3. For dressing, place 3 tablespoons of the reserved vinegar in a bowl (discard any remaining vinegar). Stir in cilantro, avocado oil, and Mexican Seasoning. Drizzle over broccoli mixture, tossing to coat.

4. Gently stir in avocado; serve immediately.

FENNEL SLAW

START TO FINISH: 20 minutes   MAKES: 4 to 6 servings

TARRAGON AND FENNEL HAVE AN ANISE OR LICORICELIKE FLAVOR. IF YOU PREFER TO HAVE A LITTLE LESS OF THAT, SUBSTITUTE SNIPPED FRESH PARSLEY FOR THE TARRAGON.

2 small fennel bulbs, ends trimmed and very thinly sliced crosswise*
2 stalks celery, very thinly sliced diagonally
1 medium red-skin apple, such as Gala or Honeycrisp, julienned
¼ cup olive oil
3 tablespoons champagne vinegar or white wine vinegar
¼ teaspoon black pepper
2 to 3 tablespoons snipped fresh tarragon

1. For slaw, in a large bowl combine fennel, celery, and apple; set aside.

2. For dressing, in a small bowl combine olive oil, vinegar, and black pepper. Pour over slaw; toss to combine. Sprinkle with tarragon and toss again.

*Tip: To very thinly slice the fennel, use a mandoline. A julienne peeler or slicer is helpful for cutting the apple into julienne strips.

CREAMY CARROT AND KOHLRABI SLAW

PREP: 20 minutes   CHILL: 4 to 6 hours   MAKES: 4 servings

KOHLRABI SEEMS TO BE IN THE SAME POSITION BRUSSELS SPROUTS WERE A FEW YEARS AGO—ON THE VERGE OF A RENAISSANCE DUE TO INNOVATIVE COOKS AND HEALTH-CONSCIOUS EATERS EVERYWHERE. THIS BULBOUS RELATIVE OF CABBAGE IS CRISP AND JUICY AND CAN BE EATEN RAW OR COOKED. HERE, IT'S SHREDDED AND TOSSED INTO A CRISP SLAW, BUT IT IS ALSO WONDERFUL COOKED WITH CELERY ROOT OR CARROTS AND PUREED—OR EVEN CUT INTO THICK STICKS LIKE HOME FRIES, FRIED IN OLIVE OIL, AND SEASONED WITH THE BLEND OF YOUR CHOICE (SEE PAGE 324).

½ cup Paleo Mayo (see recipe, page 323)
2 tablespoons apple cider vinegar
½ teaspoon celery seeds
½ teaspoon paprika
½ teaspoon black pepper
2 pounds small to medium kohlrabi, peeled and coarsely shredded
3 medium carrots, coarsely shredded
1 red sweet pepper, halved, seeded, and very thinly sliced
Snipped fresh parsley (optional)

1. In a large bowl whisk together Paleo Mayo, vinegar, celery seeds, paprika, and pepper. Gently fold in kohlrabi, carrots, and sweet pepper.

2. Cover and chill for 4 to 6 hours. Stir well before serving. If desired, sprinkle with parsley.

SPICED CARROT SLAW

pictured on page 175

pictured on page 175

START TO FINISH: **20 minutes**   MAKES: **4 servings**

THIS NORTH AFRICAN-INSPIRED CARROT SALAD COULD NOT BE SIMPLER TO MAKE, BUT THE FLAVORS AND TEXTURES ARE COMPLEX AND WONDERFUL. TRY IT WITH ROAST CHICKEN WITH SAFFRON AND LEMON (PAGE 186) OR FRENCHED LAMB CHOPS WITH POMEGRANATE-DATE CHUTNEY (PAGE 176).

¼ cup snipped fresh parsley
½ teaspoon finely shredded lemon peel
¼ cup fresh lemon juice
2 tablespoons olive oil
¼ teaspoon ground cumin
¼ teaspoon ground cinnamon
¼ teaspoon smoked paprika
¼ teaspoon crushed red pepper
2 cups coarsely shredded carrots
½ cup chopped, pitted unsweetened dates
¼ cup sliced scallions
¼ cup chopped raw unsalted pistachios

1. In a large bowl combine parsley, lemon peel, lemon juice, olive oil, cumin, cinnamon, paprika, and crushed red pepper. Add the carrots, dates, and scallions; toss to coat with dressing.

2. Just before serving, sprinkle slaw with the pistachios.

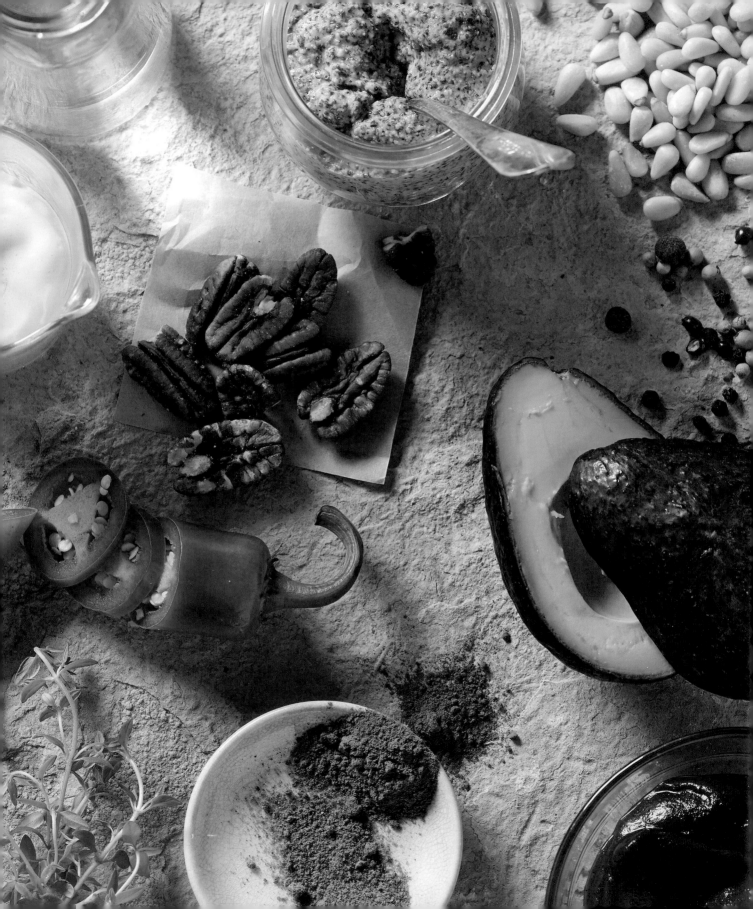

SAUCES, SALSAS, SALAD DRESSINGS & SPICE BLENDS

When some people first catch wind of The Paleo Diet®, they mistakenly believe this is a bland, boring diet that no one could possibly follow for more than a few days. How wrong they are! By now, if you have read this book from its very front cover, you totally get it: The Paleo Diet® is a mind-boggling cornucopia of almost every fruit, vegetable, nut, seed, spice, meat, fish, shellfish, and poultry that you have ever encountered in your entire life. The number of ingredients and foods found in The Paleo Diet® are as rich and varied as almost any diet on Earth. What it lacks are those same old boring and unhealthy ingredients and foods (refined sugars, refined grains, whole grains, unhealthy refined vegetable oils, salt, and dairy products) that comprise 70% of the calories in the standard American diet.

One of the greatest gifts The Paleo Diet® will give you and your family is the renovation of your palates. Living, "real" foods will gradually become more appealing as processed foods full of unnatural combinations of fat, sugar, flour, and salt are abandoned and no longer part of your daily cuisine. This transformation doesn't happen overnight. You must give it a few weeks or months as you come to know the subtle flavors and aromas of fresh veggies, fruits, herbs, and spices. Properly cooked fish and shellfish maintain delicate flavors and essences that you may have never experienced before you embarked upon The Paleo Diet®. Grass-produced meats will stun you with their rich aromas and scintillating, pungent flavors. In earlier times, you may have craved breads, cereals, pasta, chips, and french fries. In your new Paleo life, these foods will become nothing more than starchy, salty foods that cause you to feel stuffed and uncomfortable. As you become healthier and lose weight, the foods you crave will be the living, "real" food staples of The Paleo Diet.

Our excellent recipe developers have done an incredible job of creating and producing a wide lineup of sauces, salsas, salad dressings, and spice blends that emulate their conventional counterparts but without the added sugars, salt, flour, cornstarch, and bad fats. Each and every single item, ingredient, and recipe in this chapter is "pure Paleo" and conforms to the best and most accurate data underlying contemporary Paleo diets. But most of all, these Paleo condiments are tasty and appetizing and will help you to prepare recipes with many familiar condiments, dressings, and salsas.

If one of your beloved pre-Paleo dishes required mayonnaise, don't worry. We have you covered with our Paleo Mayo, along with four delicious variations: Aïoli (Garlic Mayonnaise), Herbed Mayonnaise, Wasabi Mayonnaise, and Chipotle Mayonnaise. How about traditional salt- and sugar-laden tomato ketchup? No problem—our team has created a much healthier and tastier Paleo Ketchup. Same goes for Dijon-Style Mustard. Take a look at the recipes in this chapter and note that there is an impressive lineup of delicious but also healthful pestos, salsas, vinaigrettes, and salad dressings—free of refined sugars, salt, and bad fats. Bon appétit!

PESTOS

THESE FRESH PESTOS CAN BE USED IN A MULTITUDE OF WAYS. USE THEM TO TOP A GRILLED STEAK OR STIR INTO PALEO MAYO (PAGE 323) FOR A SPREAD OR DIP. EACH ONE HAS ITS OWN UNIQUE FLAVOR. ONE FEATURES PEPPERY ARUGULA, WALNUTS, AND LEMON. ANOTHER COMBINES THE EARTHY FLAVOR OF CILANTRO WITH THE SWEETNESS OF PECANS AND ORANGE. AND THE CLASSIC IS A BLEND OF SWEET BASIL, PARSLEY, PINE NUTS, AND GARLIC.

ARUGULA PESTO

START TO FINISH: 15 minutes
MAKES: ¾ cup

- 2 cups tightly packed arugula leaves
- ⅓ cup walnuts, toasted*
- 1 tablespoon finely shredded lemon peel (from 2 lemons)
- 1 clove garlic
- ½ cup walnut oil
- ¼ to ½ teaspoon black pepper

1. In a food processor combine arugula, walnuts, lemon peel, and garlic. Pulse until coarsely chopped. With the processor running, pour the walnut oil in a thin stream into the bowl. Season with pepper.

2. Use immediately or divide into desired portions and freeze for up to 3 months in tightly covered containers.

*Tip: To toast nuts, spread in a single layer on a rimmed baking sheet. Bake in a 375°F oven for 5 to 10 minutes or until lightly toasted, stirring nuts or shaking pan once or twice. Let cool completely before using.

BASIL PESTO

START TO FINISH: 15 minutes
MAKES: 1½ cups

- 2 cups packed fresh basil leaves
- 1 cup packed fresh flat-leaf parsley
- 3 cloves garlic
- ½ cup pine nuts, toasted (see tip, below left)
- 1 cup olive oil
- ¼ teaspoon freshly ground black pepper

1. In a food processor combine basil, parsley, garlic, and pine nuts. Pulse until coarsely chopped. With the processor running, pour the olive oil in a thin stream into the bowl. Season with pepper.

2. Use immediately or freeze in desired portions for up to 3 months in tightly covered containers.

CILANTRO PESTO

START TO FINISH: 15 minutes
MAKES: ¾ cup

- 2 cups lightly packed fresh cilantro leaves
- ⅓ cup pecan halves, toasted (see tip, below left)
- 1 tablespoon finely shredded orange peel (from 1 large orange)
- 1 clove garlic
- ½ cup avocado oil
- ⅛ teaspoon cayenne pepper

1. In a food processor combine cilantro, pecans, orange peel, and garlic. Pulse until coarsely chopped. With the processor running, pour the avocado oil in a thin stream into the bowl. Season with cayenne pepper.

2. Use immediately or freeze in desired portions for up to 3 months in tightly covered containers.

SALAD DRESSINGS

ONE OF THE SIMPLEST WAYS TO EAT PALEO IS TO GRILL OR ROAST A PIECE OF MEAT AND ACCOMPANY IT WITH A BIG SALAD. COMMERCIALLY BOTTLED DRESSINGS ARE LOADED WITH SALT, SUGAR, AND ADDITIVES. THE FOLLOWING DRESSINGS ARE ALL ABOUT FRESHNESS AND FLAVOR. STORE ANY LEFTOVERS IN THE REFRIGERATOR FOR UP TO 3 DAYS—OR USE A VINAIGRETTE AS A MARINADE.

BRIGHT CITRUS VINAIGRETTE

START TO FINISH: 20 minutes
MAKES: about 2 cups

- ¼ cup minced shallots
- 2 teaspoons finely shredded orange peel
- 2 teaspoons finely shredded lemon peel
- 2 teaspoons finely shredded lime peel
- ½ cup fresh orange juice
- ¼ cup fresh lemon juice
- ¼ cup fresh lime juice
- 2 tablespoons Dijon-Style Mustard (see recipe, page 322) or 1 teaspoon dry mustard
- ⅔ cup olive oil
- ¼ cup finely snipped fresh parsley, chives, tarragon, or basil
- ½ to 1 teaspoon black pepper

1. In a medium bowl whisk together the shallots, citrus peels, citrus juices, and Dijon-Style Mustard; let stand for 3 minutes. Slowly whisk in the olive oil until emulsified. Stir in the herb and pepper.

CLASSIC FRENCH VINAIGRETTE

PREP: **5 minutes**
STAND: **15 minutes**
MAKES: **about 1¼ cups**

- 6 tablespoons fresh lemon juice
- 3 shallots, peeled and minced
- 1½ tablespoons Dijon-Style Mustard (see recipe, page 322)
- 1 cup olive oil
- 1 tablespoon finely snipped chives (optional)
- 1 tablespoon finely snipped Italian (flat-leaf) parsley (optional)
- 2 teaspoons finely snipped fresh tarragon (optional)

1. In a medium bowl combine lemon juice and shallots. Let stand for 15 minutes.

2. Whisk in Dijon-Style Mustard. Slowly whisk in olive oil in a very thin stream until mixture thickens and emulsifies. Taste vinaigrette. If it is too sharp, whisk in additional Dijon-Style Mustard or olive oil as desired.

3. If desired, before serving, whisk in herbs. When dressing salad greens with vinaigrette, add freshly cracked black pepper to the bowl and toss to coat. Store vinaigrette in a tightly covered container in the refrigerator for up to 1 week.

MANGO-LIME SALAD DRESSING

START TO FINISH: **10 minutes**
MAKES: **about 1 cup**

- 1 small ripe mango, peeled, pitted, and coarsely chopped
- 3 tablespoons walnut or coconut oil
- 1 teaspoon finely shredded lime peel
- 2 tablespoons fresh lime juice
- 2 teaspoons grated fresh ginger
  Dash cayenne pepper
- 1 tablespoon water (optional)

1. In a food processor or blender combine mango, walnut oil, lime peel, lime juice, ginger, and cayenne pepper. Cover and process or blend until smooth. If needed, thin dressing with the water to desired consistency. Cover and store for up to 1 week in the refrigerator. If using coconut oil, bring dressing to room temperature before using.

ROASTED GARLIC VINAIGRETTE

PREP: **5 minutes**
ROAST: **30 minutes**
STAND: **2 hours 5 minutes**
MAKES: **about 1¼ cups**

- 1 medium bulb garlic
- ¾ cup olive oil
- ¼ cup fresh lemon juice
- 1 teaspoon dried Greek oregano, crushed

1. Preheat oven to 400°F. Cut ¼ inch from narrow end of garlic bulb; drizzle with 1 teaspoon of the olive oil. Wrap garlic in foil. Roast for 30 to 35 minutes or until garlic is golden brown and very soft. Cool; turn upside down and squeeze garlic cloves from the bulb into a small bowl. Mash into a smooth paste.

2. In a medium bowl combine lemon juice and oregano. Let stand for 5 minutes. Whisk in remaining olive oil. Whisk in roasted garlic. Let vinaigrette stand at room temperature for 2 hours before using or refrigerating. Store in refrigerator for up to 1 week.

TOASTED PINE NUT DRESSING

PREP **10 minutes**
MAKES **about 1 cup**

- ⅔ cup pine nuts (4 ounces), toasted (see tip, page 57)
- 1 teaspoon olive oil
- ½ cup water
- ¼ cup fresh lemon juice
- 1 clove garlic, minced
- ¼ teaspoon smoked paprika
- ⅛ teaspoon cayenne pepper

1. In a blender or food processor combine pine nuts and olive oil. Cover and blend or process until smooth. Add the water, lemon juice, garlic, paprika, and cayenne pepper. Cover and blend or process until smooth.

CONDIMENTS

KETCHUP, MUSTARD, AND MAYONNAISE ARE NOT ONLY PRIZED ON THEIR OWN AS SPREADS AND DIPS, BUT THEY ARE ALSO CRUCIAL ELEMENTS IN RECIPES AS FLAVORING AGENTS AND BINDERS—BUT THE SALT, SUGAR, AND PRESERVATIVES IN COMMERCIALLY PRODUCED CONDIMENTS HAVE NO PLACE IN THE REAL PALEO DIET®. THE FOLLOWING VERSIONS ARE PERFECTLY PALEO AND FULL OF FLAVOR. NO SUMMER WOULD BE COMPLETE WITHOUT A BACKYARD BARBECUE AND SOME SMOKY GRILLED MEAT, SO WE'VE INCLUDED A SALT- AND SUGAR-FREE BBQ SAUCE AS WELL. HARISSA IS A FIERY SAUCE FROM TUNISIA. CHIMICHURRI IS A FLAVORFUL HERB SAUCE FROM ARGENTINA.

DIJON-STYLE MUSTARD

PREP: 10 minutes
STAND: 48 hours
MAKES: 1¾ cups

- ¾ cup brown mustard seeds
- ¾ cup unsweetened apple juice or cider
- ¼ cup white wine vinegar
- ¼ cup dry white wine or water
- ½ teaspoon turmeric
- 1 to 2 tablespoons water

1. In a glass bowl stir together mustard seeds, apple juice, vinegar, wine, and turmeric. Cover tightly and let stand at room temperature for 48 hours.

2. Transfer mixture to a high-powered blender.* Cover and blend until smooth, adding enough of the water to make desired consistency. If air bubbles form, stop and stir mixture. For a smoother texture, press the finished mustard through a fine-mesh sieve.

3. Use immediately or store in the refrigerator in a tightly covered container for up 1 month. (The flavor will mellow with storage.)

*Note: You may use a regular blender and process on high speed; the texture of the mustard will not be as smooth.

HARISSA

PREP: 20 minutes
STAND: 20 minutes
MAKES: about 2 cups

- 8 guajillo chiles, stemmed and seeded (see tip, page 56)
- 8 ancho chiles, stemmed and seeded (see tip, page 56)
- ½ teaspoon caraway seeds
- ¼ teaspoon coriander seeds
- ¼ teaspoon cumin seeds
- 1 teaspoon dried mint
- ¼ cup fresh lemon juice
- 3 tablespoons olive oil
- 5 cloves garlic

1. Place guajillo and ancho chiles in a large bowl. Add enough boiling water to cover peppers. Let stand for 20 minutes or until soft.

2. Meanwhile, in a small skillet combine caraway seeds, coriander seeds, and cumin seeds. Toast spices over medium heat for 4 to 5 minutes or until very fragrant, shaking skillet frequently. Let cool. Transfer toasted seeds to a spice grinder; add mint. Grind to a powder. Set aside.

3. Drain chiles; transfer chiles to a food processor. Add ground spices, lemon juice, olive oil, and garlic. Cover and process until smooth. Transfer to a tightly sealed glass or nonreactive container. Store in refrigerator for up to 1 month.

PALEO KETCHUP

PREP: 10 minutes
STAND: 10 minutes
COOK: 20 minutes
COOL: 30 minutes
MAKES: about 3½ cups

- ½ cup raisins
- 1 28-ounce can no-salt-added tomato puree
- ½ cup cider vinegar
- 1 small onion, chopped
- 1 clove garlic, chopped
- ¼ teaspoon ground allspice
- ¼ teaspoon ground cinnamon
- ⅛ teaspoon ground mace
- ⅛ teaspoon ground cloves
- ⅛ teaspoon cayenne pepper
- ⅛ teaspoon black pepper

1. In a small bowl cover raisins with boiling water. Let stand for 10 minutes; drain.

2. In a medium saucepan combine raisins, tomato puree, vinegar, onion, garlic, allspice, cinnamon, mace, cloves, cayenne pepper, and black pepper. Bring to boiling; reduce heat. Simmer, uncovered, for 20 to 25 minutes or until onion is tender, stirring frequently to keep mixture from burning. (Be careful; mixture will spatter as it cooks.)

3. Remove from heat. Let cool about 30 minutes or until just slightly warm. Transfer to a high-power blender* or food processor. Cover and process or blend to desired consistency.

4. Divide between two clean pint glass jars. Use immediately or freeze for up to 2 months. Store in refrigerator for up to 1 month.

*Note: You can use a regular blender, but the consistency won't be as smooth.

BBQ SAUCE

START TO FINISH: **45 minutes**
MAKES: **about 4 cups**

2 pounds ripe roma tomatoes, quartered lengthwise and seeded
1 large sweet onion, cut into thin wedges
1 red sweet pepper, halved and seeded
2 poblano peppers, halved and seeded (see tip, page 56)
2 teaspoons Smoky Seasoning (see recipe, page 324)
2 tablespoons olive oil
½ cup fresh orange juice
⅓ cup raisins
3 tablespoons cider vinegar
2 tablespoons tomato paste
1 tablespoon minced garlic
⅛ teaspoon ground cloves

1. In an extra-large bowl combine tomatoes, onion, sweet pepper, poblano peppers, Smoky Seasoning, and olive oil. Place vegetables in a grill basket. For a charcoal or gas grill, place grill basket on a grill rack directly over medium heat. Cover and grill for 20 to 25 minutes or until very tender and charred, stirring occasionally; remove from grill and cool slightly.

2. In a small saucepan heat orange juice until simmering. Remove saucepan from heat and add the raisins; let stand for 10 minutes.

3. In a food processor or blender combine the grilled vegetables, raisin mixture, vinegar, tomato paste, garlic, and cloves. Cover and process or blend until very smooth, scraping sides as needed. Transfer vegetable mixture to a large saucepan. Bring to simmering; cook to desired consistency.

CHIMICHURRI SAUCE

START TO FINISH: **20 minutes**
MAKES: **about 2 cups**

2 cups lightly packed fresh Italian (flat-leaf) parsley
2 cups lightly packed cilantro
½ cup lightly packed mint
½ cup chopped shallots
1 tablespoon minced garlic (6 cloves)
⅓ cup red wine vinegar
2 dried unsulfured apricots, finely chopped
⅛ teaspoon crushed red pepper
¾ cup olive oil

1. In a food processor or blender combine all ingredients. Cover and blend or process until ingredients are finely chopped and combined, scraping sides as necessary.

PALEO MAYO

PREP: **45 minutes**
STAND: **45 minutes**
MAKES: **3½ cups**

1 large or extra-large egg
1 tablespoon fresh lemon juice or white wine vinegar
½ teaspoon dry mustard
1 cup walnut, avocado, or olive oil, at room temperature*

1. Let egg stand at room temperature for 30 minutes.

2. Crack egg into a tall, narrow glass jar (a wide-mouth pint canning jar works well). Add lemon juice and dry mustard.

3. Carefully pour in oil. Let egg settle down to the bottom of the jar, under the oil.

4. Insert an immersion blender and push it all of the way to the bottom of the jar. Turn power on high and let it run for 20 seconds without moving it. The mayonnaise will start forming and rising to the top of the jar. Slowly start raising the blender until it reaches the top of the jar. Use mayonnaise immediately or store in the refrigerator for up to 1 week.

Paleo Aïoli (Garlic Mayo): Add 1 clove minced garlic with lemon juice and mustard in Step 2.

Herbed Paleo Mayo: Fold 2 tablespoons snipped fresh herbs into finished mayonnaise. Good choices include chives, parsley, tarragon, and basil—solo or in any combination.

Wasabi Paleo Mayo: Add 1 teaspoon all-natural, preservative-free wasabi powder with the lemon juice and mustard in Step 2.

Chipotle Paleo Mayo: Add 2 to 3 teaspoons chipotle powder with lemon juice and mustard in Step 2.

*Note: If you use extra virgin olive oil, the olive flavor will come through in the mayonnaise. For a milder flavor, use walnut or avocado oil.

SEASONING BLENDS

THESE VERSATILE BLENDS ARE ENTIRELY SALT-FREE AND OFFER A WIDE RANGE OF FLAVORS.

LEMON-HERB SEASONING

START TO FINISH: **5 minutes**
MAKES: about ½ cup

6 tablespoons dried lemon peel
1 tablespoon herbes de Provence
2 teaspoons onion powder
1 teaspoon black pepper

1. In a small bowl combine lemon peel, herbes de Provence, onion powder, and pepper. Store in an airtight container at room temperature up to 6 months. Stir or shake before using.

MEDITERRANEAN SEASONING

START TO FINISH: **10 minutes**
MAKES: about ⅓ cup

2 teaspoons fennel seeds
1 teaspoon dried rosemary
1 tablespoon dried oregano
1 tablespoon dried thyme
2 teaspoons preservative-free granulated garlic
1 teaspoon dried lemon peel

1. In a dry small skillet toast fennel seeds over medium-low heat for 1 to 2 minutes or until fragrant, shaking skillet occasionally. Remove from the heat; cool about 2 minutes. Transfer seeds to a spice grinder; grind to a powder. Add rosemary; grind until rosemary is coarsely ground. Transfer fennel and rosemary to a small bowl. Stir in oregano, thyme, garlic,

and lemon peel. Store in an airtight container at room temperature up to 6 months. Stir or shake before using.

MEXICAN SEASONING

START TO FINISH: **5 minutes**
MAKES: about ¼ cup

1 tablespoon cumin seeds
4 teaspoons paprika
1 tablespoon preservative-free granulated garlic
1 teaspoon dried oregano
½ to 1 teaspoon ground chipotle pepper or cayenne pepper (optional)
½ teaspoon ground cinnamon
¼ teaspoon ground saffron

1. In a dry small skillet toast cumin seeds over medium-low heat for 1 to 2 minutes or until fragrant, shaking skillet occasionally. Remove from the heat; cool about 2 minutes. Transfer seeds to a spice grinder; grind the cumin. Transfer cumin to a small bowl. Stir in paprika, garlic, oregano, chipotle pepper (if using), cinnamon, and saffron. Store in an airtight container at room temperature up to 6 months. Stir or shake before using.

SMOKY SEASONING

START TO FINISH: **5 minutes**
MAKES: about ½ cup

¼ cup smoked paprika
4 teaspoons dried orange peel
2 teaspoons garlic powder
1 teaspoon onion powder
1 teaspoon ground cloves
1 teaspoon dried basil

1. In a small bowl combine smoked paprika, orange peel, garlic powder, onion powder, cloves, and dried basil. Store in an airtight container at room temperature up to 6 months. Stir or shake before using.

CAJUN SEASONING

START TO FINISH: **5 minutes**
MAKES: about ⅓ cup

2 tablespoons paprika
1 tablespoon garlic powder
1 tablespoon onion powder
2 teaspoons dried thyme, crushed
2 teaspoons white pepper
1½ teaspoons black pepper
1 teaspoon cayenne pepper
1 teaspoon dried oregano, crushed

1. In a small bowl combine the paprika, garlic powder, onion powder, thyme, white pepper, black pepper, cayenne pepper, and oregano. Store in an airtight container up to 6 months. Stir or shake before using.

JAMAICAN JERK SEASONING

START TO FINISH: **5 minutes**
MAKES: about ¼ cup

1 tablespoon onion powder
1 tablespoon dried thyme, crushed
1½ teaspoons ground allspice
1 teaspoon black pepper
½ teaspoon ground nutmeg
½ teaspoon ground cinnamon
½ teaspoon ground cloves
¼ teaspoon cayenne pepper

1. In a small bowl stir together onion powder, thyme, allspice, black pepper, nutmeg, cinnamon, cloves, and cayenne pepper. Store in an airtight container in a cool, dry place for up to 6 months. Stir or shake before using.

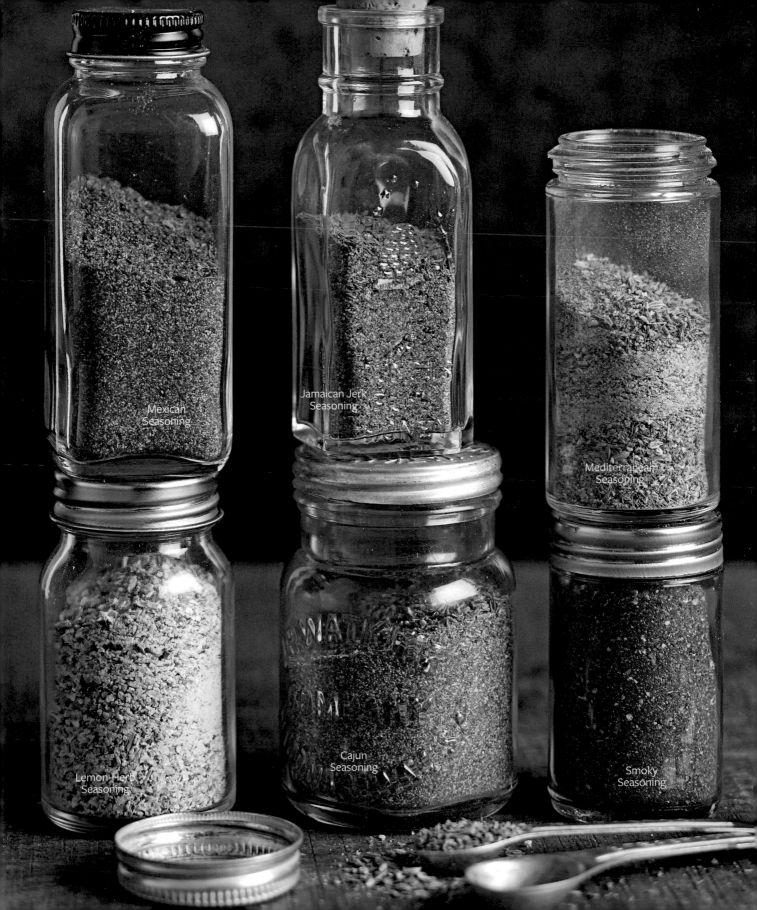

Mexican
Seasoning

Jamaican Jerk
Seasoning

Mediterranean
Seasoning

Lemon-Herb
Seasoning

Cajun
Seasoning

Smoky
Seasoning

SALSAS

RIPE CHOPPED TOMATO, CHILE, LIME, AND CILANTRO IS A CLASSIC, BUT THESE FRESH COMBINATIONS OF FRUITS, VEGETABLES, AND HERBS ENCOURAGE YOU TO GET OUT OF YOUR SALSA PARADIGM. ON A BUSY WEEKNIGHT, ALL YOU NEED TO DO TO MAKE A GREAT DINNER IS GRILL A PIECE OF MEAT, POULTRY, OR FISH AND TOP IT WITH SALSA. ALTHOUGH THERE ARE NO HARD AND FAST RULES FOR COPACETIC COMBINATIONS, WE SUGGEST THE FOLLOWING: FISH OR CHICKEN WITH CITRUS-FENNEL SALSA OR SWEET ONION-CUCUMBER SALSA WITH MINT AND THAI CHILE; BEEF WITH CRUNCHY AVOCADO SALSA; AND PORK WITH GRILLED PINEAPPLE SALSA VERDE OR RUBY RED BEET SALSA.

CITRUS-FENNEL SALSA

START TO FINISH: 20 minutes
MAKES: about 3½ cups

- 1 cup orange segments* or sliced kumquats (2 small oranges)
- 1 cup red grapefruit segments* (1 to 2 small grapefruits)
- ¾ cup shaved fennel** (about ½ a bulb)
- ½ cup pomegranate seeds or diced sweet red pepper
- ¼ cup chopped fresh tarragon or basil
- ¼ cup chopped fresh parsley
- ¼ teaspoon black pepper

1. In a large bowl gently toss together orange, grapefruit, fennel, pomegranate seeds, tarragon, parsley, and pepper until combined. Serve salsa with poached or grilled fish, seafood, or chicken.

*Tip: To segment citrus, trim the top and bottom off a whole piece of fruit. Place a cut side on a cutting board and use a paring knife to trim off the peel, following the natural curve of the fruit. After removing the peel, hold the fruit over a bowl and slice on either side of the membranes to release the segments into the bowl. After the segments have been removed, squeeze the membrane over the bowl to extract the juice. Discard the membrane.

**Tip: To shave fennel, trim off the stalks of a fennel bulb and cut bulb in half from top to bottom. Cut out the triangular-shape core. Using a mandoline or very sharp chef's knife, slice fennel as thinly as possible.

CRUNCHY AVOCADO SALSA

START TO FINISH: 20 minutes
MAKES: about 1½ cups

- ½ teaspoon finely shredded lime peel
- 2 tablespoons fresh lime juice
- 1 tablespoon avocado oil or olive oil
- ¼ teaspoon ground cumin (optional)
- ¼ teaspoon ground coriander (optional)
- 1 avocado, peeled, seeded, and diced*
- ½ cup seeded and diced English cucumber
- ½ cup diced red radishes
- ¼ cup thinly sliced scallions
- ¼ cup snipped fresh cilantro
- ½ to 1 jalapeño or serrano chile, seeded and minced (see tip, page 56)

1. In a medium bowl whisk together lime peel, lime juice, oil, and, if desired, cumin and coriander. Add avocado, cucumber, radishes, scallions, cilantro, and chile. Gently stir until evenly coated and combined.

*Tip: To neatly dice the avocado, halve and seed the fruit. Using a small paring knife, cut crisscross lines into the flesh of each half down to the skin to create small squares. Using a spoon, gently scoop the cut flesh into the bowl. You should have small cubes of avocado.

SWEET ONION-CUCUMBER SALSA WITH MINT AND THAI CHILE

PREP: 20 minutes
CHILL: 2 hours
MAKES: about 1½ cups

- ½ of a seedless cucumber, finely chopped
- 1 small sweet onion, finely chopped
- 1 or 2 fresh Thai chiles, minced (see tip, page 56), or dried Thai chiles, crushed
- ¼ cup snipped fresh mint
- ½ teaspoon finely shredded lime peel
- 2 tablespoons fresh lime juice
- 2 tablespoons snipped fresh cilantro
- ½ teaspoon ground coriander

1. In a medium bowl combine cucumber, onion, chile(s), mint, lime peel, lime juice, cilantro, and coriander. Toss gently to combine.

2. Cover and chill for at least 2 hours before serving.

GRILLED PINEAPPLE SALSA VERDE

PREP: 15 minutes
GRILL: 5 minutes   MAKES: 4 cups

- ½ of a peeled and cored fresh pineapple
- 10 fresh medium tomatillos, husked and cut in half

½ cup chopped green or red sweet pepper

¼ cup snipped fresh cilantro

3 tablespoons chopped red onion

2 tablespoons fresh lime juice

1 jalapeño, seeded and chopped (see tip, page 56)

1. Cut the pineapple into ½-inch slices. For a charcoal or gas grill, place pineapple on a grill rack directly over medium heat. Cover and grill for 5 to 7 minutes or until pineapple is lightly charred, turning once halfway through grilling. Cool pineapple completely. Chop pineapple; measure 1½ cups, reserving any extra for another use.

2. Finely chop the tomatillos in a food processor fitted with a chopping blade. Place chopped tomatillos in a medium bowl. Stir in sweet pepper, cilantro, onion, lime juice, and jalapeño. Stir in the 1½ cups grilled pineapple. Cover and chill for up to 3 days.

RUBY RED BEET SALSA

PREP: 20 minutes
ROAST: 45 minutes
COOL: 1 hour   CHILL: 1 hour
MAKES: about 5 cups salsa

1½ pounds small beets

2 teaspoons olive oil

1 ruby red grapefruit or 2 blood oranges, sectioned (see tip, page 326) and chopped

½ cup pomegranate seeds

1 small shallot, finely chopped

1 serrano chile, seeded and finely chopped (see tip, page 56)

½ cup snipped fresh cilantro

1. Preheat oven to 400°F. Cut off the tops and root ends from the beets; place in the center of a large piece of foil. Drizzle with olive oil. Bring up ends of foil and fold to seal. Roast for 45 to 50 minutes or until tender. Let cool completely. Peel and finely chop beets.

2. In a medium bowl combine the chopped beets, grapefruit, pomegranate seeds, shallot, cilantro, and serrano chile. Chill for at least 1 hour before serving.

CREAMS & BUTTERS

ALTHOUGH THE PALEO DIET® DOESN'T INCLUDE DAIRY PRODUCTS, THERE ARE OCCASIONS WHERE A TOUCH OF SOMETHING COOL AND CREAMY ADDS A LOT TO A RECIPE. CASHEW CREAM IS THE SOLUTION. IT'S MADE BY SOAKING RAW, UNSALTED CASHEWS IN WATER—PREFERABLY OVERNIGHT—AND PUREEING THEM WITH FRESH WATER IN A BLENDER UNTIL VERY SMOOTH. THE RESULT IS INCREDIBLY VERSATILE. IT CAN BE INFUSED WITH LIME AND CILANTRO AND DRIZZLED OVER TACOS OR STIRRED TOGETHER WITH CINNAMON AND VANILLA EXTRACT AND USED AS A TOPPER FOR WARM ROASTED FRUIT. THE PINE NUT BUTTER IS A GOOD SUBSTITUTE FOR TAHINI IN DRESSINGS AND SAUCES.

CASHEW CREAM

PREP: 5 minutes
STAND: 4 hours to overnight
MAKES: about 2 cups

1 cup raw unsalted cashews
Water

1. Rinse cashews; drain and place in a bowl or jar. Add enough water to cover by about 1 inch. Cover and let stand at room temperature at least 4 hours and preferably overnight.

2. Drain cashews; rinse under cold water. Place cashews in a high-power blender* and add 1 cup of water; process until smooth, scraping down the sides.

3. Store cashew cream in an airtight container in the refrigerator for up to 1 week.

***Note:** You may use a regular blender and process on high; the texture of the cream will not be as smooth.

PINE NUT BUTTER

START TO FINISH: 10 minutes
MAKES: 1 cup

2 cups pine nuts

3 tablespoons avocado oil

1. In a large skillet toast pine nuts over medium heat for 5 to 8 minutes or until golden brown, stirring frequently. Cool slightly. Place nuts and oil in a high-power blender. Process until smooth. Store in an airtight container in the refrigerator for up to 2 weeks.

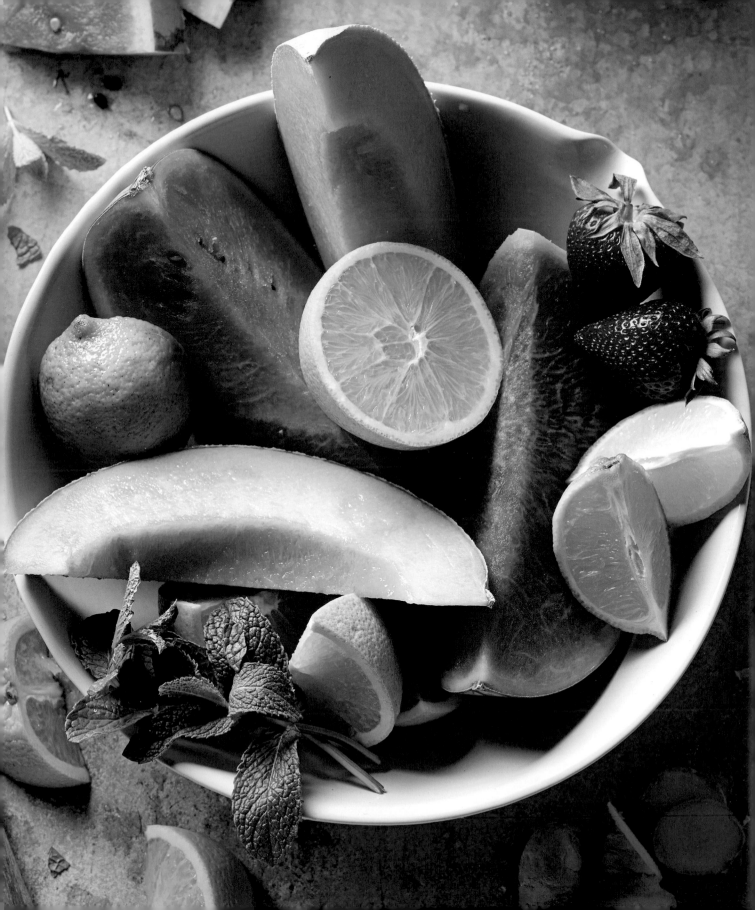

TREATS

We all deserve to treat ourselves and our families once in a while by enjoying sweets and "comfort" foods. Paleo dieters do, too, except that Paleo treats are nutritious, healthy, and contain no concentrated refined sugars, honey, grains, or bad fats. One item in this list that needs further explanation is honey. Most of us believe that honey is a "natural" sugar that is healthier than manufactured, processed sugar because it is produced by bees. There is absolutely no doubt that our hunter-gatherer ancestors would have voraciously consumed honey whenever and wherever it was available. Does this mean that we should follow suit? Absolutely not. For our foraging ancestors, honey would have only been available seasonally. Consequently, it was impossible to consume year-round. If we would like to, we could consume honey every day, all year long, and in effect eat a contemporary Paleo diet that would maintain very non-Paleo nutritional characteristics by having such a high sugar intake.

It is frequently assumed by some segments of the Paleo community that honey is "natural" and is somehow healthier than regular table sugar or high-fructose corn syrup. Truth be known, honey is a mixture of two sugars (fructose and glucose) that is virtually identical to high-fructose corn syrup in its concentrations of these two simple sugars. In our bodies, honey produces the same adverse spikes in blood sugar and insulin as do table sugar and high-fructose corn syrup. If you enjoy honey, use it sparingly and consistent with the guidelines I have outlined in Paleo Principles and the 85:15 rule (page 14).

The basis for the delectable recipes in this chapter comes from clever and judicious blends of fresh fruits, nuts, freshly squeezed fruit juices, and dried fruits in conjunction with spices and extracts, which enhance flavors and aromas. These seasonings include allspice, anise, caraway seeds, cardamom, cinnamon, cloves, ginger, mace, mint, nutmeg, vanilla beans, and almond, lemon, orange, rum, and vanilla extracts.

Paleo desserts may be served any time and don't necessarily need to be included at the end of a meal. However, if you are overweight, obese, or have one or more elements of the metabolic syndrome (high blood cholesterol, high cholesterol, heart disease, or type 2 diabetes), you should be cautious when eating any fruit—particularly dried fruit. As per my recommendations in Paleo Principles, people with health complications should limit their fruit consumption to fruits that are very low, low, or moderate in total sugars.

CHOCOLATE-COVERED APPLE CHIPS

PREP: 15 minutes   BAKE: 2 hours   STAND: 1 hour 30 minutes   MAKES: 6 to 8 servings

HIGHLY PROCESSED CHOCOLATE LOADED WITH SUGAR IS NOT A PALEO INGREDIENT. BUT CHOCOLATE MADE ONLY FROM CACAO AND VANILLA BEANS IS PERFECTLY ACCEPTABLE. THE NATURAL SWEETNESS OF THE FRUIT COMBINED WITH THE RICH FLAVOR OF THE CHOCOLATE MAKES THESE CRISP, PAPER-THIN CHIPS A REAL TREAT.

2   Honeycrisp or Fuji apples, cored*

3   ounces unsweetened chocolate, such as Scharffen Berger 99% cacao bar, chopped

½   teaspoon unrefined coconut oil

¼   cup finely chopped walnuts or pecans, toasted (see tip, page 57)

1. Preheat oven to 225°F. Line two large baking sheets with parchment paper; set aside. Using a mandoline, thinly slice apples crosswise. Lay apple slices in a single layer on prepared sheets. (You should have about 24 slices total.) Bake apple slices for 2 hours, turning once halfway through baking time. Turn off oven; let apple slices stand in oven for 30 minutes.

2. In a small saucepan heat chocolate and coconut oil over low heat, stirring constantly until smooth. Drizzle apple slices with the melted chocolate. Sprinkle with nuts. Let stand at room temperature about 1 hour or until chocolate is set.

*Tip: You can cut the core out using a paring knife, but an apple corer makes this job much easier.

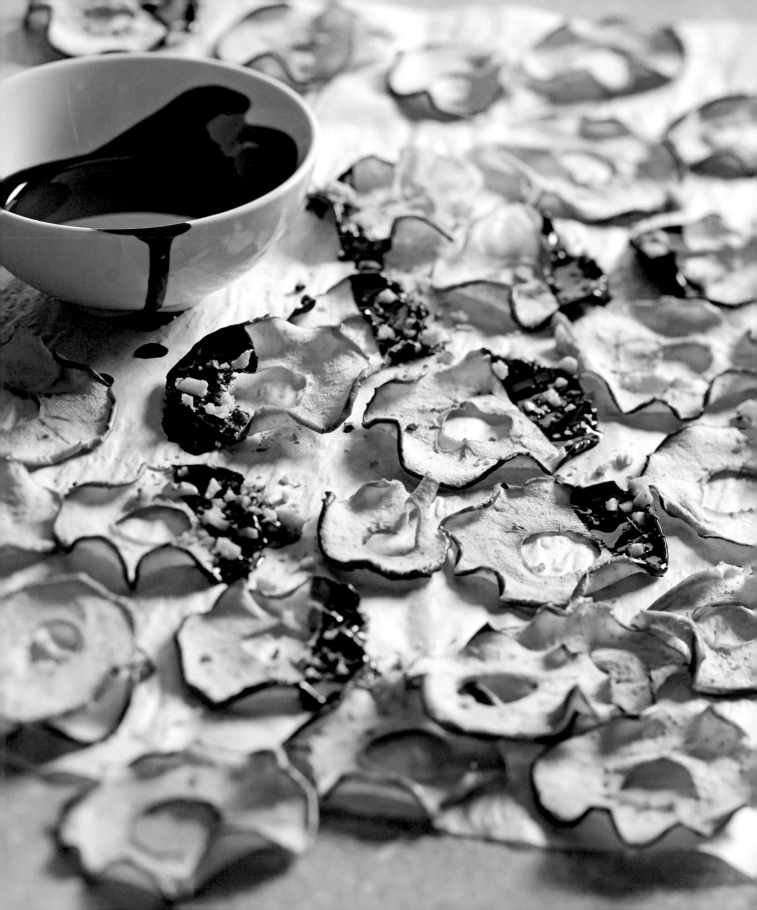

CHUNKY CHUTNEY-STYLE APPLESAUCE

PREP: 15 minutes   COOK: 15 minutes   COOL: 5 minutes   MAKES: 4 servings

THE APPLE VARIETIES LISTED BELOW TEND TO BE FAIRLY SWEET RATHER THAN TART AND ARE CONSIDERED TO BE GOOD "SAUCE" APPLES. IF YOU'D LIKE, YOU CAN SUBSTITUTE ¾ CUP GREEN TEA FOR THE APPLE CIDER AND WATER.

5 apples (such as Jonathon, Fuji, McIntosh, Braeburn, and/or Yellow Delicious)

½ cup apple cider

¼ cup water

2 star anise

3 cup raisins

1 tablespoon balsamic vinegar

½ teaspoon apple pie spice

¼ cup chopped walnuts or pecans, toasted (see tip, page 57)

¼ teaspoon pure vanilla extract

1. Peel and core the apples; cut into 1-inch chunks. In a large saucepan combine apple chunks, cider, the water, and star anise. Bring just to boiling over medium-high heat, stirring frequently. Reduce heat to low. Cover and cook for 10 minutes. Stir in raisins, vinegar, and pie spice. Cover and cook for 5 to 10 minutes more or until apples are soft. Remove from heat. Uncover and cool for 5 minutes.

2. Remove star anise from apple mixture. Using a potato masher, mash to desired consistency. Stir in nuts and vanilla. Serve apple warm or cover and refrigerate for up to 5 days.

ROASTED PEAR CRUMBLE

PREP: 20 minutes   BAKE: 15 minutes   MAKES: 4 servings

THIS AUTUMNAL DESSERT IS A MIXTURE OF TEXTURES AND TEMPERATURES. WARM AND TENDER OVEN-ROASTED PEARS ARE TOPPED WITH A COOL ORANGE-AND-VANILLA-INFUSED CASHEW CREAM—AND FINISHED WITH A SPRINKLE OF CRUNCHY SPICED NUTS.

2 ripe, firm Anjou or Bartlett pears, halved and cored

2 teaspoons coconut oil or walnut oil

1 tablespoon coconut oil or walnut oil

¼ cup unsalted whole almonds, coarsely chopped

¼ cup unsalted pepitas

¼ cup shaved coconut

¼ teaspoon freshly grated nutmeg

¼ cup Cashew Cream (see recipe, page 327)

½ teaspoon finely shredded orange peel

¼ teaspoon pure vanilla extract
   Freshly grated nutmeg

1. Preheat oven to 375°F. Place pears, cut sides up, on a baking pan; drizzle with the 2 teaspoons oil. Roast about 15 minutes or until soft. Let cool slightly.

2. Meanwhile, for nut crumble, in a medium skillet heat the 1 tablespoon oil over medium heat. Add almonds and pepitas; cook and stir for 2 minutes. Add coconut; cook and stir for 1 minute or until nuts and coconut are toasted. Sprinkle with the ¼ teaspoon nutmeg; stir and let cool.

3. For sauce, in a small bowl combine Cashew Cream, orange peel, and vanilla. Place pears on individual serving plates. Sprinkle with additional nutmeg. Drizzle pears with sauce and sprinkle with nut crumble.

Green Tea-Ginger Poached Pears with
Orange-Mango Puree, *recipe page 338*

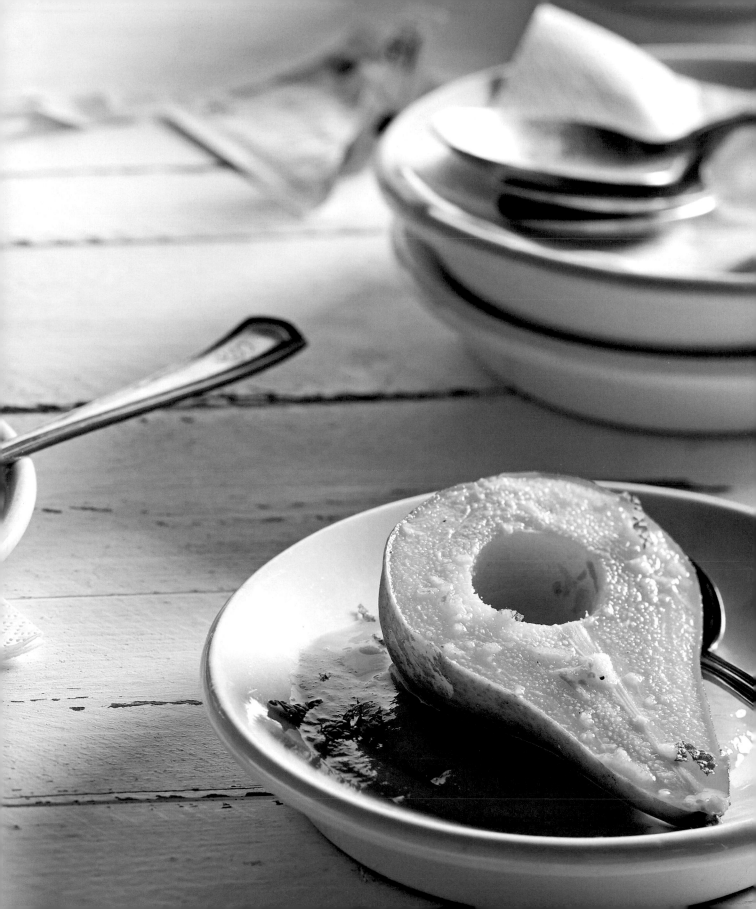

GREEN TEA-GINGER POACHED PEARS WITH ORANGE-MANGO PUREE

pictured on page 336

PREP: 30 minutes   COOK: 10 minutes   MAKES: 8 servings

THIS RECIPE IS A GOOD EXAMPLE OF ONE IN WHICH YOU WILL GET THE BEST RESULTS USING A HIGH-PERFORMANCE BLENDER. A REGULAR BLENDER WILL WORK FINE, BUT A HIGH-PERFORMANCE BLENDER WILL MAKE THE ORANGE-MANGO SAUCE AS SMOOTH AS SILK.

2 cups fresh orange juice
2 cups water
2 tablespoons loose green tea leaves or 3 bags green tea
4 medium Bosc or Anjou pears, halved lengthwise and cored
2 tablespoons minced fresh ginger
2 teaspoons finely shredded orange peel
2 mangoes, peeled, seeded, and chopped
   Snipped fresh mint

1. In a medium saucepan combine orange juice and the water. Bring to boiling. Remove from heat. Add the green tea. Let steep for 8 minutes. Strain mixture and return to saucepan. Add the pear halves, ginger, and 1 teaspoon of the orange peel. Return mixture just to boiling; reduce heat. Simmer, uncovered, about 10 minutes or just until pears are tender. Using a slotted spoon, remove pears, reserving poaching liquid. Let pears and liquid cool to room temperature.

2. In a food processor or blender combine the mangoes, 2 tablespoons of the poaching liquid, and the remaining 1 teaspoon orange peel. Cover and process or blend until smooth, adding more poaching liquid, 1 tablespoon at a time, as necessary to reach desired consistency.

3. Place 1 pear half on each of eight serving plates; spoon some of the mango puree over each serving. Sprinkle with snipped fresh mint.

PERSIMMONS WITH CINNAMON-PEAR SAUCE

PREP: 20 minutes   COOK: 10 minutes   MAKES: 4 servings

PERSIMMONS ARE IN GENERALLY IN SEASON FROM OCTOBER THROUGH FEBRUARY, DEPENDING ON WHERE YOU LIVE. BE SURE TO PURCHASE FUYU—NOT HACHIYA—PERSIMMONS. THE SKINS OF FUYU PERSIMMONS CAN BE TOUGH. IF SO, SIMPLY PEEL THEM USING A VEGETABLE PEELER.

2 ripe Bartlett pears, peeled, cored, and chopped
⅓ cup water
1 teaspoon fresh lemon juice
½ teaspoon ground cinnamon
1 whole vanilla bean
3 ripe Fuyu persimmons
⅓ cup chopped walnuts, toasted (see tip, page 57)
⅓ cup apple juice-sweetened dried cranberries or currants

1. In a small saucepan combine the pears, the water, lemon juice, and cinnamon; set aside.

2. Slice the vanilla bean in half lengthwise. Save one half for another use. Using the back of a paring knife, scrape the seeds from the remaining half of the vanilla bean and add to the pear mixture.

3. Cook pear mixture over medium-low heat for 10 to 15 minutes or until pears are very soft, stirring occasionally. (Cooking time will depend on how ripe your pears are.) Using an immersion blender, puree the mixture in the saucepan until smooth. (If you don't have an immersion blender, transfer mixture to a regular blender; cover and blend until smooth.) Transfer to a bowl; cover and refrigerate until completely cooled.

4. To prepare the persimmons, cut off and discard the stem ends. Slice in half horizontally and remove any seeds. Cut persimmons into ½-inch pieces.

5. To serve, divide pear puree among four serving bowls. Top with persimmons, walnuts, and cranberries.

GRILLED PINEAPPLE WITH COCONUT CREAM

CHILL: 24 hours   PREP: 20 minutes   GRILL: 6 minutes   MAKES: 4 servings

YOU'LL NEED TO PLAN AHEAD A BIT BEFORE MAKING THIS SIMPLE FRUIT DESSERT. REFRIGERATING THE CAN OF COCONUT MILK UPSIDE DOWN IN THE REFRIGERATOR OVERNIGHT ALLOWS THE COCONUT-MILK SOLIDS TO SOLIDIFY SO YOU CAN BEAT THEM WITH AN ELECTRIC MIXER UNTIL THEY ARE LIGHT AND FLUFFY.

1 13.5-ounce can natural full-fat coconut milk (such as Nature's Way)
1 pineapple, peeled, cored, and cut into four 1-inch rings
Fresh lime juice
Snipped fresh mint and mint sprigs (optional)

1. Refrigerate the can of coconut milk upside down for at least 1 day before you plan to serve this dish.

2. For a charcoal or gas grill, place pineapple rings on a grill rack directly over medium heat. Grill for 6 to 8 minutes or until lightly charred, turning once halfway through cooking. Transfer pineapple to a platter. Drizzle lime juice over pineapple.

3. For coconut cream, turn the chilled can of coconut milk right side up and open the can. Pour off the liquid portion of the coconut milk, reserving it to use in smoothies or sauces. Transfer the coconut milk solids to a deep mixing bowl. Beat with an electric mixer on medium until light and fluffy, about 5 to 6 minutes. Serve the pineapple with a spoonful of coconut cream. If desired, sprinkle with snipped fresh mint and garnish with fresh mint sprigs.

COCONUT-MANGO MOUSSE-FILLED TARTLETS

PREP: 40 minutes   CHILL: overnight   COOK: 6 minutes   MAKES: 6 tartlets

THESE INDIVIDUAL TARTS ARE A BIT FUSSY TO MAKE, BUT THEY WILL WOW YOUR GUESTS—ESPECIALLY CONSIDERING THAT THEY CONTAIN NO WHEAT OR GRAINS, PROCESSED SUGAR, OR DAIRY. THE NUT AND DRIED-FRUIT CRUSTS AND THE MANGO MOUSSE FILLING NEED TO BE REFRIGERATED OVERNIGHT—SO THEY ARE EASILY MADE AHEAD.

CRUSTS
- 1½ cups raw macadamia nuts
- 1¼ cups pitted unsweetened Medjool dates
- 2 tablespoons unsweetened shredded coconut
- ¼ teaspoon ground ginger
- ¼ teaspoon ground cinnamon
- ⅛ teaspoon ground cloves
- ⅛ teaspoon freshly grated nutmeg

FILLING
- 1½ cups cubed ripe mango
- 1 teaspoon finely shredded lime peel
- 2 tablespoon fresh lime juice
- 4 eggs, separated
- 1 14.5-ounce can full-fat coconut milk
- ¾ cup coconut shards, toasted (optional)
  Fresh raspberries (optional)

1. For the crust, in a food processor or blender process or blend macadamia nuts until finely ground. (Be careful not to overprocess or you'll wind up with nut butter.) Add dates, coconut, ginger, cinnamon, cloves, and nutmeg. Process until dates are finely chopped, incorporated, and mixture forms a ball.

2. Divide nut mixture evenly into six portions. Press each portion into a 4-inch tart pan with removable bottom. Cover tart shells and refrigerate overnight.

3. Pour coconut milk into a small bowl. Cover and refrigerate overnight.

4. For filling, in a food processor or blender, combine mango, lime peel, and lime juice. Cover and process or blend until smooth. Transfer puree to a double boiler* placed over simmering water. Whisk in egg yolks. Cook and stir for 6 to 8 minutes or until mixture thickens. Remove from heat; cool slightly. Cover and refrigerate filling overnight. (Refrigerate egg whites in a tightly sealed container overnight.)

5. The next day, remove egg whites from the refrigerator and let stand at room temperature for 30 minutes. Remove the layer of solidified coconut cream from the top of the refrigerated coconut milk. (Reserve thin liquid for another purpose.)

6. In a medium mixing bowl combine coconut cream and chilled mango mixture. Beat with an electric mixer on medium until well combined; set aside. Wash beaters well; dry thoroughly.

7. In another clean medium mixing bowl beat egg whites on high until soft peaks form, 4 to 5 minutes. Using a rubber spatula, fold beaten egg whites into coconut-mango mixture.

8. Pile filling into refrigerated tart shells. Refrigerate until serving time. Carefully remove tart pan sides by pushing up on the bottom of each tart. (The bottoms should stay in place for serving.) If desired, garnish tartlets with coconut shards and fresh raspberries.

***Tip:** If you don't have a double boiler, you can create one. Set a stainless-steel or glass bowl on top of a saucepan with simmering water in it. The water shouldn't touch the bottom of the bowl, but there should be a tight seal so that the steam is trapped in the pan and heats the contents of the bowl.

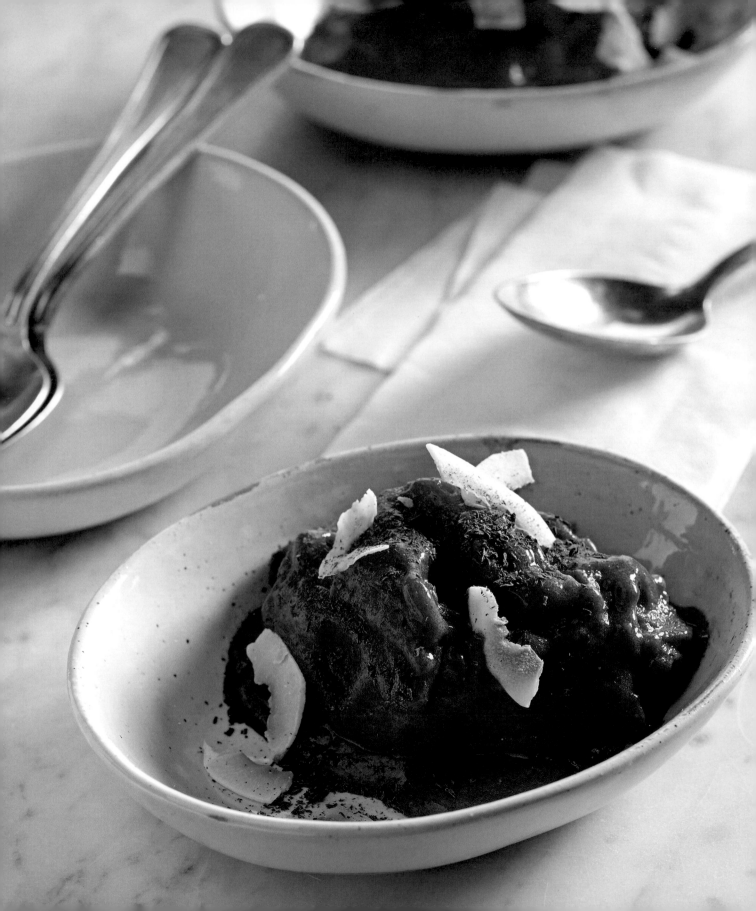

SOFT-SERVE RASPBERRY-BANANA SORBET

PREP: 15 minutes   FREEZE: 1 hour   CHILL: 30 minutes   MAKES: 4 servings

YOU CAN USE PACKAGED FROZEN RASPBERRIES OR YOU CAN FREEZE YOUR OWN: WASH AND DRAIN FRESH RASPBERRIES AND PLACE IN A SINGLE LAYER ON A LARGE RIMMED BAKING PAN LINED WITH WAXED PAPER. COVER LOOSELY AND FREEZE FOR SEVERAL HOURS OR UNTIL VERY FIRM. TRANSFER THE FROZEN RASPBERRIES TO AN AIRTIGHT CONTAINER AND KEEP FROZEN FOR UP TO 3 MONTHS.

1 medium banana, cut into ½-inch slices
¾ cup fresh orange juice
2½ cups frozen unsweetened raspberries
Grated unsweetened chocolate (such as Scharffen Berger 99% cacao bar), toasted unsweetened coconut chips, and/or toasted slivered almonds

1. Place banana on a small baking pan lined with waxed paper. Cover loosely with another sheet of waxed paper. Freeze for 1 to 2 hours or until completely firm.

2. Meanwhile, in a small saucepan bring orange juice to boiling. Boil gently, uncovered, for 5 to 8 minutes or until reduced to ⅓ cup. Pour juice into a heatproof bowl. Chill for 30 to 60 minutes or until cold.

3. In a food processor combine frozen banana slices, the reduced orange juice, and frozen raspberries. Cover and process until well combined but still frozen, stopping to stir often. Sorbet will be very thick. Immediately spoon into chilled serving bowls. Serve immediately. (Or place the filled bowls in the freezer until serving time; let stand at room temperature for 5 minutes before topping and serving.) Sprinkle sorbet with chocolate, coconut chips, and/or almonds just before serving.

GRAPEFRUIT-BASIL GRANITA WITH RIESLING

PREP: 10 minutes   COOK: 15 minutes   FREEZE: 3 hours   MAKES: 6 to 8 servings

THIS IS THE MOST REFRESHING FINISH TO A MEAL YOU CAN IMAGINE—PERFECT FOR A HOT SUMMER NIGHT. IT REQUIRES A BIT OF JUICING (3 CUPS OF FRESH GRAPEFRUIT JUICE!), SO BE SURE TO HAVE A GOOD JUICER ON HAND.

1 cup fresh orange juice
2 tablespoons snipped fresh basil
3 cups fresh grapefruit juice
   (ruby red or pink)
½ cup Riesling wine
1 tablespoon snipped fresh basil

1. In a small saucepan combine orange juice and the 2 tablespoons basil. Bring to boiling over medium heat. Reduce heat to low. Simmer, uncovered, until reduced by half, about 15 minutes.

2. Strain orange juice mixture through a fine-mesh sieve into a large bowl, pressing on the basil with the back of a spoon. Stir grapefruit juice and wine into orange juice in bowl.

3. Pour mixture into a 13×9-inch glass or other nonreactive rectangular dish. Freeze about 1 hour or until edges are frozen. Remove from freezer; scrape frozen mixture with a fork, pulling from the edges to the center. Return to the freezer. Freeze about 3 hours or until texture of shaved ice, scraping with fork from edges to center every 30 minutes.

4. To serve, spoon granita into small bowls and sprinkle with fresh basil; serve immediately.

STRAWBERRY-CANTALOUPE SOUP WITH LIME AND MINT

PREP: 10 minutes   CHILL: 4 to 24 hours   MAKES: 4 to 6 servings

COOLING FRUIT SOUPS ARE POPULAR IN EASTERN EUROPEAN AND SCANDINAVIAN CUISINES. GET THE RIPEST FRUIT YOU CAN FIND FOR THIS MELANGE OF STRAWBERRIES, CANTALOUPE, LIME, MINT, AND GINGER.

4 cups cubed ripe cantaloupe
1½ cups ripe strawberries, hulled
1 cup fresh orange juice
½ cup dry white wine
2 tablespoons fresh lime juice
1 teaspoon finely chopped fresh ginger
2 tablespoons snipped fresh mint
Sliced strawberries and mint leaves (optional)

1. In a food processor or blender combine cantaloupe, strawberries, orange juice, wine, lime juice, and ginger. Process until smooth.

2. Pour into a large bowl or container. Cover and refrigerate for at least 4 hours or overnight.

3. To serve, stir snipped mint into soup. Divide soup among serving bowls. If desired, garnish with sliced strawberries and mint leaves.

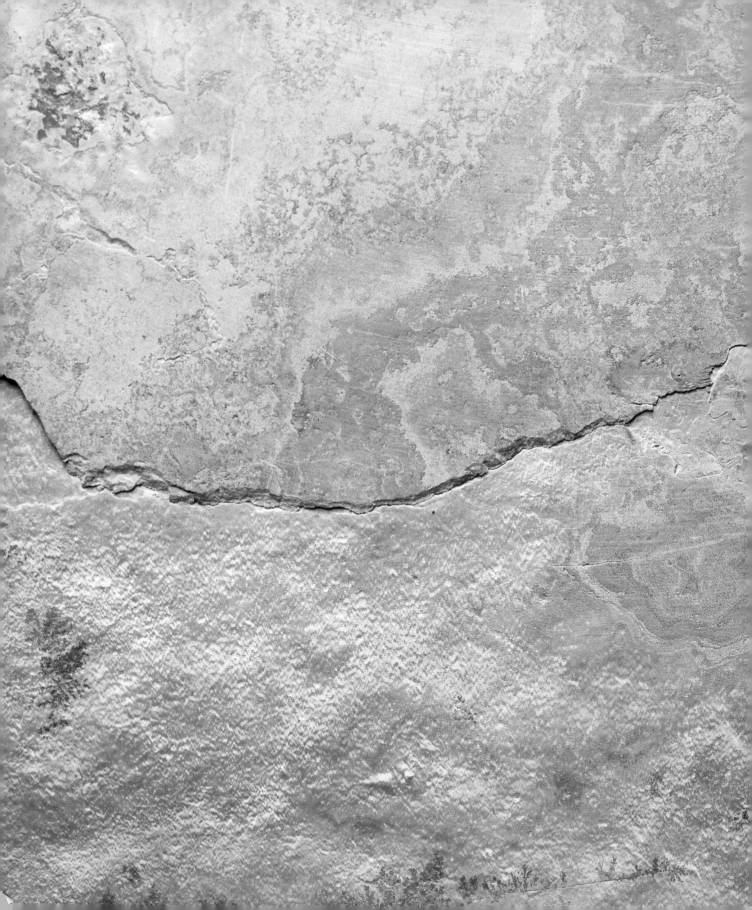